ATLAS OF FOOT

RADIOLOGY

ATLAS OF FOOT RADIOLOGY

Jacques MONTAGNE, M.D.

Alain CHEVROT, M.D.

Jean-Marie GALMICHE, M.D.

English translation edited by

Neil CHAFETZ, M.D.

Assistant Professor of Radiology
University of California School of Medicine
San Francisco, California

MASSON Publishing USA, Inc.

New York • Paris • Barcelona • Mexico City • Milan • Rio

Original French Edition : Atlas de Radiologie du pied
© Masson, Paris, 1980.

ISBN : 0-89352-097-7

Library of Congress Catalog Card Number : 80-83859

Printed in France

PREFACE

In recent years, several radiological atlases of the hand have appeared in the medical book market.

Some of these are works of reference to which we resort when a difficulty arises in the interpretation of radiographs of the hand, this pre-eminently noble organ.

Now the ill-loved, despised, underrated foot, often martyred by current activities, professionnal life, sport or... fashion, has not until now benefited from any radiological atlas devoted to itself.

The present work, the first of its kind, comes at the right time to fill this gap.

In order to achieve its purpose, it is essentially composed of plates accompanied by detailed and accurate legends.

When it deals with rare or little-known diseases, a short statement precedes the iconography : specific symptoms of the disease, frequency, etiology... etc.

However, the originality of this major contribution by three radiologists, consists chiefly in the classification of the chapters : after having studied the normal radiological aspect in adult and child, together with the statics of the foot, the book carries on with a semeiotic scheme, starting from a given picture to run through the differential diagnoses which could produce similar or closely related radiological characteristics.

Though the study of bones and joints is prominent, the other foot components are not neglected : their reactions are analyzed, including... their relations with the shoe !

So conceived, this thorough atlas ought to make the information required rapidly accessible, and it should find its place, as a work of reference, in the library of all the physicians whose specialization leads them to interpret foot radiographs, particularly radiologists, rheumatologists and orthopedic surgeons.

Pr GUY PALLARDY, M.D.
Head of Department Radiology B
Cochin Hospital, Paris

INTRODUCTION

Forsaken for a long time, by most authors including Destot, Lejars, Hohmann, the foot is the last arrival in the bone and joint medical literature.

In 1958, the International College of Podology (C.I.P.) was founded by J. Lelievre who, as early as 1952, published at Masson's his first treatise, which in numerous editions has become the basic work for this very special science. At the same time, R. Meary became interested in the foot and, when he was named chairman of the orthopedic surgical clinic at the Cochin Hospital, this pathology had definitively found its place in the University and the scientific societies : symposium on the flatfoot of the French Society of Orthopedic Surgery and Traumatology (1976), joint meeting of the C.I.P. and the American Orthopedic Foot Society in Dallas (1978) ; joint meeting with the French Society of Rheumatology (1979).

Unfortunately, R. Meary and J. Lelievre died untimely. The relay was taken by P. Maurer and B. Tomeno at Cochin Hospital, and by P. Galmiche who founded in 1969 the French Society of Foot Medicine and Surgery, of which J. Benassy, J. Schnepp and L. Simon have been the successive chairmen.

On an international level, A. Viladot y Perice (Spain), A. de Wulff (Belgium), P. Chiappara (Italy) followed each other as heads of the International College of Podology, the International Congresses of which have sustained their rythm and their interest, owing to the active devotion of their General Secretary, J. Montagne, and his successor, S. Braun. The latter started in 1976, in the Cochin Hospital, the teaching of « Podology », the study of which has been certified since 1978 by an official certificate issued by Paris V University. This teaching has been a succes.

Thus, from 1952 to 1978, medico-surgical podology has achieved a first rank. This multi-disciplinary science, which includes orthopedics and rheumatology along with dermatology, angiology, neurology..., has now come of age. It leads to rational therapeutics where as, up to 1952, the treatment of foot diseases was « too frequently run in a merely empirical way » according to R. Merle d'Aubigne.

This new science is based, of course, on anatomy, physiology and biology like any other medical specialization, but radiology is prominent in the examination of the diseased foot.

The radiology investigation is a difficult one, because, it requires careful technique and has no recourse to artificial contrast. In order to obtain a valid interpretation of the radiographs, these have to be perfect, in the photographic quality as well as in the precision of the incidence of the beam. Here again, foot radiology has long been a poor relation, except for some innovators, like A. Djian. In 1977, the G.E.T.R.O.A. (Group of Study and Work in Osteo-Articular Radiology) animated by C. Massare, M. Bard, M. Lequesne etc. reserved to Foot Pathology its annual course in specialization.

The book by J. Montagne, A. Chevrot and J.M. Galmiche comes to fill a gap, and will no doubt be a work of reference. As it is written by radiologists, it starts, not from the diagnosis to show the correlated pathologic pictures, but from the specific radiographic appearance : cyst-like lytic bone lesion, condensation, demineralization..., to lead to the diagnosis.

The abundance in documents is considerable (more than 1 500 plates), the text being purposely limited to commented legends to the pictures. Published simultaneously in French, and in English in the U.S., this work is intended for a very wide public of specialists. We are glad to introduce it to the reader.

Paul Galmiche, M.D.
Chairman and Founder of the French
Society of Foot Medicine and Surgery.
Vice Chairman of the International College of Podology.

FOREWORD

The framework consists in the gathering together of radiographic likenesses, and the approach to diagnosis through pattern analysis (except in chapter one, the subject of which is the normal radiologic anatomy). We have reproduced radiographs consecutive to trauma or surgery, but fractures and surgical procedures will be found developed in other specialized books.

The plates represent purposely the right ankle or the right foot with the heel on the left side and the toes upward.

The legends, as detailed as necessary, are occasionally supplemented by a short clinical review. The lists of differential diagnoses originate, for the most part, from M.M. REEDER and B. FELSON'S Gamuts.

Our thanks are due :

To our colleagues, who have made us free to use their collections : P.-CH. ACHACH, Paris ; B. AMOR, Paris ; R. ANDRE, Marly-le-Roi ; Ph. AGNARD, Orléans ; Ph. BAUDOIN, Orléans ; J. BENASSY, Paris ; J. BENNET, Paris ; G.-C. BERARDI, Gênes ; P. BERTRAND, Paris ; J. BIENAYME, Paris ; F. BIRBEAU, Orléans ; A. BONNIN, Paris ; S. BRAUN, Paris ; J.-M. BURUTARAN, San Sebastian ; J.-P. CARRET, Lyon ; G. CHATIGNOUX, Paris ; J.-C. CHENARD, Orléans ; M.-C. CHENARD, Orléans ; O. CHEREAU, Paris ; L. CHEVROT, Marseille ; A. CHEVROT-VINENT, Paris ; P. CHIAPPARA, Gênes ; C. CHIPPAUX, Marseille ; G. CORREAS, Paris ; R.-P. DELAHAYE, St Mandé ; F. DELBARRE, Paris ; J. DELPLACE, Orléans ; A. DENIS, Paris ; G. DESSE, Paris ; J. DUBOUSSET, Paris ; A.-M. FOURNIER, Marseille ; F. GACHE, La Varenne St-Hilaire ; G. GAIZLER, Budapest ; B. GALMICHE-ZELLER, Evreux ; B. GARBAY, Cannes ; R. GARELLI, Moncalieri ; M. GENTILINI, Paris ; H.-A. GHARDI, Tunis ; R. GORIN, Paris ; J. GOUGEON, Reims ; J. GRELLET, Paris ; J. GUIVARCH, Roscoff ; M. JEDDI, Sousse ; M. KATZ, Paris ; M. KERBOUL, Paris ; M. LAVAL-JEANTET, Paris ; J.-P. LEBARD, Paris ; G. LEDOUX-LEBARD, Paris ; A. LEDUC, Bruxelles ; J.-M. LEFUR, Brest ; P. LOUYOT, Nancy ; J. MARIE, Paris ; P. MAROTEAUX, Paris ; M. MARTINI, Alger ; J. MARTORELL-MARTORELL, Barcelone ; P. MAURER, Paris ; D. MAZARGUIL, Orléans ; Ch. MENKES, Paris ; E. MONTAGNE, Paris ; J. MONTAGNE, Brouzet-les-Alès ; G. MOSTINI, Morlaix ; J. MOUTOUNET, Paris ; M. OGRIZEK, Mossendjo ; P.-P. PETIT, Paris ; G. PISANI, Alba ; J. POLGE, Provins ; M. POSTEL, Paris ; G. RAMELA, Paris ; R. REGAL, Montpellier ; B. REGNAULD, Nantes ; Ch RENON, Paris ; P. RIGAULT, Paris ; C. ROHR, Paris ; J.-P. ROUX, Paris ; J. SAUVEGRAIN, Paris ; M. SERVELLE, Paris ; I. STROESCU, Bucarest ; P.-I. TEMESVARY, Budapest ; B. TOMENO, Paris ; M. TONNELIER, Paris ; M. TRICOIT, Orléans ; H. TRISTANT, Paris ; J.-F. VIALA, Orléans ; A. VILADOT, Barcelone ; A. VOLTE, Orléans ; H. VOUTEY, Dijon ; J. WITVOET, Paris.

To Professor J. ANTHONY and to Mr. L. GINSBURG, from the National Museum of Natural History in Paris, for their assistance in the chapter on the evolution of the foot.

To the physicians in various hospital clinical departments, who have committed to us their patients.

To the technicians of our departments of Radiology, Mrs : J. AKAYA, A.-M. AMELINE, F. BAKIR, J. BARBERI, F. BEZIER, S. DESMOLIN, C. DUDILLEUX, E. DUFOUR, D. DURAND, M. LANDAIS, M. LANGLOIS, M.-C. LE DALLOUR, B. LEGIOT, M. MARSAT, M.-P. MESSAGER, I. MICHAU, I. PAUDECERF, T. PILLOT, P. QUETELART, C. REAU, Ch. SANCEAUME, Ch. THOREZ. MM : Y. DIBOU, A. FERACCI, P. HELENON, J.-L. HERMAN, Y. MENGELLE, J.-L. PETETIN, B. SERAPIGLIA, M. STEPHANT, H. TALLON, A. WAHL.

To Mrs. F. CALAFAT for her advice on ortheses.

To Mrs M.-J. ZELLER who took charge of the secretariat.

To Mrs D. PARDIEU, responsible for the documentation.

To Mr and Mrs F. LEFEVRE for their drawings and diagrams.

To Mrs M. BAILLARGE who designed the make-up.

To Dr P. DE LA JUDIE who assumed the translation in English.

To the GUERBET Laboratory.

To the AGFA-GEVAERT Company.

CONTENTS

1

THE NORMAL FOOT OF THE ADULT

RADIOGRAPHIC METHODOLOGY AND ANATOMY

RADIOGRAPHY OF BOTH FEET IN THE ANTEROPOSTERIOR POSITION

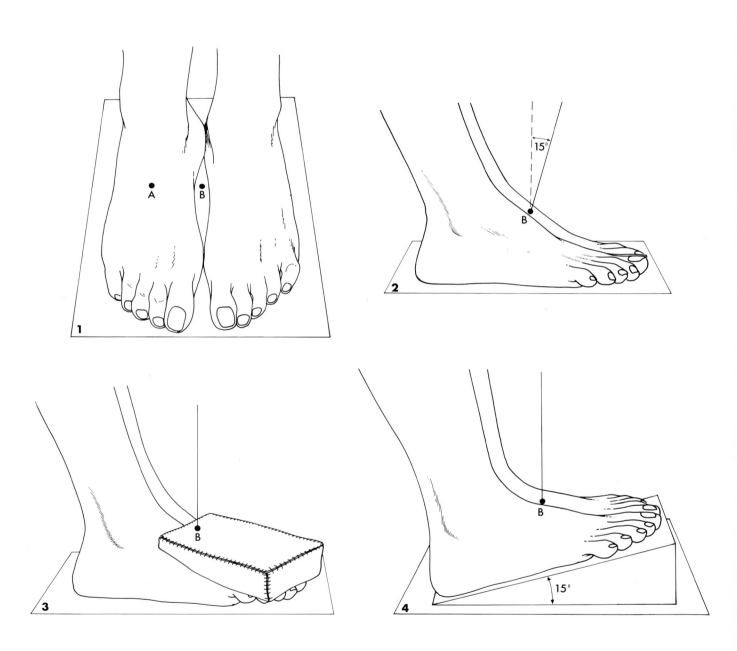

1, 2, 3, 4. Schemas of the incidences

Position : the patient is recumbent in the supine position with the knees flexed ; the feet are placed with the plantar aspect in contact with the film on the flat table (**1**).

Direction of the X-ray beam : the central ray from the X-ray tube is at right angles to the dorsum of the foot and angled 15 degrees toward the ankle joint (dorsiplantar projection) (**2**).

Center : to expose both feet separately (A) ; between the feet (B), to expose them simultaneously. To avoid excessive contrast in density between the thick and thin portions of the foot, the Clark's graduated thickness wedge (**4**) or a flour-bag (**3**) are employed. Center with the tube straight.

An electrostatically charged selenium plate (*xeroradiography*) softens the contrast between the bones and soft tissues (**5**). However, the standard X-ray film is preferred for an optimum image of bone cortex and medullary space trabeculae.

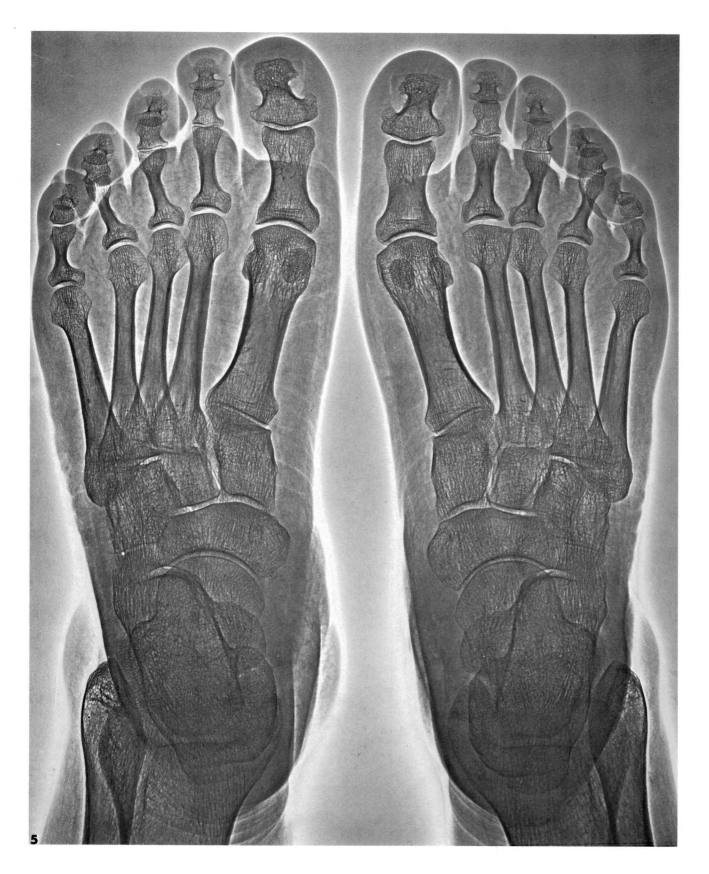

5. Xeroradiograph of both feet in the dorsiplantar position

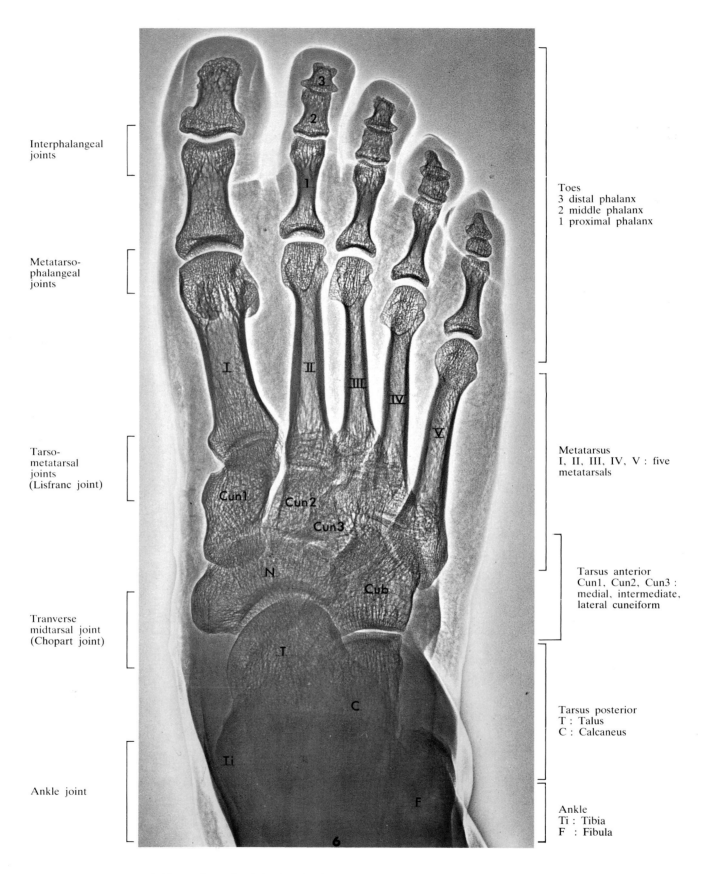

Interphalangeal
joints

Metatarso-
phalangeal
joints

Tarso-
metatarsal
joints
(Lisfranc joint)

Tranverse
midtarsal joint
(Chopart joint)

Ankle joint

Toes
3 distal phalanx
2 middle phalanx
1 proximal phalanx

Metatarsus
I, II, III, IV, V : five
metatarsals

Tarsus anterior
Cun1, Cun2, Cun3 :
medial, intermediate,
lateral cuneiform

Tarsus posterior
T : Talus
C : Calcaneus

Ankle
Ti : Tibia
F : Fibula

6. Xeroradiograph of the foot in the dorsiplantar position : the principal regions

Phalanges and metatarsals

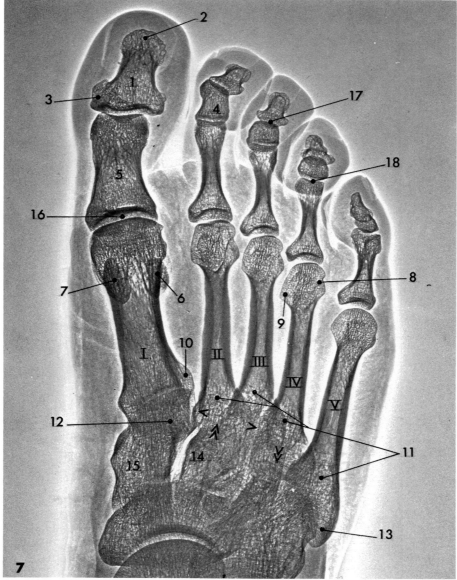

7. Xeroradiograph

1 : distal phalanx ; 2 : tuft of the terminal phalanx ; 3 : tubercle of insertion of the flexor hallucis longus tendon ; 4 : middle phalanx ; 5 : proximal phalanx ; 6 : lateral sesamoid bone ; 7 : medial sesamoid bone ; 8 : pit and tubercle for ligamentous insertion ; 9 : head of the metatarsal and articular condyle ; 10 : lateral side of the metatarsal diaphysis of the great toe ; 11 : metatarsal bases : they join laterally with each other (>) and posteriorly (>>) with the tarsus anterior bones (Lisfranc joint) ; 12 : pyramidal process of the base first metatarsal for insertion of the peroneus longus tendon ; 13 : styloid apophysis of the fifth metatarsal ; 14 : intermediate cuneiform ; 15 : medial cuneiform ; 16 : metatarsophalangeal joint ; 17 : distal interphalangeal joint ; and 18 : proximal interphalangeal joint, between the head of the phalanx with double articular trochlea and the base of the phalanx with double articular glenoid surface ; I, II, III, IV, V, first, second, third, fourth, fifth metatarsal shafts.

Tarsus

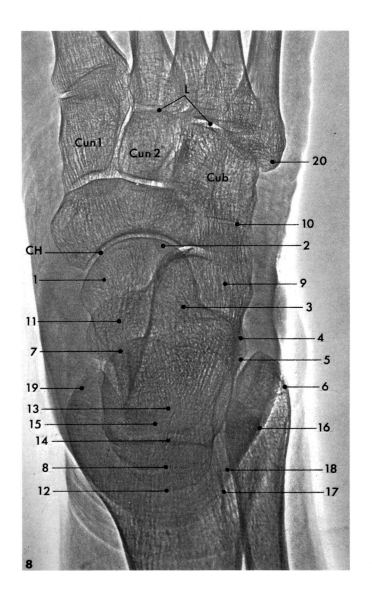

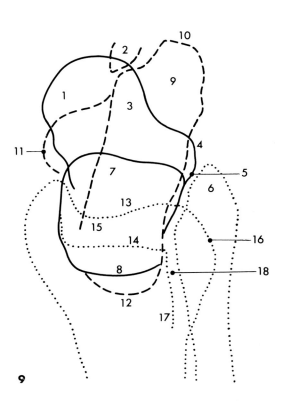

8, 9. Xeroradiograph and diagram. CH : Chopart joint ; Cub : cuboïd ; Cun 1 : medial cuneiform ; Cun 2 : intermediate cuneiform ; L : Lisfranc joint. Only two joint spaces are clearly defined and the lateral cuneiform is overshadowed.

1 : head of the talus ; 2 : pyramidal apophysis of the cuboid ; 3 : neck of the talus ; 4 : external process of the talus ; 5 : articular facet of the lateral malleolus ; 6 : tip of the lateral malleolus ; 7 : trochlear surface of the talus ; 8 : posterior margin of the talus ; 9 : great process of the calcaneus ; 10 : calcaneo-cuboid joint ; 11 : sustentaculum tali ; 12 : posterior tuberosity of the calcaneus ; 13 : anterior margin of the tibial mortice and the talotrochlear surface ; 14 : posterior margin of the mortice ; 15 : tibial mortice ; 16 : anterior tibial tubercle ; 17 : posterior tibial tubercle ; 18 : distal tibiofibular joint ; 19 : medial-malleolus ; 20 : styloid tuberosity of the base of the fifth metatarsal.

RADIOGRAPHY OF THE FOOT IN THE LATERAL POSITION

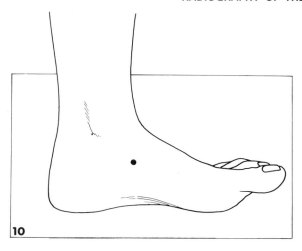 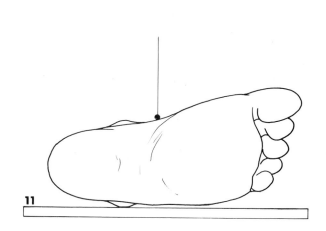

10, 11. Schemas of the incidence.

Position : the patient is in the lateral position with the plantar aspect of the foot at right angles to the film (**10**).

Center : with the cube directly over the navicular bone (**11**).

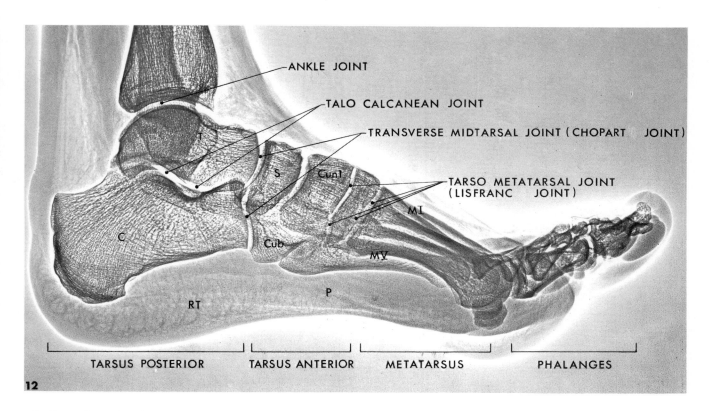

12. Xeroradiograph : the principal regions.

C : calcaneus ; Cub : cuboid bone ; Cun 1 : medial cuneiform ; M I : shaft of the first metatarsal ; M V : shaft of the fifth metatarsal ; P : plantar aponeurosis ; T : talus ; R T : rete plantar of Lejars.

Tarsus

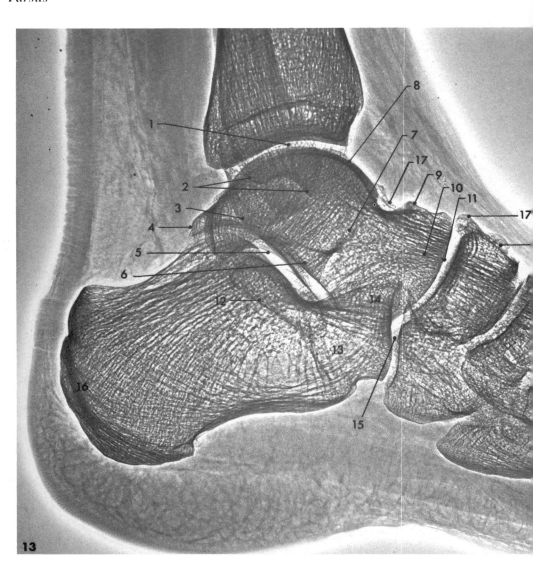

13. Xeroradiograph.

1 : ankle joint ; 2 : medial malleolus ; 3 : lateral malleolus ; 4 : posterior process of the talus and os trigonum ; 5 : subtalar joint ; 6 : external process of the talus ; 7 : neck of the talus ; 8 : trochlear surface of the talus ; 9 : Farabeuf triangle (see page 30) ; 10 : head of the talus ; 11 : talonavicular joint ; 12 : sustentaculum tali ; 13 : great apophysis of the calcaneus ; 14 : beak of the great process of the calcaneus ; 15 : calcaneocuboid joint ; 16 : posterior tuberosity of the calcaneus ; 17 : osteophyte or supernumerary bone.

Forefoot

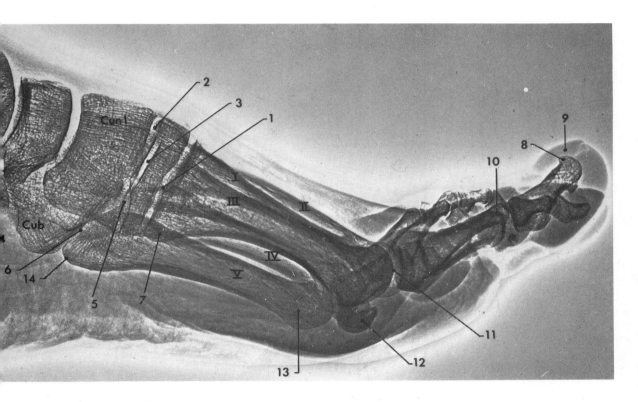

14. Xeroradiograph.

Cub : cuboid ; Cun 1 : medial cuneiform ; I, II, III, IV, V : metatarsal shafts ; 1 : medial cuneiform - first metatarsal joint ; 2 : intermediate cuneiform - second metatarsal joint ; 3 : lateral cuneiform - third metatarsal joint ; 4 : pyramidal process of the cuboid bone ; 5 : cuboid - fourth metatarsal joint ; 6 : cuboid - fifth metatarsal joint ; 7 : pyramidal process of the base of the first metatarsal ; 8 : subungual exostosis ; 9 : nail ; 10 : overshadowing phalanges ; 11 : overshadowing metatarsal heads ; 12 : sesamoid bones ; 13 : head of the fifth metatarsal ; 14 : styloid tuberosity of the fifth metatarsal.

RADIOGRAPHY OF THE FOOT IN THE OBLIQUE POSITION

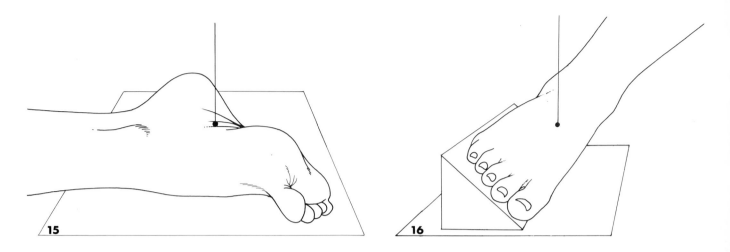

15, 16. Schemas of the incidences.

15. Oblique.

— The patient is lying in the lateral position and the plantar aspect of the foot is oblique in relation to the X-ray table.
— Direct the beam to the navicular bone, with the tube straight.

16. Dorsi-plantar oblique.

— The patient is in the supine position with the knee flexed ; the plantar aspect of the foot is placed on a balsa wood wedge (angle block of 45°).
— Center in the mid-plane of the dorsal surface of the foot, with the tube straight.

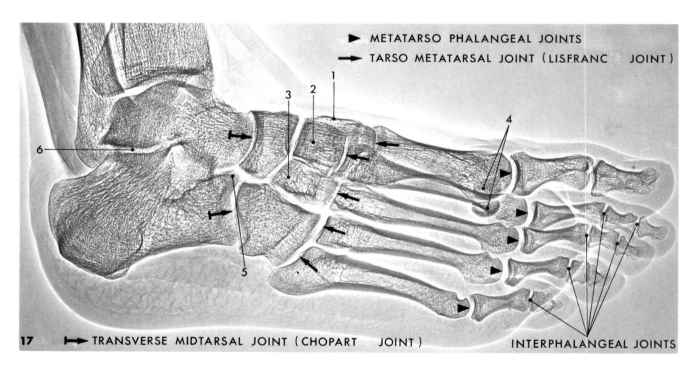

17. Xeroradiograph. The lateral positions with the plantar aspect of the foot right angles to the film, gives a true lateral projection of the tarsal bones and the five metatarsals which overshadow each other. Whith the foot placed in dorsi-plantar oblique position, the radiograph shows good separation of the tarsus and metatarsus, with clearly defined tarsometatarsal and metatarsophalangeal joints.

1 : medial cuneiform ; 2 : intermediate cuneiform ; 3 : lateral cuneiform ; 4 : sesamoid bones ; 5 : beak of the great apophysis of the calcaneus ; 6 : posterior subtalar joint.

RADIOGRAPHY OF THE FOOT IN PLANTAR-DORSAL OBLIQUE POSITION

The plantar-dorsal position tends to give a more satisfactory projection of the tarsus bones and tarso-metatarsal joints than the reverse dorsi-plantar oblique position.

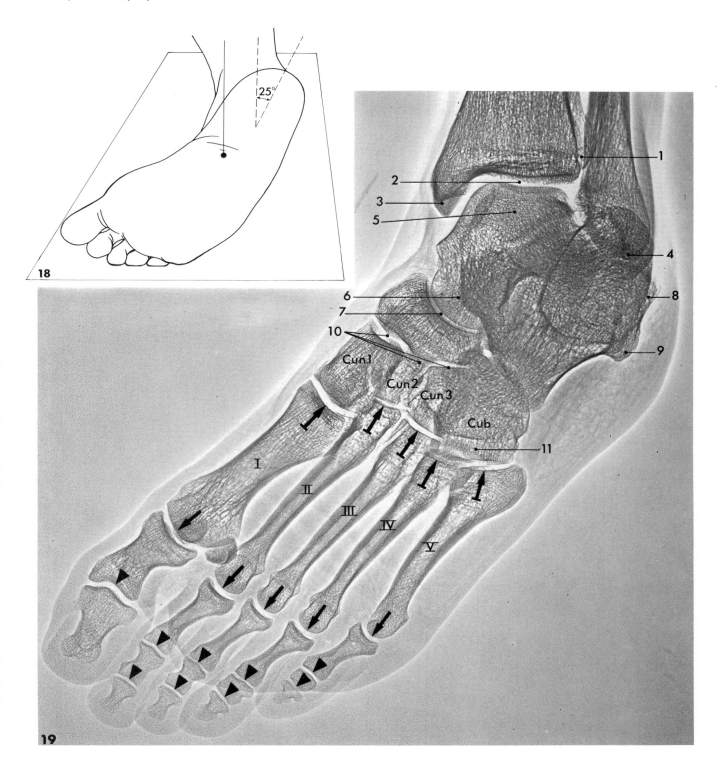

18. Schema of the incidence.

Position : The patient is prone on the X-ray table with the dorsum of the foot in contact with the film, the heel angled 25⁰ from the vertical line.

Center : With the tube straight or angled perpendicular to the general concavity of the plantar surface of the foot.

19. Xeroradiograph.

Cub : cuboid ; Cun 1 : medial cuneiform ; Cun 2 : intermediate cuneiform ; Cun 3 : lateral cuneiform ; I, II, III, IV, V : metatarsal shafts ; 1 : distal tibiofibular joint ; 2 : ankle joint ; 3 : medial malleolus ; 4 : lateral malleolus ; 5 : trochlear surface of talus ; 6 : head of the talus ; 7 : talonavicular joint ; 8-9 : posterior tuberosity of the calcaneus with lateral tubercle (8) and medial tubercle (9) ; 10 : cuneiform navicular joints ; 11 : groove of cuboid for the peroneus longus tendon ; tarsometatarsal joints (→) ; metatarsophalangeal joints (→) ; interphalangeal joints (▶).

RADIOGRAPHY OF THE ANKLE JOINT IN THE ANTERO-POSTERIOR POSITION

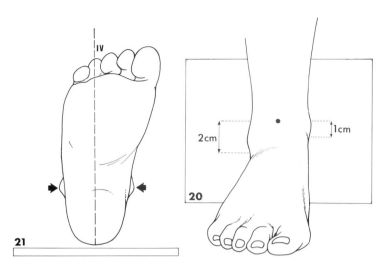

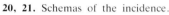

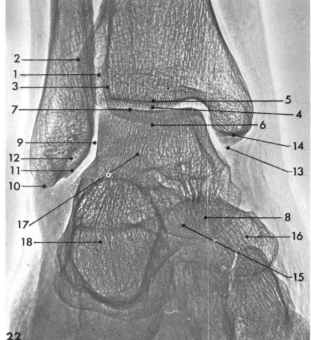

20, 21. Schemas of the incidence.

Position : the patient is in the supine position with the back of the heel in contact with the film. The ankle is supported in flexion and the limb is rotated medially until the medial and lateral malleoli are equidistant from the film. In this position, the axis of the fourth metatarsal shaft is, in general, at right angles to the film (**21**).

Center : with the tube straight, 1 cm above the tip of the medial malleolus or 2 cm above the tip of the lateral malleolus (**20**).

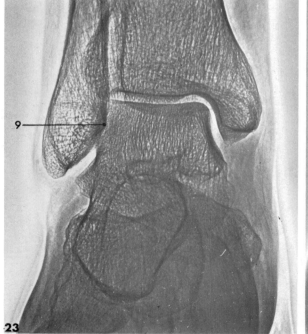

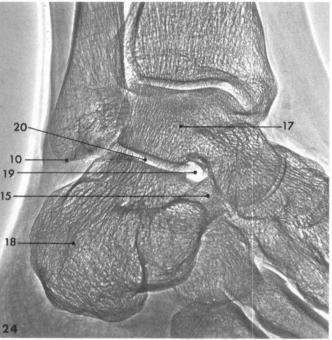

22, 23, 24. Xeroradiographs.

22. The limb is rotated medially until the intermalleolar line is paralled to the film, thus ensuring a clear joint space between fibula and talus.

1 : distal tibiofibular joint ; 2 : anterior tubercle of tibia ; 3 : posterior tubercle of tibia ; 4 : ankle joint ; 5 : anterior margin of the tibia ; 6 : promontory of the tibia ; 7 : trochlear surface of talus ; 8 : head of the talus ; 9 : talofibular ; 10-11 : tip of the lateral malleollus (10) ; posterior tubercle projecting lower than the anterior tubercle (11) ; 12 : malleolar fossa ; 13-14 : tip of the medial malleolus (13) ; anterior tubercle projecting lower than the posterior tubercle (14) ; 15 : sustentaculum tali ; 16 : navicular ; 17 : talus ; 18 : calcaneus.

23. The limb is not rotated enough : the distal tibio-fibular joint is overshadowed.

24. The limb rotated medially (45°) with such an oblique position, the tip of the lateral malleolus is cleared.

19 : tarsal sinus ; 20 : posterior talocalcanean joint.

RADIOGRAPHY OF THE ANKLE IN THE LATERAL POSITION

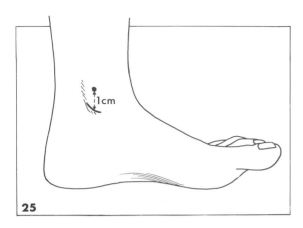

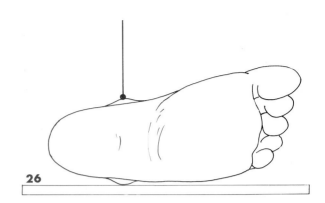

25, 26. Schemas of the incidence

Position : the patient is placed in the true lateral position with the medial malleolus (mediolateral position) or the lateral malleolus (lateromedial position) in contact with the film. In both positions it is essential that the axes of the malleoli be perpendicular to the cassette.

Center : with the tube straight, 2 cm above the tip of the lateral malleolus (lateromedial position) or 1 cm above the tip of the medial malleolus (mediolateral position).

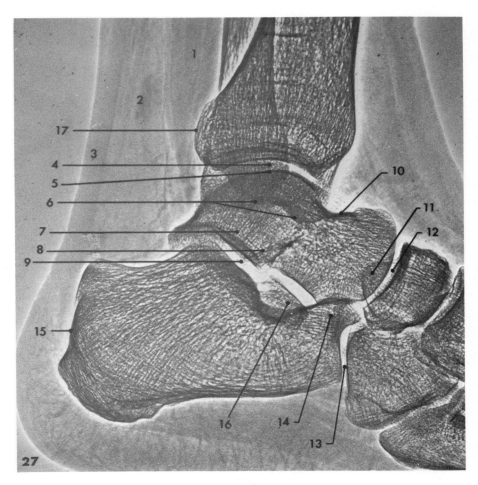

27. Xeroradiograph.

1 : Flexor tendons ; 2 : Kager triangle (adipose tissue) ; 3 : Achilles tendon ; 4 : ankle joint ; 5 : trochlear surface of talus ; 6 : medial malleolus (anterior and posterior tubercles) ; 7 : lateral malleolus ; 8 : lateral talar process ; 9 : posterior subtalar joint ; 10 : neck of the talus ; 11 : pyramidal process of the navicular ; 12 : talonavicular joint ; 13 : calcaneocuboid joint ; 14 : beak of the great apophysis of the calcaneus ; 15 : tuber calcanei ; 16 : sustentaculum tali ; 17 : Destot malleolus.

RADIOGRAPHY OF THE SESAMOIDS

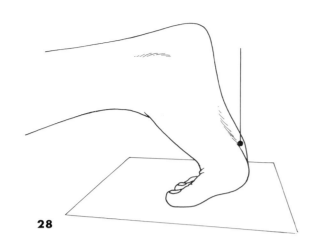

28

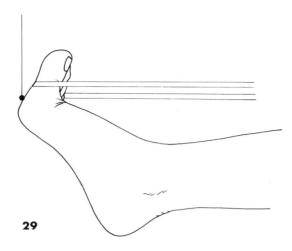

29

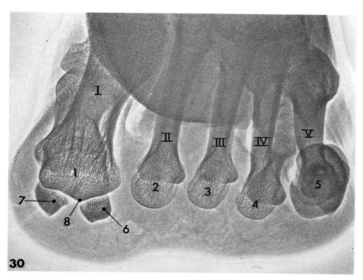

30

28, 29. Schemas of the incidences.

Position : flexion at the first metatarsophalangeal joint is aided with the patient sitting, by a tight bandage passed around the toe **(29)** and, with the patient in the prone position, by pressing the plantar aspect of the phalanges against the film **(28).**

Center : through the sesamoid bones with the tube straight.

30. Xeroradiograph with the patient in prone position.

I, II, III, IV, V : metatarsal shafts ; 1, 2, 3, 4, 5, : metatarsal heads ; 6 : lateral sesamoid bone ; 7 : medial sesamoid bone : 8 : first metatarsal head and median ridge between articular surfaces of sesamoids.

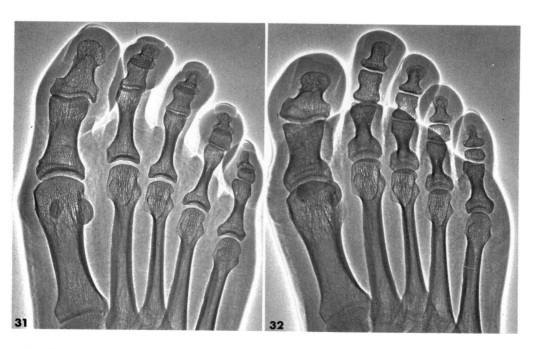

31   **32**

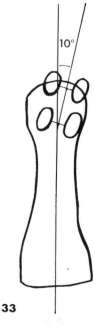

33

31, 32. Comparative dorso-plantar radiographs of the foot in weight-supporting position with the toes either lying flat in relaxation on the X-ray table **(31)** or in active dorsi-flexion **(32).** Note the change in the radiographic appearances of the metatarso-phalageal joints.

The sesamoid bones move forward along the median ridge of the first metatarsal head.

33. At the time the toes are actively flexed, the sesamoids move forward about 10 to 12 mm along an axis that coincides with the line passing through the median ridge of the first metatarsal head. This axis and the midshaft tend to form an acute angle of approximately 10°.

RADIOGRAPHY OF THE CALCANEUS IN THE AXIAL POSITION

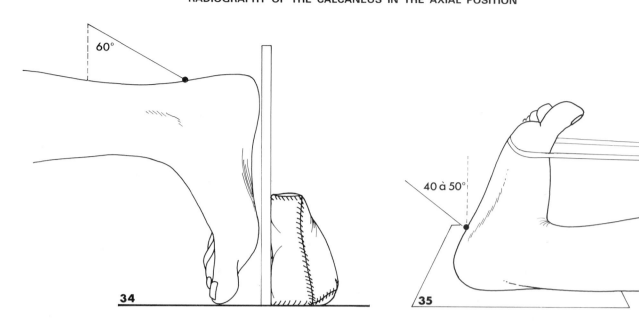

34, 35. Schemas of the incidences

34. Downward posterior tibial angle.

Position : the patient is prone, with the sole of the foot pressing the film, which is supported in the vertical position.

Center : over the posterior aspect of the heel with the tube angled 60° from the vertical.

35. Upward posterior tibial angle.

Position : the patient is seated or recumbent, with the ankles in the antero-posterior position and maintained in position by extending a bandage round the forepart of the sole of the foot ; the film is placed under the back of the heel.

Center : to the plantar aspect of the foot, with the tube angled at 40° to 50° from the vertical.

36. Xeroradiograph.

1 : anterior subtalar joint ; 2 : posterior talocalcanean joint ; 3 : sustentaculum tali ; 4 : styloid tuberosity of the fifth metatarsal ; 5 : calcanean groove ; 6 : posterior tuberosity of calcaneus ; 7 : trochlear process.

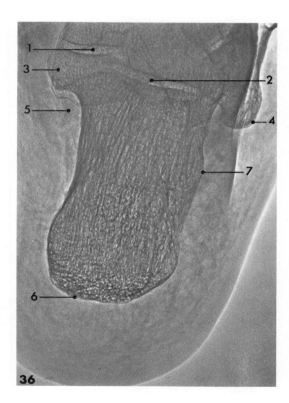

NORMAL VARIANTS

SESAMOID BONES

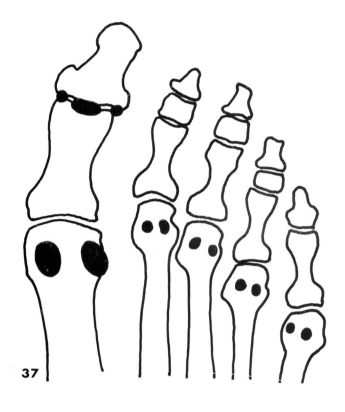

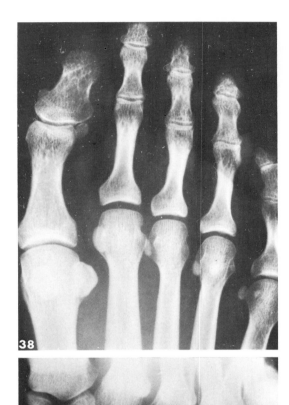

37. Schematic diagram of the forefoot sesamoids. The medial and lateral sesamoids of the great toe are constant.

38, 39. Sesamoids on all the metatarsal heads.

Interphalangeal sesamoid bones of the great toe

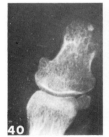 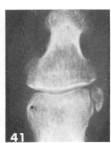 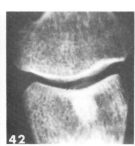 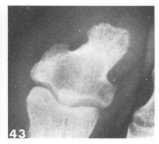 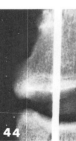 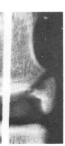

40. Sesamoid in lateral position.

41. Sequela of fracture.

42. Solitary osteosclerotic bone island.

43. Medial and internal sesamoid bones.

44. Irreducible fracture. Dislocation of the interphalangeal joint due to interposition of the sesamoid.

Metatarso-phalangeal sesamoid bones of the great toe

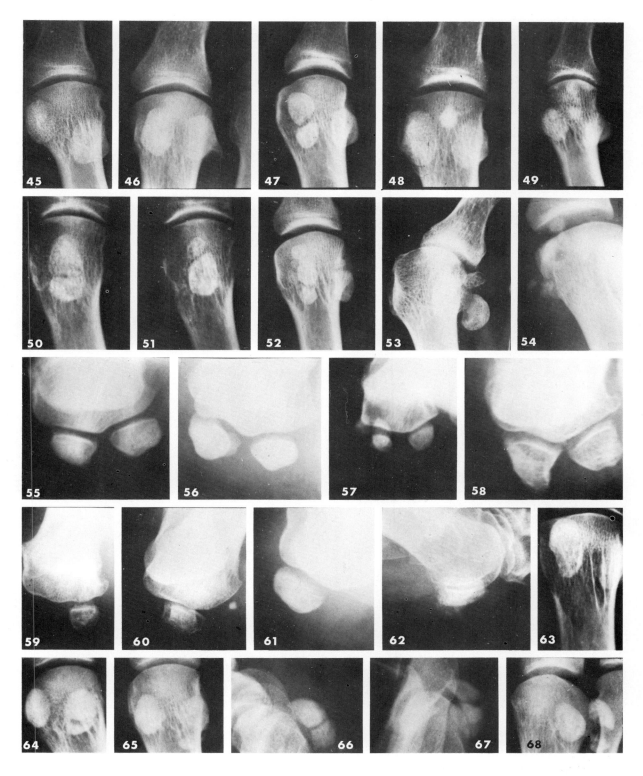

45. Sesamoids in asymmetrical relationship.
46. Lateral sesamoid spur formation.
47. Bipartite medial sesamoid bone.
48. Bone island.
49. Osteopoikilosis.
50, 51. Hypoplasia and aplasia of a sesamoid.
52. Multipartite sesamoid bones.
53. Osteochondromatosis.
54. Comminuted fracture of the medial sesamoid.
55. Axial projection. Normal view.
56. Medial bipartite sesamoid.
57. Lateral multicentric sesamoid.
58. Medial sesamoid conical-shaped by osteophytosis.

59. Aplasia of the medial sesamoid.
60. Hypoplasia of the lateral sesamoid.
61. Surgical ablation of the lateral sesamoid (McBride procedure).
62. Spur formation of the medial sesamoid.
63. Bone crest.
64. Fracture of the lateral sesamoid : irregular fracture line.
65. Same case, six months later, widening of the clearing space between the fragments : pseudoarthrosis.
66. Bipartite sesamoid.
67. Same as 64.
68. Same as 65.

Sesamoid bones of the peroneus longus tendon

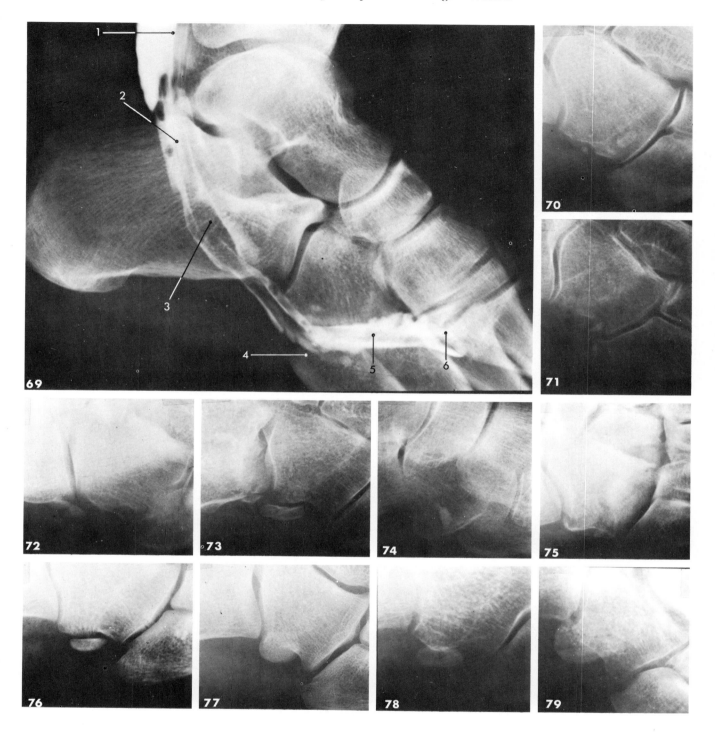

69. Peroneal tenography. An opaque medium is injected into the synovial sheaths of the peroneal muscles close to the posterior aspect of the lateral malleolus (1). The sheaths (2) are parted by the calcaneus : the peroneus brevis tendon passes above the peroneal trochlea (3) and is attached to the tuberosity of the fifth metatarsal (4) ; the peroneus longus tendon passes under the peroneal trochlea, runs in a groove (5) of the cuboid, and is attached to the plantar tuberosity (6) of the first metatarsal.

The ankle joint is never connected with the synovial sheaths of the peroneal tendons, except in case of rupture of the articular capsule (see **1431**). Hence the value of radiography of the peroneal muscle tendons for the differential diagnosis of severe ankle sprain.

70. Multicentric os peroneum set at the margin of the cuboid groove and inside it.

71. Fracture of the cuboid.

72. Bipartite os peroneum.

73. Os peroneum and fracture of the great calcaneal apophysis.

74. Bone island.

75. Fracture of the cuboid.

76, 77, 78. Variations in appearances of the os peroneum.

79. Fracture of the cuboid.

SUPERNUMERARY BONES

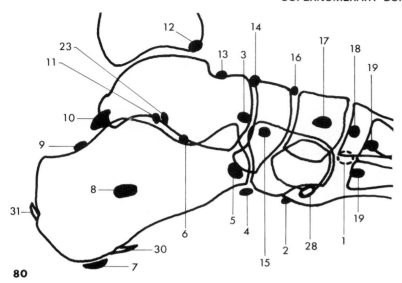

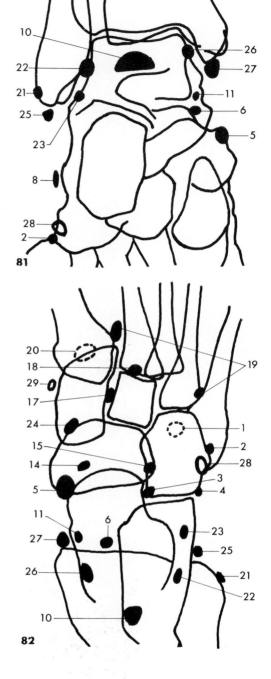

80, 81, 82. Schematic diagram of the supernumerary bones of the foot (after Komler A. and Zimmer E.A.). The most common of these ossicles are italicized.

1 : processus uncinatus (plantar surface) ; 2 : os vesalianum ; 3 : secondary calcaneus ; 4 : accessory cuboid ; 5 : *os tibiale externum* ; 6 : os sustentaculum tali ; 7 : os subcalcis ; 8 : os trochleare calcanei ; 9 : os supracalcis ; 10 : *os trigonum* ; 11 : accessory talus ; 12 : os talotibiale ; 13 : os supratalare ; 14 : *os supra naviculare* ; 15 : cuboides secondarium ; 16 : os infranaviculare ; 17 : os intercuneiform ; 18 : intercuneo-second metatarsal bone ; 19 : *os intermetatarseum* ; 20 : pars peronea metatarsalia I ; 21 : os retinaculi ; 22 : intercalary fibular bone ; 23 : talus secondarius ; 24 : intercuneo-navicular bone ; 25 : *os subfibulare* ; 26 : intercalary tibial bone ; 27 : *os subtibiale* ; 28 : *os pereoneum or sesamoid bone of the peroneus longus tendon* ; 29 : sesamoid bone of the tibialis anterior tendon ; 30 : plantar calcaneal spur ; 31 : posterior calcaneal spur.

83, 84. Diagram showing avulsion fractures simulating accessory ossicles.

83. Lateral view. 1 : avulsion of the posterior malleolus of the tibia ; 2 : Cloquet Shepherd fracture ; 3 : dorsum of the talus ; 4,5 : dorsum of the navicular ; 6 : base of the navicular ; 7 : dorsum of the cuboid ; 8 : calcaneal beak ; 9 : base of the cuboid ; 10 : base of the fifth metatarsal.

84. Dorsoplantar view. 1 : tip of the medial malleolus ; 2 : tip of the lateral malleolus ; 3 : medial border of the talus ; 4 : medial border of the navicular ; 5 : proximal medial tip of the cuboid ; 6 : proximal lateral border of the cuboid ; 7 : base of the fifth metatarsal.

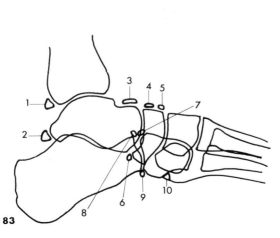

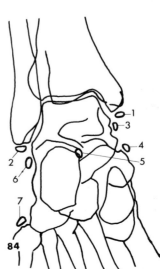

Os trigonum

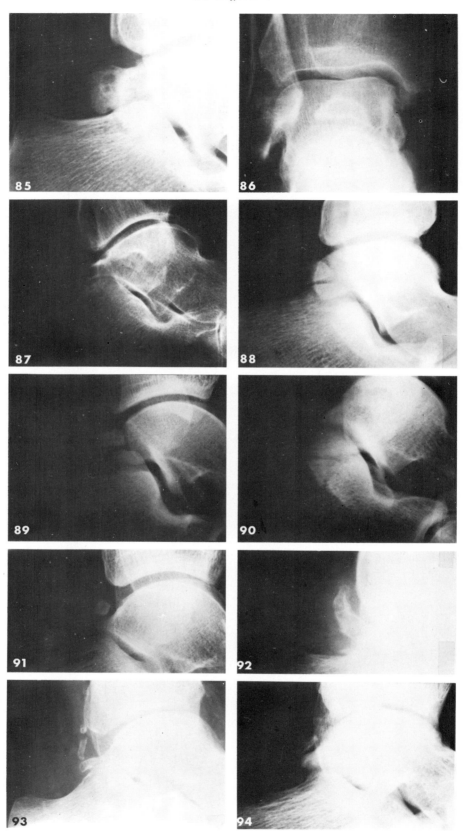

85. Complete fusion of the os trigonum to the talus.
86. Os trigonum : frontal view.
87. Complete fusion of the os trigonum to the talus.
88, 89. Os trigonum : lateral view.
90. Fracture of the sustentaculum tali.

91. Osteochondromatosis of the ankle joint.
92. Horn-like hypertrophic spur formation on the posterior aspect of the talus.
93. Arterial calcification.
94. Arterial calcification and os trigonum.

Os supratalare (Pirie bone)

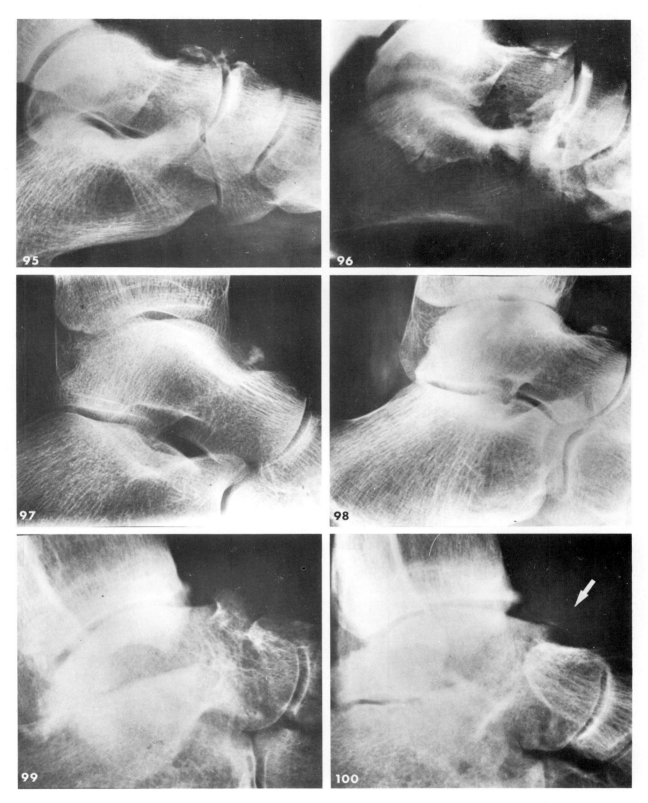

95. Avulsion from the neck of the talus.
96. Fracture.
97. Osteoid osteoma of the talar neck.
98. Os supratalare.
99. Talar beak.
100. Os supratalare.

Navicular

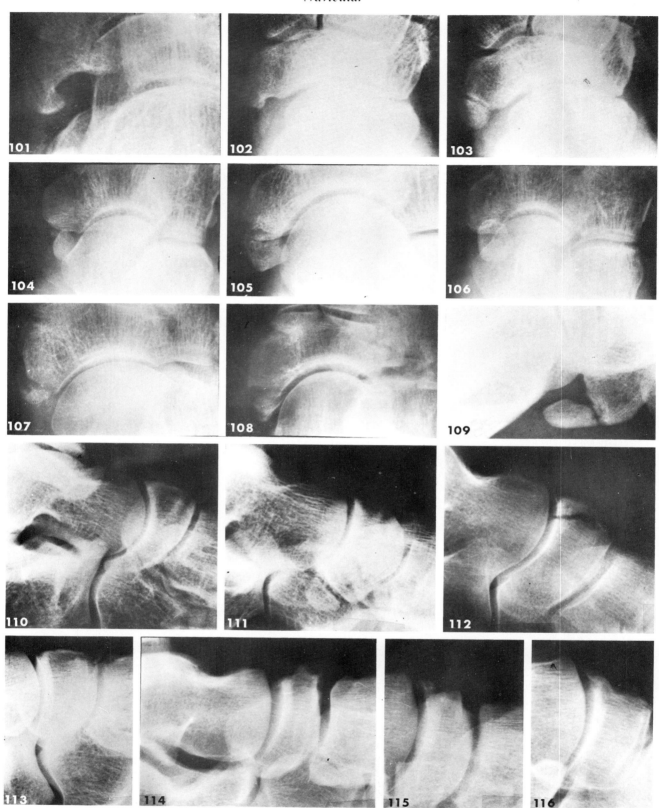

101, 102. Navicular cornutum.

103. Incomplete fusion of the os tibiale externum to the navicular.

104, 105, 106. Os tibiale externum : frontal view.

107, 108. Fracture of the navicular bone.

109. Os tibiale externum : lateral oblique view.

110. Complete fusion of the os tibiale externum to the navicular bone (lateral view).

111. Os tibiale externum : lateral view.

112. Fracture of the navicular bone.

113. Avulsion of the medial cuneiform.

114. Navicular bone exostosis.

115. Small fragment avulsed from the navicular.

116. Os supranaviculare.

Various supernumerary bones of the foot

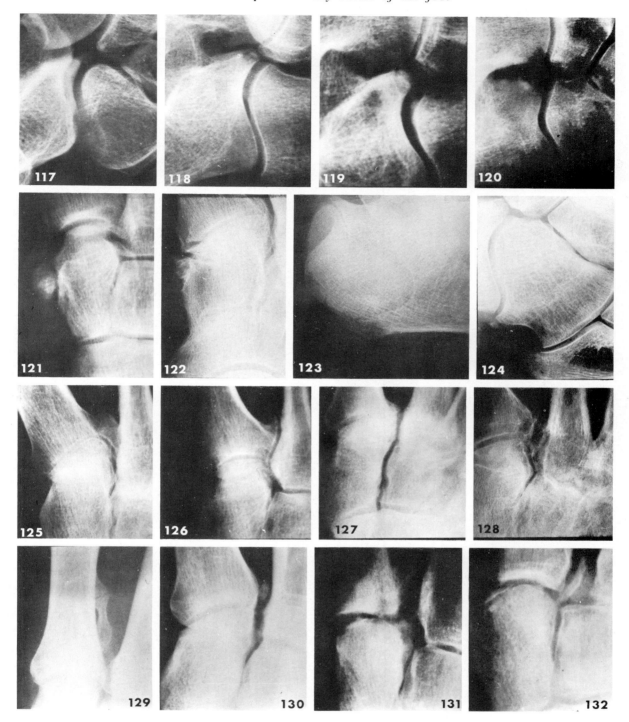

117. Calcaneus secondarius.

118, 119. Fracture of the beak of the tuber calcanei.

120. Calcaneus secondarius : identical radiographic image on the opposite foot.

121. Sesamoid bone in the tibialis anterior tendon.

122. Bone spur formation.

123. Os subcalcis.

124. Accessory cuboid.

125. Os intermetatarsum.

126. Bone spur formation.

127. Normal spacing between the first and second cuneiforms.

128. Pseudogout.

129. Supernumerary metatarsal.

130. Vascular calcification.

131. Bone spur formation.

132. Avulsion (Lisfranc dislocation).

Supernumerary bones of the ankle joint

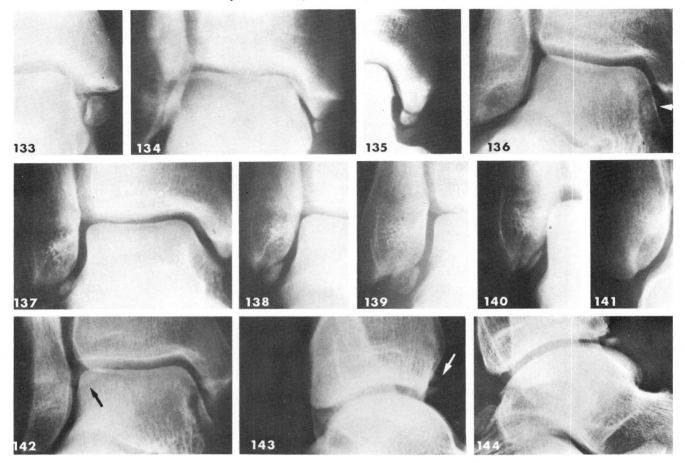

133, 134. Os subtibiale.

135. Os subtibiale and accessory talus.

136. Intercalary tibial bone.

137, 138, 139. Os subfibulare.

140. Avulsion of the lateral malleolus.

141. Malleolar fossa.

142. Intercalary fibular bone.

143. Bone spur formation or os talotibiale ?

144. Os talotibiale, os trigonum, talar beak.

SYNOSTOSES

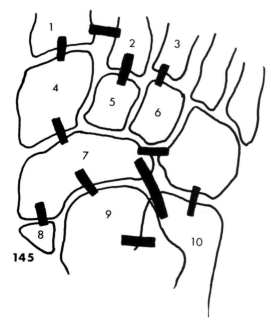

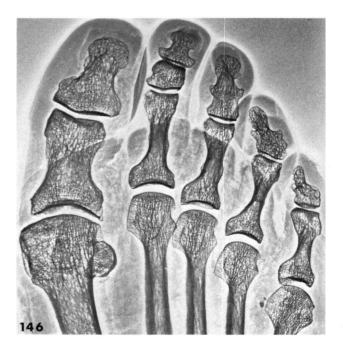

145. Diagram to illustrate the synostoses. One complete fusion between two bones may be considered a normal variant. On the other hand, multiple coalitions are pathological (dysostis).

1, 2, 3 : basis of the first, second and third metatarsal ; 4, 5, 6 : medial, intermediate and lateral cuneiform ; 7 : navicular ; 8 : os tibiale externum ; 9 : talus ; 10 : calcaneus.

146. Xeroradiograph. The distal interphalangeal coalition is most frequent : two phalanged third, fourth and fifth toes.

Congenital tarsal synostoses

The frequency of tarsal fusion with clinical signs in the population, is 1 % (statistics of 2 000 cases, Vaughan and Segal, 1953). The incidence of congenital tarsal synostoses is greater as 76 % of all synostoses are asymptomatic. This abnormality is doubtless hereditary (40 % of Leonard's patients). The calcaneonavicular fusion is most frequent : 50 % of cases (statistics of Meary-Roger, 1969) ; talocalcaneal coalition : 40 % ; other coalitions : 10 %.

Calcaneo-navicular fusion : it is characterized by a bone bridge between the superior and medial extremity of the calcaneal great apophysis and the posteroinferior margin of take navicular. This bridge may be cartilaginous or fibrous tissue and its ossification at the time of puberty initiates or increases symptoms and clinical signs. As the bridge grows and ossifies, it pushes the talar head inward, causing the medial arch to sag ; hence a flat foot appears. In the dorsal aspect of the foot, the navicular-calcaneal fusion produces an exostosis of the talar head (talar-beak).

Talocalcaneal coalition : the fusion may be complete or incomplete (often anterior and medial). The bone bridge between the sustentaculum tali and the talar inferior surface may be seen in the lateral radiograph of the foot (**155**). It will be confirmed by the calcaneal axial projections (Harris). Tomography may be necessary to exclude to coalition, especially of the anterior talocalcaneal joint (Conway and Cowell, 1969).

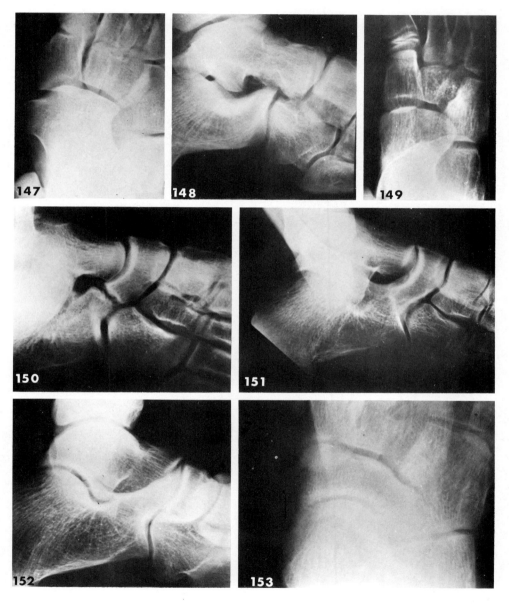

148. Talonavicular coalition.

Talonavicular coalition with congenital aplasia of the fifth arsal : dysostis.

150. Incomplete calcaneonavicular coalition.

151, 152, 153. Calcaneonavicular coalition. **151.** Radiograph in the oblique position. **152.** Radiograph in the lateral position. **153.** Anteroposterior view.

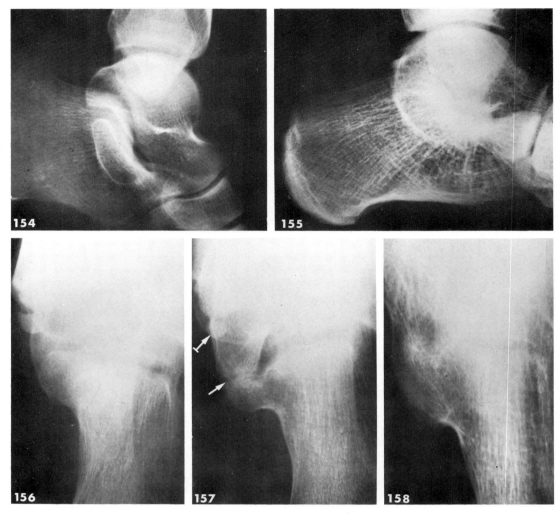

154. Normal radiographic appearance of the sustentaculum tali in the lateral position.

155. Talocalcaneal coalition : in the lateral view, the contour of the trochlear surface of the talus extends without any gap to the lower cortex of the sustentaculum.

156. Radiograph of the calcaneus in the axial projection : normal appearance of the anterior talocalcanean joint.

157. Incomplete talocalcaneal coalition. See the os tibiale externum (↦).

158. Complete talocalcaneal coalition.

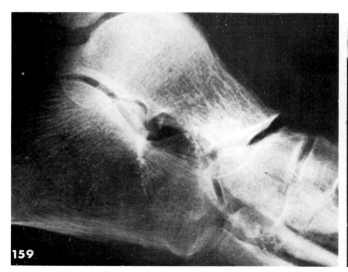

159. Talonavicular and calcaneocuboid coalition : dysostis.

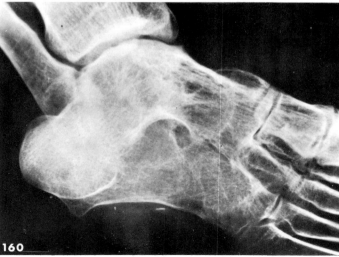

160. Rheumatoid arthritis : fusion of the tarsus posterior.

RADIOGRAPHY OF THE CUNEIFORM JOINTS

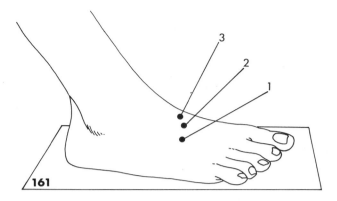

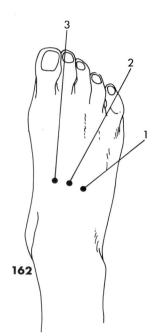

161, 162. Schematic diagram of the Chaumet-Hirtz-Didiée projections.

Position : the patient is in the supine or semirecumbent position, the knee is flexed with the plantar aspect of the foot in contact with the film.

Three directions of the X-ray beam are used, with varying tube angulation toward the ankle and the lateral margin of the foot.
Center in the axis of the interdigital space.

Radiography of the cuneal joints can be done as well in the dorsi-plantar projection. The foot should be rotated medially to a pronation of 10 degrees to the X-ray table top to radiograph the joint between the medial and intermediate cuneiform, to a supination of 20^0 for the joint between the intermediate and the lateral cuneiform, and to a supination of 50^0 for the joint between the lateral cuneiform and the cuboid.

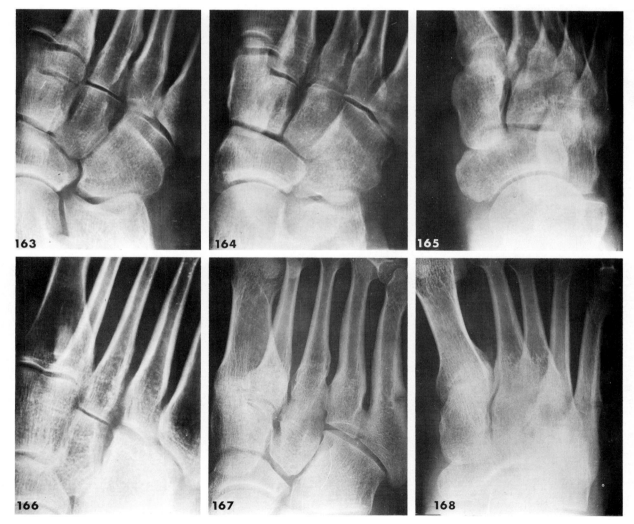

163. Cuneocuboid joint (1).

164. Joint between the lateral and intermediate cuneiforms (2).

165. Joint between the medial and intermediate cuneiforms (3).

166, 167, 168. Same patient. The three lateral oblique projections, after Chaumet, are necessary to document a false synostosis (note the fatigue fracture of the shaft of the fifth metatarsal).

FIFTH METATARSAL

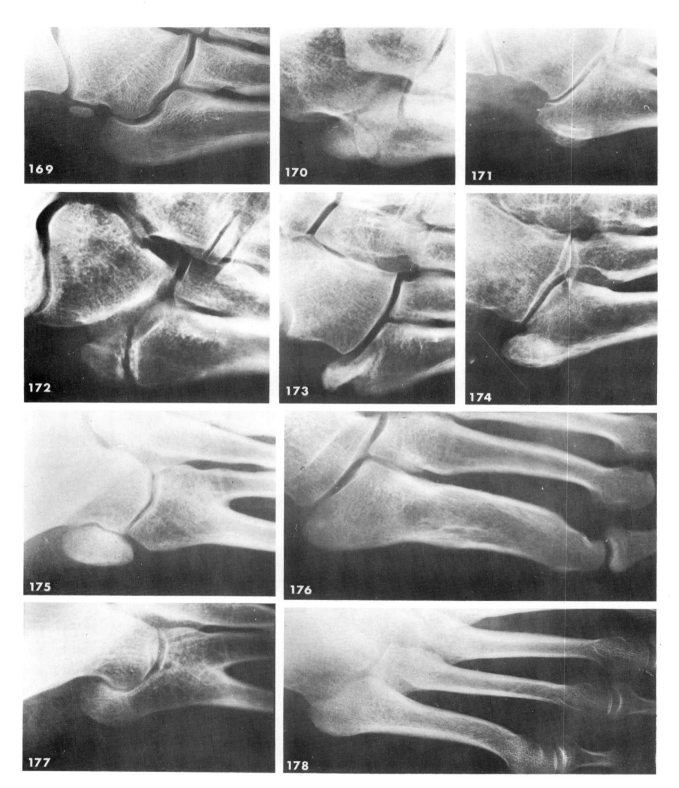

169. Surrounding styloid process and os peroneum.

170. Incomplete fusion of the fifth metatarsal styloid.

171. Hyperostosis of the fifth metatarsal styloid.

172. Pseudarthrosis.

173. Old fracture.

174. Rheumatoid arthritis : osteosclerosis at the insertion of the peroneus brevis muscle on the styloid tuberosity of the fifth metatarsal, due to a reactive bone formation secondary to rheumatoid synovitis.

175. Supernumerary bone and complete fusion of the fourth and fifth metatarsal bases (in an Apert syndrome).

176. Pagetoid changes of the fifth metatarsal.

177. Same patient as 175 : surrounding styloid apophysis, complete fusion of the fourth and fifth metatarsal bases.

178. Exaggeration of the normal curvature of the fifth metatarsal shaft.

CALCANEUS

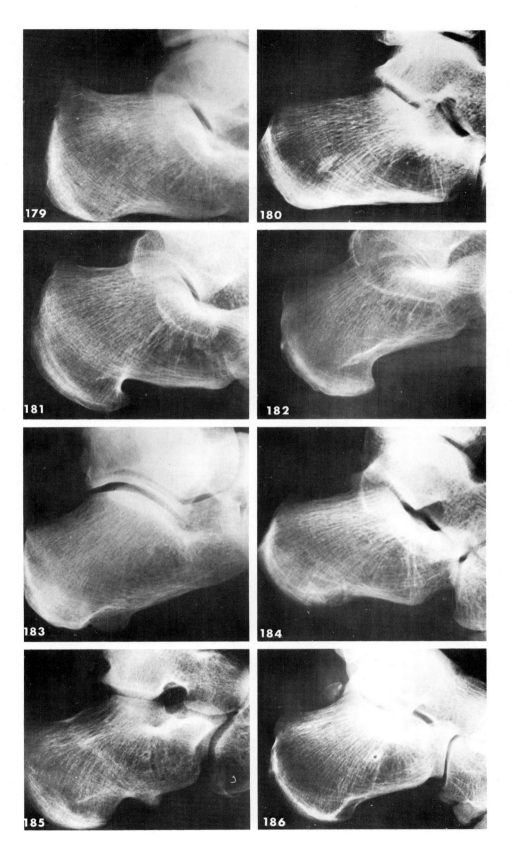

179. Calcaneus high and sharp (Haglund calcaneus). Note the erosion due to rheumatoid arthritis.

180. Calcaneus flat, with the inferior aspect horizontal.

181, 182. Hypertrophic posterior tuberosity of the calcaneus.

183. Nontangential view of calcaneus : tubercle of the posterior tuberosity is shown.

184. Fracture of the posterior tuberosity.

185. Calcaneal osteotomy (Dwyer procedure).

186. Nutrient foramen and os trigonum.

TALUS

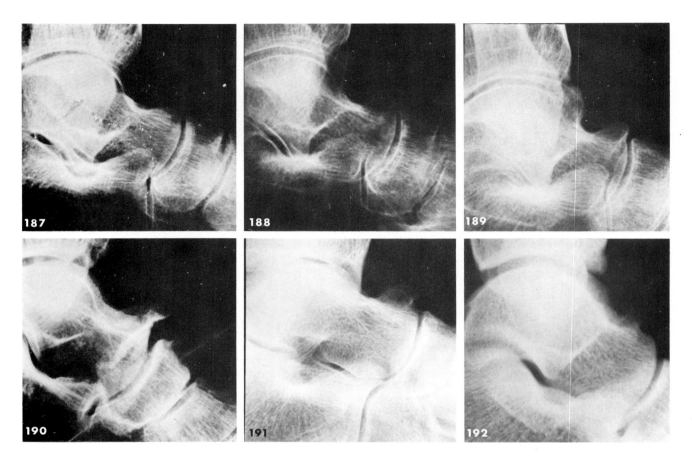

187, 188, 189. Growing talar beak : same patient, one year between each radiograph.

190. Osteophyte.
191, 192. Talar beak.

ANGIOGRAPHY

FOOT ARTERIES

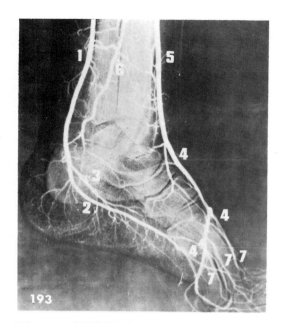

193. General and normal radiographic anatomy.

1 : posterior tibial artery ; 2 : medial plantar artery ; 3 : lateral plantar artery ; 4 : dorsalis pedis artery and deep plantar arch ; 5 : anterior tibial artery ; 6 : peroneal artery ; 7 : plantar metatarsal arteries.

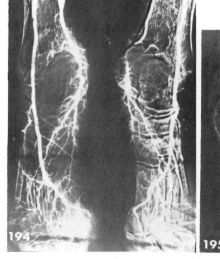

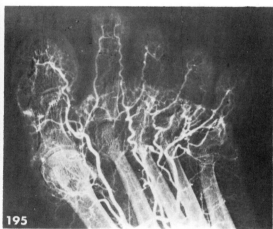

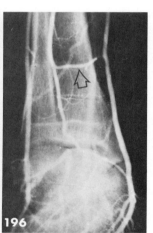

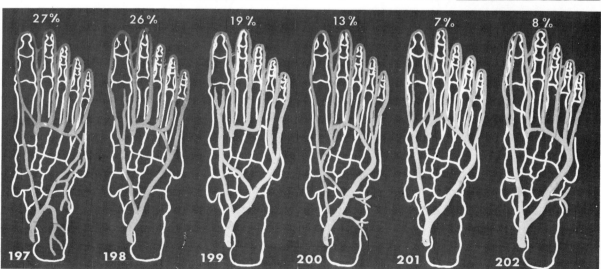

194 → 202. Arterial anatomic variants.

194. Predominant dorsalis pedis artery.

195. Common arterial network : two proper plantar digital arteries for the 2nd toe, one lateral artery for the great toe, one medial artery for the third, fourth and fifth toes.

196. Anastomosis between peroneal and posterior tibial arteries.

197 → 202. Anatomic variants of the plantar arterial network (after Dubreuil-Chambardel).

ARTERIAL TARSUS VASCULATURE

(after J.P. CARRET)

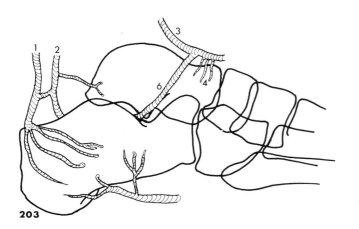

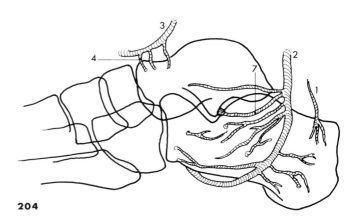

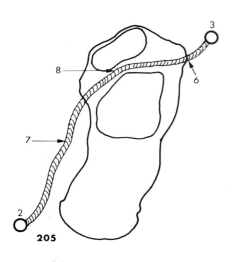

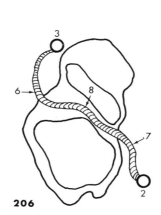

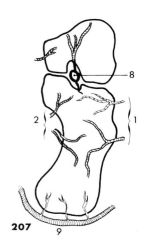

203 → 207. Diagrams to illustrate the posterior tarsus vasculature.

203. Lateral view.

204. Medial view.

205. Superior view of the right calcaneus.

206. Inferior view of the right talus.

207. Frontal section.

1 : peroneal artery ; 2 : posterior tibial artery ; 3 : dorsalis pedis artery ; 4 : arteries of the talar neck ; 5 : lateral plantar artery ; 6 : tarsal sinus artery ; 7 : tarsal canal artery ; 8 : tarsal sinus arch ; 9 : underlying calcaneal arch.

ARTERIAL TALAR VASCULATURE

(after J.P. CARRET)

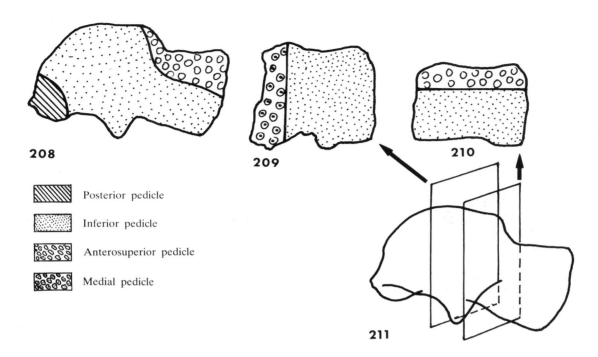

208 **209** **210** **211**

▨ Posterior pedicle

▩ Inferior pedicle

▨ Anterosuperior pedicle

▨ Medial pedicle

208 → 211. Schematic diagrams of the talar arterial networks. The arch of the tarsal sinus carries the most important vascular flow and is not to be cut during surgical operation of the subtalar joint.

However the posterior pedicle is not essential. Cutting it during osteosynthesis by the posterior approach will not impair bone vasculature.

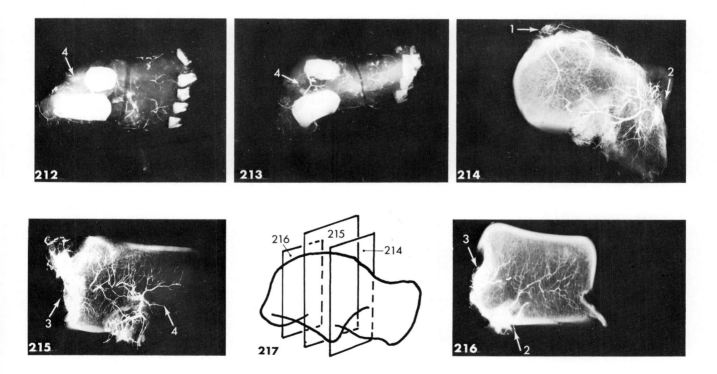

212 **213** **214** **215** **216** **217**

212, 213. Microangiographs of the posterior tarsus arteries of a fetus (anatomical specimens). Arch of the tarsal sinus comparatively wider than in the adult.

214, 215, 216. Microangiographs with injection of the arterial pedicles in an adult (anatomical specimens) according to frontal sections of the talus on the diagram **217.** The calcaneus is mostly vascularized by arteries passing through the lateral and medial aspects.

1 : anterosuperior blood supply ; 2 : inferior blood supply ; 3 : medial blood supply ; 4 : arch of tarsal sinus.

217. Diagram of frontal sections.

ARTERIAL CALCANEAL VASCULATURE

(after J.C. CARRET)

The vasculature of the calcaneus arises principally from perforating branches of its medial and lateral sides.

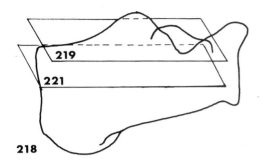

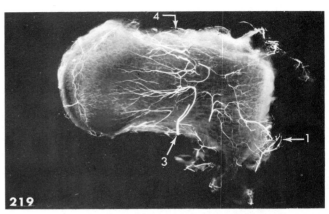

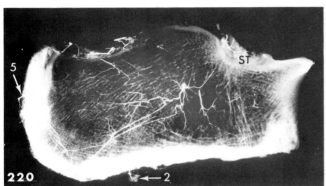

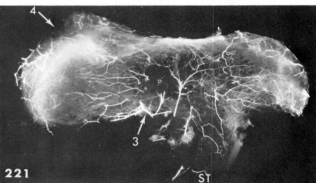

218. Diagram of transverse sections corresponding to the following microangiographs.

219, 220, 221. Microangiographs of the left calcaneus in the adult (anatomical specimens).

219. Superior transverse section. **220.** Median sagittal section. **221.** Inferior transverse section.

1 : anterosuperior blood supply ; 2 : inferior blood supply ; 3 : medial blood supply ; 4 : lateral blood supply ; 5 : posterosuperior blood supply ; ST : sustentaculum tali.

ANGIOGRAPHY OF THE SOLE OF THE FOOT

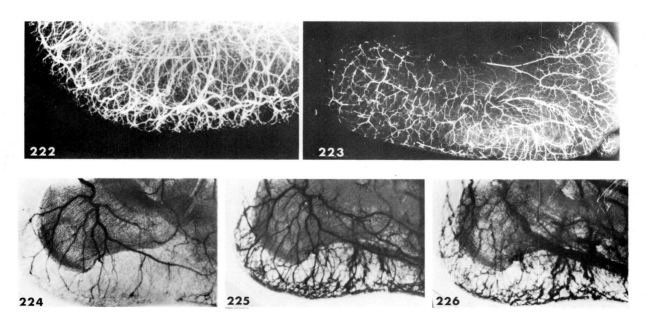

222, 223. Anatomical specimens.

222. Lateral view of the posterior aspect of the heel.

223. « Scalp » of the sole of the foot.

224, 225, 226. Arteriograms.

224. Arterial phase.

225. Arteriolar phase.

226. Venous phase.

ARTERIAL VASCULATURE OF THE TOES

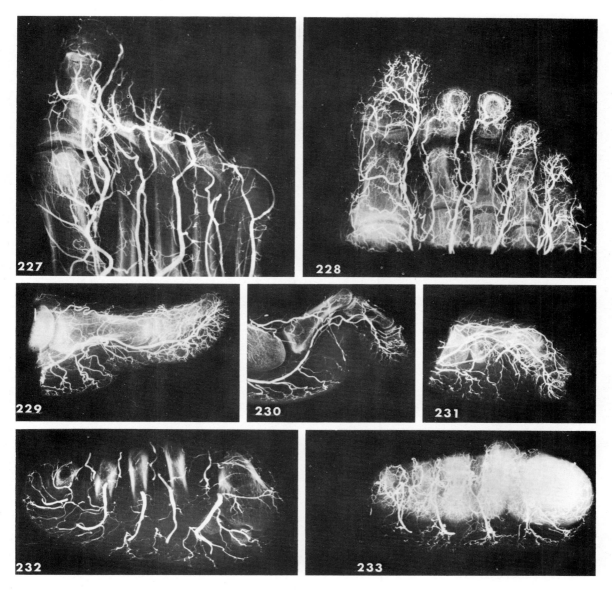

227 → 233. Anatomical specimens : predominant plantar arterial network.

VENOGRAPHY

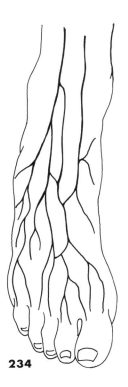
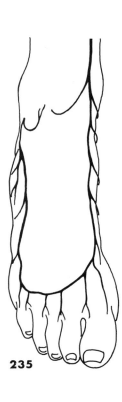
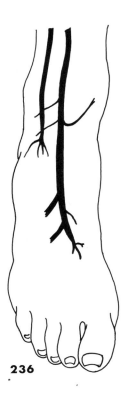
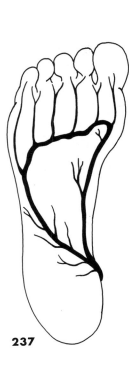

234   **235**   **236**   **237**

234 → 238. Normal venography of the foot (after J. Chermet).

The veins of the foot constitute five networks : a dorsal subcutaneous network ; a dorsal venous arcade anastomosing the great saphenous vein with the small one (between superficial and deep aponeurosis) ; a deep network accompanying arteries and including dorsalis-pedis veins and plantar veins ; a superficial plantar network ; perforating veins.

234. Superficial dorsal veins.

235. Dorsal venous arcade.

236, 237. Deep venous network with dorsal veins (**236**) and plantar veins which form an arcade in the sole of the foot (**237**).

238. Superficial plantar veins which connect to the deep plantar veins and also dorsal superficial veins and the saphenous veins.

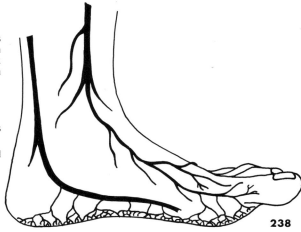

238

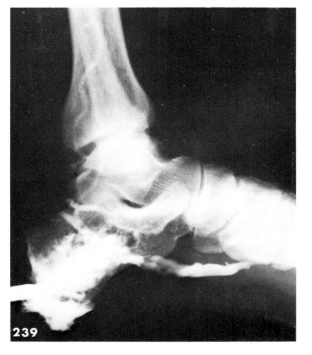

239. Transosseous calcaneal venography (J. Benassy procedure). The radiopaque contrast medium injected in the spongy bone drains via the deep venous satellites of the arteries. The author recommends this study in severe and chronic talalgia, arguing from premises that the pain is due to venous stasis. Percalcaneal venography : unsatisfactory filling of the venous network, stasis of the contrast medium and reflux.

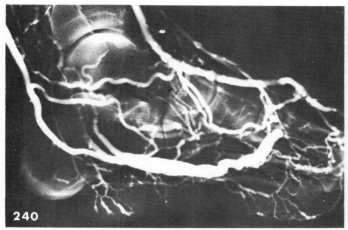 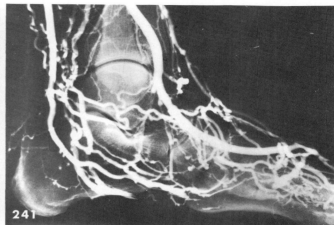

240, 241. Normal venography of the foot by injection in a dorsal digital vein of the great toe.

240. Nonweight-bearing lateral oblique venogram with the patient recumbent : filling of the plantar veins.

241. Weight-bearing lateral venogram : the compressed plantar veins have emptied.

THERMOGRAPHY

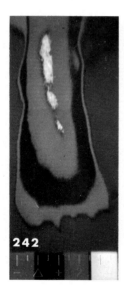 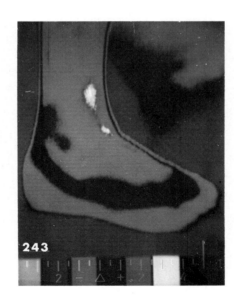 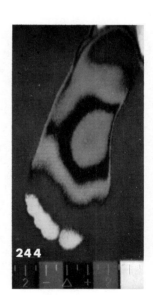

242 → 244. Normal infrared thermograms of the foot.

242. Dorsal aspect of the foot.

243. Lateral aspect.

244. Plantar surface.

The dark zones show the warmest areas, viz the best vascularized.

SCINTIGRAPHY

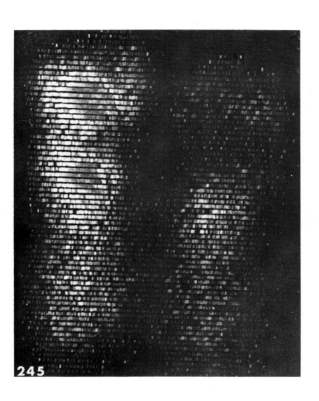

245

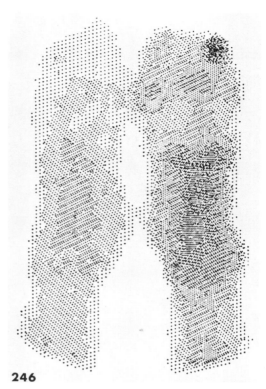

246

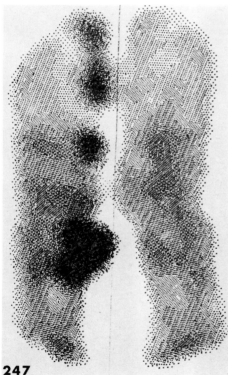

247

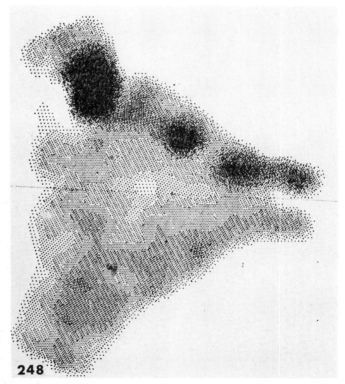

248

245. Scintigram 5 months after a surgical intervention : alignment and embedding of the second, third and fourth metatarsal heads (B. Regnauld's procedure) : intense accumulation in the left tarsus and the second, third and fourth metatarso-phalangeal joints. Normal uptake in the right foot.

246. Scan of both feet (view from above) : on the left, normal scan ; on the right, increased uptake in distal phalanx of the fourth toe. Note a general increase in osseous metabolism.

247, 248. Scintigram from the same patient as in figure **1381**.

247. Frontal view : in the left, areas of increased uptake in the first digit and the ankle joint. Normal right foot.

248. Lateral view, patient with the soles of the feet facing each other. Bottom, normal foot.

2

THE FOOT IN STANDING

COMPARATIVE ANATOMY* : EVOLUTION OF THE AUTOPODIUM

THE ORIGINS

Various types of pelvic fins

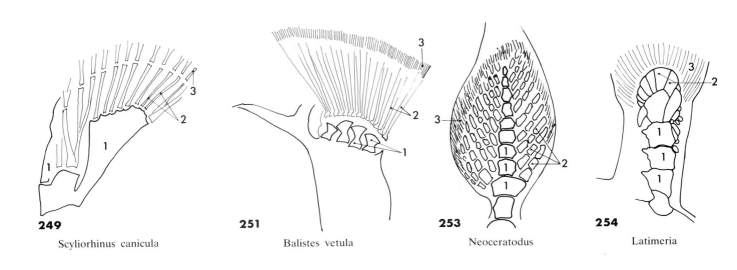

249   **251**   **253**   **254**
Scyliorhinus canicula   Balistes vetula   Neoceratodus   Latimeria

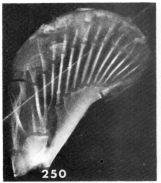 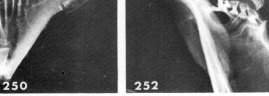

250   **252**

Scyliorhinus canicula   Balistes vetula

249 → 254. Present fishes : schematically, the skeleton of a fin consists of basic laminae on which are inserted numerous cartilaginous rays, called pterygophores, which are extended by the lepidotrichiae, dermal parts forming the framework of the fin.

249 → 252. Early structures : **249.** In a chondrychthian, *Scyliorhinus canicula* ; **250.** Life size radiograph ; **251.** In a teleostean, *Balistes vetula* ; **252.** Life-size radiograph.

253. Diagrams after Jollie : *Neoceratodus,* dipneuste : the basic laminae are along a straight line ; **254.** *Latimeria,* coelacanthimorph : the lepidotrichiae are set laterally.

255. Fossil fish : *Eusthenopteron,* rhipidistian, diagram after Jarvik : the paired tibia (T) - fibula (P) appears under a femur (F). This laying out fortetokens the limb of the tetrapod *Ichthyostega* (**256**). The skeleton of the tetrapod's limb consists of three segments : the stylopodium, always formed by a single bone (humerus or femur), articulates the limb with the girdle ; the zeugopodium formed by two bones (radius and ulna, or tibia and fibula) ; the autopodium which consists of two parts : the basipodium constituted by the bones of the hand or the foot ; and the acropodium which composes the skeleton of digits.

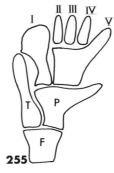 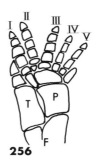 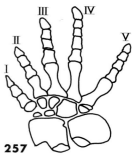

255   **256**   **257**
Eusthenopteron   Ichthyostega   Ophiacodon

Originating in water

256. *Ichthyostega,* primitive quadruped (diagram after Jarvik) : the fin is changed into a weight-bearing horizontal limb ; the autopod lies flat on the ground to support, at best, the weight of the body (upper Devonian, 350 million years or so ago). However, the amphibians spend the beginning of life within waters, but at the upper carboniferous (300 million years or so ago) appears in the captorhinomorph reptiles, the amnionic egg with a protective shell : whence the final escape out of the waters. The body rises, the limbs are held in a vertical and parasagittal posture with rotation and abduction of the autopodium ; so, the tibia becomes medial and the acropod anterior. This change in posture modifies the tarsus : an ankle joint appears between the pair tibia-fibula and a protarsus formed by the talus and the calcaneus united transversally ; this arrangement persists in birds (**259**) an crocodiles (**258**). This vertical position of the limb has proceeded by stages : in the pelycosaurs (**257**) which originate from the captorhinomorphs, only the zeugopod is vertical ; the stylopod is still horizontal.

257. Foot of *Ophiacodon mirus* (diagram after Romer and Price), pelycosaur of the lower Permian (about 280 million years ago).

* All the pictures in this chapter have been reproduced from radiographs of anatomical specimens graciously forwarded by Professor J. Anthony, Director of the Laboratory of Comparative Anatomy of the Museum of Natural History in Paris. We would like to thank G. Desse M.D. whose work has inspired us for this chapter.

The complete verticality appears in the middle or upper Permian in mammalian reptiles (Therapsides) which have followed the pelycosaurs about 200 million years ago.

At the lower Jurassic (about 170 million years ago), originating from the mammalian reptiles, appear the mammalia which, owing to their homeothermy, are able to live in countless surrounding mediums. The autopodium specializes itself in particular types : shovel, oar, etc. but always the disposition of the original tetrapod will be found (256).

258. Crocodile.

259. *Anhima cornuta (Kamachi cornu).*

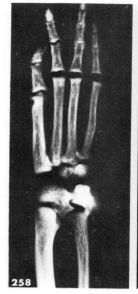
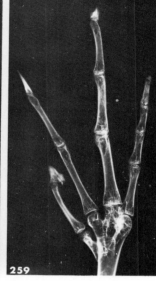

258 Crocodile   259 Kamachi

THE ADAPTATION

Specialization of the autopodium in the mammals and marsupals.

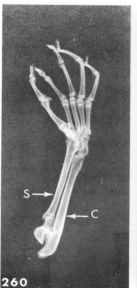
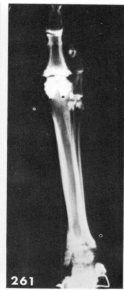
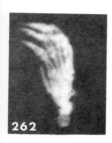

262 Mole

260 Galago   261 Kangaroo

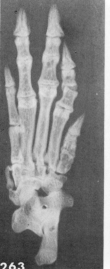
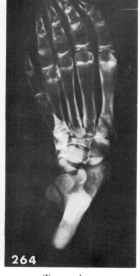

263 Armadillo   264 Tamandua

The jumpers

260. *Galago senegalensis* (life-size), type of tree-living jumper : lengthening of the calcaneus (C) and navicular (S) which became as long as a tibia.

261. *Macropus rufus* (Kangaroo) lengthening of the foot, especially of the tuber calcanei constituting a big lever-arm with a long fourth metatarsal, the other metatarsals being atrophied.

The fossorials

262. *Talpa talpa,* insectivorous (Mole, life-size) ; shovel-like widening of the autopodium with pre-hallux.

263. *Dasypus,* edentate (Armadillo, life-size), prehallux, heavy phalanges with a distal phalanx splitted into a groove.

The climbers and the hangers

264. *Myrmecophaga jubata* (Tamandua) : distal phalanges with huge claws which also serve to rip the ant-hills. One may see also hocked phalanges with claws and suckers in the climber and hanger monkeys, eg.

265. *Hylobates* (Gibbon).

266. *Bradypus* edentate (Ai) (three-toed sloth) : tarsal and metatarsal coalition forming a bone block on which hook-like claws insert.

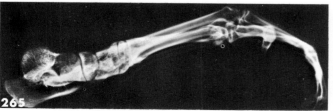

265 Gibbon

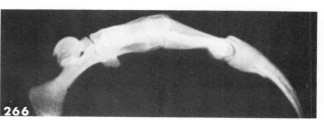

266 Ai

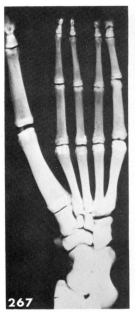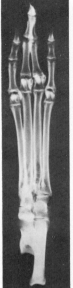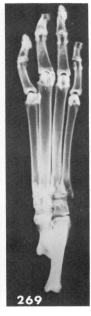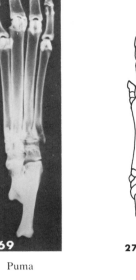

Otary   Wolf   Puma

Decrease of the lateral rays.

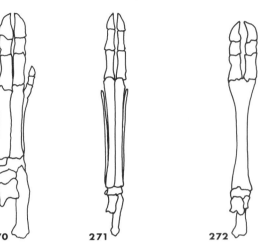

In ungulate paraxonic

The swimmers

267. *Otaria jubata* (Otary) : Oar-like widening of the autopodium, of which the plantar aspect is lateral with talus and calcaneus on a same horizontal level ; lengthening of the nails.

The runners

268. *Canis lupus* (Wolf) ; **269.** *Felis prima*, felid, (puma) : narrowing of the foot ; lengthening of the metatarsus with disappearance of the first ray. **270***. *Sus scrofa* (Wild boar), ungulate paraxonic, viz the functional axis of the limb passes between the third and fourth metatarsals, which are separated. **271.** In *Tragulus*, these metatarsals join in a single bone (shank bone) where one may still discern the junction line. The reindeer lowers the remaining second and fifth rays as brakes in the snow. **272.** *Bos taurus* (Ox) : these metatarsals join entirely and the second and fifth rays disappear.

Same adaptation to running in the mesaxonic ungulates, viz the functional axis of the limb passes through the third metatarsal (like in **273**, *Elephas* or **274**, *Tapirus*), this metatarsal remaining alone in the present genus *Equus* **(275).**

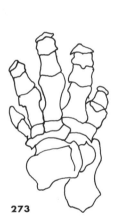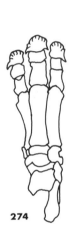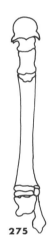

In ungulate mesaxonic

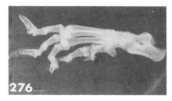

Hedgehog

The walkers or plantigrades

276. *Erinaceus europaeus*, insectivore (hedgehog, life-size) not adapted to walking, but it has a predominant posterior limb, like the bear and the man.

277 → 288. The primates, plantigrades highly adapted to walking.

277. *Papio papio*, cynomorph (baboon) narrow and long foot (40 % of the length of the limb), short tarsus (30 % of the length of the foot). In man, the foot is short (24 % of the length of the lower limb) and the tarsus is long (52 % of the length of the foot) (see **282, 283, 284**). The baboon is a poor walker. It leans on the medial side of the everted foot ; the calcaneus does not press on the ground ; it is slender, horizontal, and without a posterior tuberosity **(285)**.

* Figures 270 to 275 are reproduced from the *Traité de Zoologie*, by P.P. Grassé, Masson Ed., Paris, 1967.

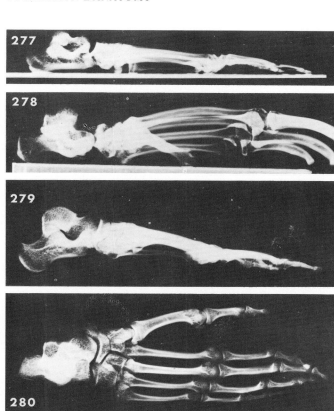

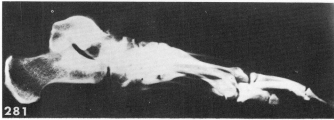

From top to bottom : Baboon, Orang, Chimpanzee, Chimpanzee, Gorilla.

Evolution of the respective lengths of the tarsus, metatarsus and phalanges, in relation to the entire length of the foot.

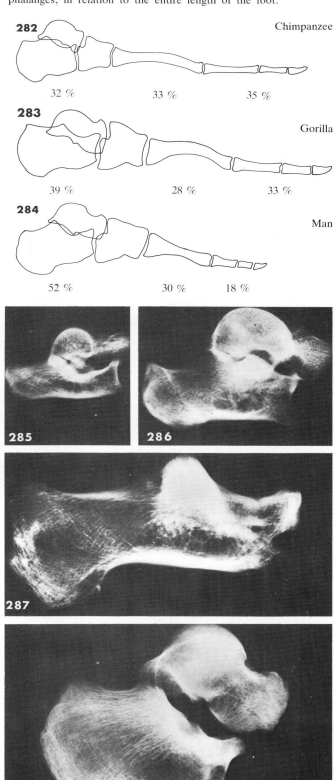

282   Chimpanzee

32 %   33 %   35 %

283   Gorilla

39 %   28 %   33 %

284   Man

52 %   30 %   18 %

285   **286**

287

288

Evolution of the calcaneal anatomy in relation to the erect position : Baboon, Chimpanzee, Gorilla, Man.

278. Pongo pygmaeus (orangoutan) ; **279, 280.** *Pan troglodytes* (chimpanzee) ; **281.** *Gorilla gorilla* (gorilla) : these monkeys stand like men, and have a long narrow foot with a short everted tarsus, like the baboon (see **282, 283, 284**). But the weight-bearing base of the foot progressively becomes more nearly perfect up to the gorilla : the calcaneus straightens, little by little, with the appearance of differentiated arciform bony tuberculae along lines of highest resistance, transmitting the weight of the body. The calcaneus becomes quite vertical in man, showing a large posterior tuberosity (**285, 286, 287, 288**). The talus overlaps the calcaneus and a longitudinal plantar arch appears. Another most important change : man places the foot in the prone position, the functional axis of the foot becoming antaxonic, viz medial, passing through the second metatarsal. The monkeys' toes are long, the greatest being the third toe, and the toe-pattern is 3>4>5>2>1, whereas in man the first toe is prominent (see p. 47).

The hallux of the monkey is divergent and adducent. In man, on the other hand, the hallux lies alongside the second metatarsal ; the metatarsals tighten and the toes shorten ; the foot of our hominian ancestors was similar to this pattern, which is our own*.

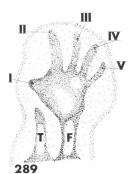

289. Foot of a human embryo 15 mm long (T : tibia ; F : fibula).

* Note of the authors : To describe the metatarsus varus or brevis, the terms « prehistoric foot », « ancestral foot », « Neanderthal foot » are improper. It would be more accurate to speak of « fetal foot », or « immature foot » (Georges Desse). Bardeen has actually shown that the human embryonal foot (**289**) keeps the fibula and the calcaneus in close contact up to the 49th day, without any joint at the level of the ankle, and it has a short and very divergent hallux.

RADIOGRAPHIC TECHNIQUES - MARKINGS AND MEASUREMENTS

The strain due to the body weight and applied to the foot bones and joints is radiographically apparent only on weight-bearing films (294). The foot of the patient in erect positioning is radiographed successively according to the three planes of symmetry of the body : dorsi-plantar radiograph (horizontal plane of the foot), lateral radiograph (median sagittal plane) and, for the frontal plane, antero-posterior radiograph of the ankle.

On these graphs, lines and angles are drawn for the measurements.

HORIZONTAL PLANE

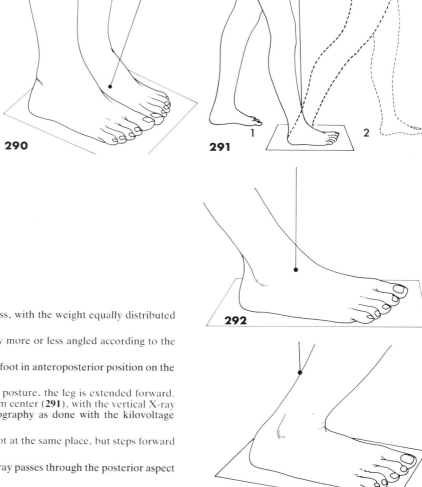

RADIOGRAPHY OF THE WEIGHT-BEARING FOOT IN ANTERO POSTERIOR POSITION

The dorsoplantar radiography of both feet of a patient in upright posture (290) meets two requirements :

1) The X-ray beam must be as close as possible to the vertical axis : too marked an inclination of the tube will cause distorsion of the radiographic image (295, 296).

2) An equal contrast between fore and hind-foot is necessary (297, 298) to obtain good quality radiographs. For this purpose, the double exposure technique is very satisfactory (299), but this method is difficult to perform (291).

The xeroradiograph (301) gives as good information as the bifocal radiograph (300), the posterior tarsus being visible through the tibia, and any measurement of the foot can be taken with the shoe on (302).

290 → 293. Schemas of the incidences.

290. Frontal radiography of weight-bearing feet.

Position : the patient is in the erect posture, motionless, with the weight equally distributed between both feet.

Center : to the dorsum of the foot with the central ray more or less angled according to the stoutness of the subject.

291, 292, 293. Double exposure of the weight-bearing foot in anteroposterior position on the same film.

First exposure : position 1 : the patient is in upright posture, the leg is extended forward. The plantar aspect of the foot is in contact with the film center (291), with the vertical X-ray beam centered over the ankle joint (292). The radiography as done with the kilovoltage required for tarsus anterior.

Second exposure : position 2 : the patient keeps his foot at the same place, but steps forward with the opposite limb (291).

The X-ray tube is not displaced ; therefore the central ray passes through the posterior aspect of the ankle (293).

The radiograph is taken with the kilovoltage required for the tarsus posterior.

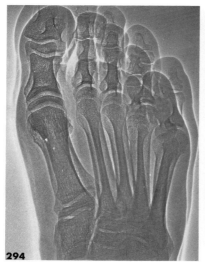

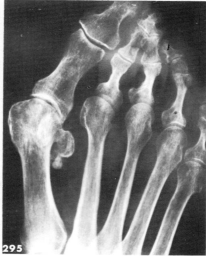

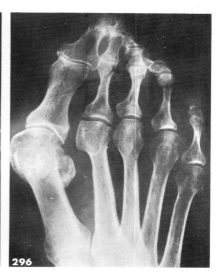

294. Successive exposures, on the same film, of a weight-bearing foot and the same foot relaxed : the pictures are dissimilar : elongation (1 cm) of the fore foot, widening of the metatarsus (7 to 9 cm), broadening of the metatarsus varus (6 to 10°).

295, 296. Dorsoplantar radiograph of the weight-bearing foot : 295. X-ray beam very much angled : apparent subluxation of the second and third metatarsophalangeal joints ; 296. Vertical X-ray beam : same patient, no subluxation (note a sequela of Freiberg's disease).

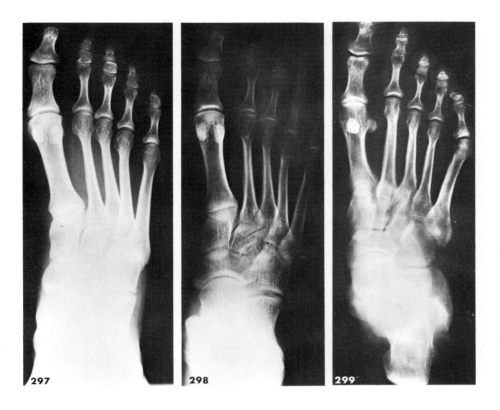

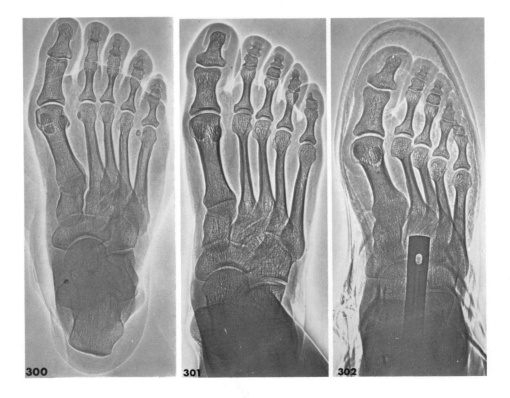

297. Radiography of the foot in the frontal projection with adequate penetration of the forefoot.

298. Frontal radiography of foot in the antero-posterior position with adequate penetration of the hindfoot.

299. Frontal radiography of foot by the double exposure technique.

300. Frontal xeroradiography of the foot by the bifocal technique.

301. Frontal xeroradiography of the foot in anteroposterior position.

302. Frontal xeroradiography of the foot, with the shoe on, in anteroposterior position.

ROENTGENOGRAPHIC MEASUREMENTS IN THE HORIZONTAL PLANE

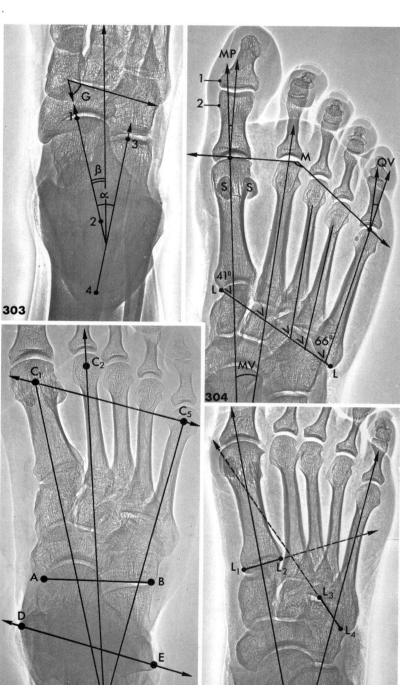

303. The axis of the talus extends from the middle point of the anterior margin (1) to the middle point of the posterior margin (2) of the talus. The axis of the calcaneus extends from the midpoint of the anterior aspect of the great apophysis (3) to the midpoint of the posterior tuberosity (4). These two axes form an angle α, the *talocalcaneal divergence* of 15-25°. Usually, the midtalar line and the line through the shaft of the second metatarsal form an acute angle β of 5 to 10° (G. Lang). *Giannestra's angle* $\widehat{G}$ is the angle between the midtalar line and the line producing the axis of the intermediate cuneiform-navicular joint : normal value 60° to 80°.

304. The axes of the shafts of the distal (1) and proximal (2) phalanges of the great toe form a straight line.

The axes of the shafts of the first phalanx of the great toe and the first metatarsal form an angle $\widehat{MP}$ from 8 to 12°, the metatarsalphalangeal angle.

The axes of the shafts of the first phalanx of the fifth toe and the fifth metatarsal form an angle $\widehat{QV}$ of 8-10°.

The sesamoid bones (SS) of the big toe are normally projected on a radiograph exactly on the head of the first metatarsal.

The axes of the shafts of the first and second metatarsals form an angle $\widehat{MV}$ of 5-10° *(normal physiologic metatarsus varus)*.

An acute angle (>) is formed by the axis of the shaft of each metatarsal with the midtarsal joint. These angles increase progressively : 41° for the first metatarsal to 66° for the fifth metatarsal. They decrease in the pes adductus and increase in the flat foot and the pes supinatus.

The tangent of the first to second metatarsal heads and the tangent of the second to fifth metatarsal heads form a normal angle of 140°. This *Meschan's angle* $\widehat{M}$ is less than 135° in case of shortening of the first metatarsal.

305. The anteroposterior axis of the foot extends from the center of the second metatarsal head to the midpoint C of the posterior tuberosity of the calcaneus. This is the *anatomical axis* of the foot.

The mechanical and kinetic axis of the foot generally coincide with the midshaft line of the first metatarsal. The three bony points supporting the weight of the body are the centers C_1 and C_5 of the head of the first and fifth metatarsals and the middle C of the calcaneal tuberosity. Thus, the supporting surface is in the form of a *triangle*.

The transverse cuboid-navicular line A.B extends from the medial extremity of the talonavicular joint to the lateral extremity of the cuboid-calcaneal joint. This line is usually divided in two equal segments by the anteroposterior axis C_2C of the foot. Unequal segments characterize an exaggerated supination or pronation of the forefoot.

The line passing through the medial and the lateral malleoli D.E. and a second line drawn through the centers of the first and fifth metatarsal heads C_1-C_5 are parallel or slightly convergent laterally. Any increase in this lateral convergency characterizes the pes abductus ; any medial convergency is typical of adduction.

Abduction and pronation denote a pes valgus, adduction and supination a pes varus.

306. The axis of the shafts of the first and fifth metatarsals form an angle ω of 20-28°, named spreading out angle or *opening angle of the foot*.

The straight line drawn from the medial portion of the tarsometatarsal joint L_1-L_2 passes through the middle of the fifth metatarsal shaft.

The straight line drawn from the lateral portion of the tarsometatarsal joint L_3-L_4 passes through the first metatarsal head.

TOE PATTERN*

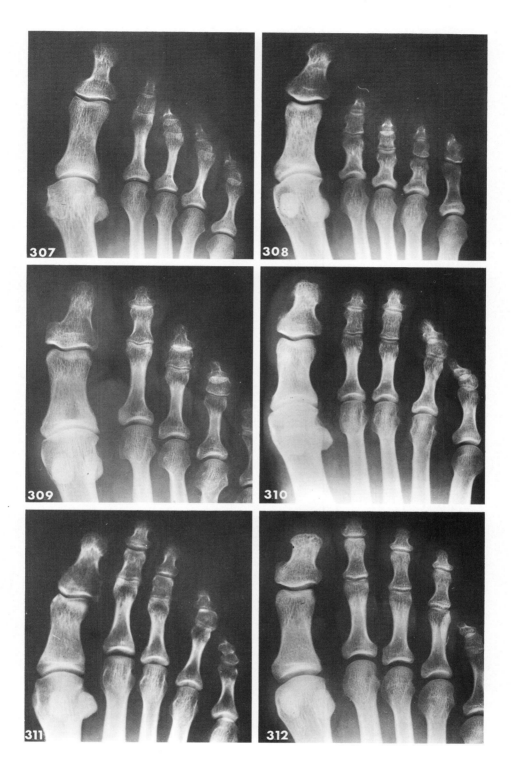

307, 308. *Egyptian foot :* first toe longer than the second (1>2) 50 %.
Two variants : **307.** 48,5 % 1>2>3>4>>5.
308. 1,5 % 1>>2>3>4>>5 (hallomegaly).

309, 310. *Square foot :* first toe of the same length as the second (1 = 2) 27 %.
Two variants : **309.** 23,5 % 1 = 2>3>4>>5.
310. 3,5 % 1 = 2 = 3>4>>5.

311, 312. *Greek foot :* first toe shorter than the second (1<2) 23 %.
Two variants : **311.** 13,5 % 2>1>3>4>>5.
312. 9,5 % 2>3>1>4>>5.

The standard woman's shoe fits only the Greek foot which is, however, far less common than the Egyptian type.

METATARSAL PATTERN

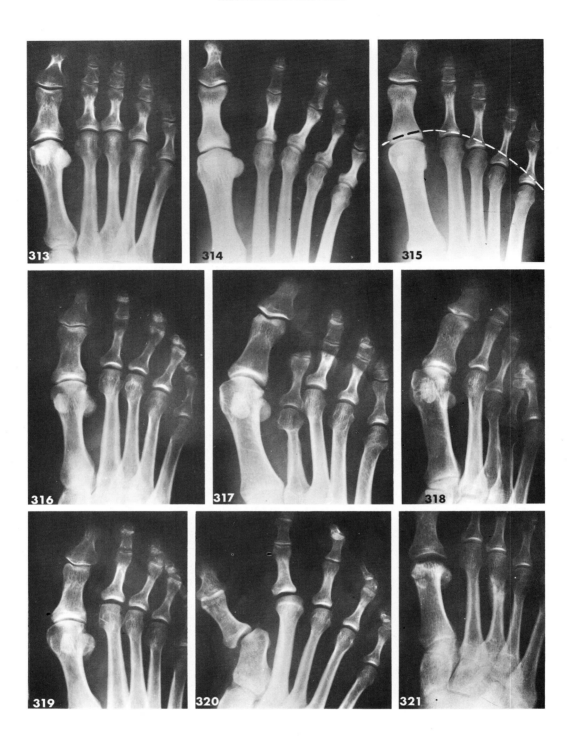

313. Compressed metatarsus.

314. Spreading metatarsus.

315. Ideal metatarsal pattern (J. Lelievre's parabola).

Many metatarsalgia are caused by the breaking of this parabola due to shortening of the metatarsals, particulary of the first one. The shortening of the first metatarsal, the causes of which may be congenital (**316-319**), dysplasic (**320**) or surgical (**321**) conveys the body weight on the second metatarsal head. Such an overloaded head is exposed to dislocation (**389**), arthrosis (**1371**) or stress fracture (**321**).

316. Congenital shortening of the first metatarsal.

317. Short second metatarsal.

318. Short third and fourth metatarsals.

319. Congenital shortening of the first metatarsal : early hallux valgus.

320. Dysostosis of the first metatarsal.

321. Sequela of the Hueter-Mayo surgical procedure : overload fracture of the second metatarsal shaft.

SAGITTAL PLANE

RADIOGRAPHY OF THE WEIGHT-BEARING FOOT IN THE LATERAL POSITION

The standard film (324) gives a satisfactory radiographic picture of bone density of the ankle, the posterior and the anterior tarsus. With xeroradiography (325, 326), the phalanges and the soft tissues are most easily revealed, even through the shoe.

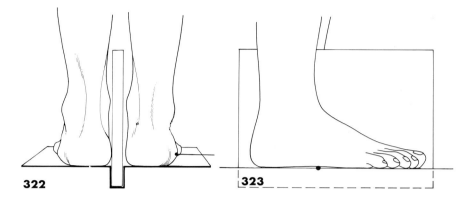

322

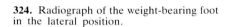

323

322, 323. Schemas of the incidence.

Position : the patient is in the erect position, standing on both feet, with the film placed vertically between the feet and ankles.

Center : to the lateral aspect of the foot using horizontal tube projection.

324. Radiograph of the weight-bearing foot in the lateral position.

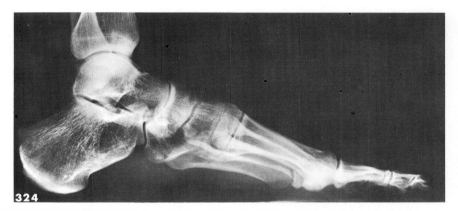

324

325. Xeroradiograph of the weight-bearing foot in the lateral position.

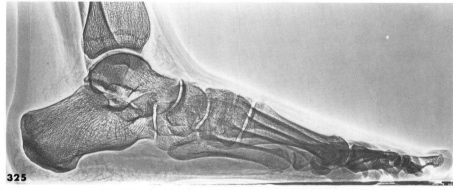

325

326. Lateral xeroradiograph of the foot, erect and weight-bearing, with the shoe on. All the shoe components and the orthosis are obvious. 1 : orthopedic insole ; 2 : sole wedge ; 3 : cambrion.

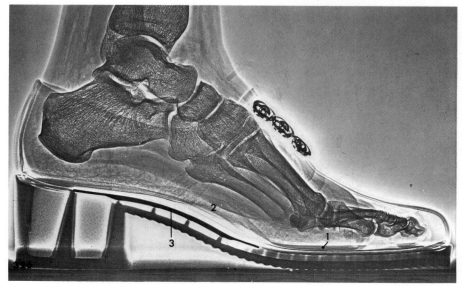

ROENTGENOGRAPHIC MEASUREMENT IN THE SAGITTAL PLANE

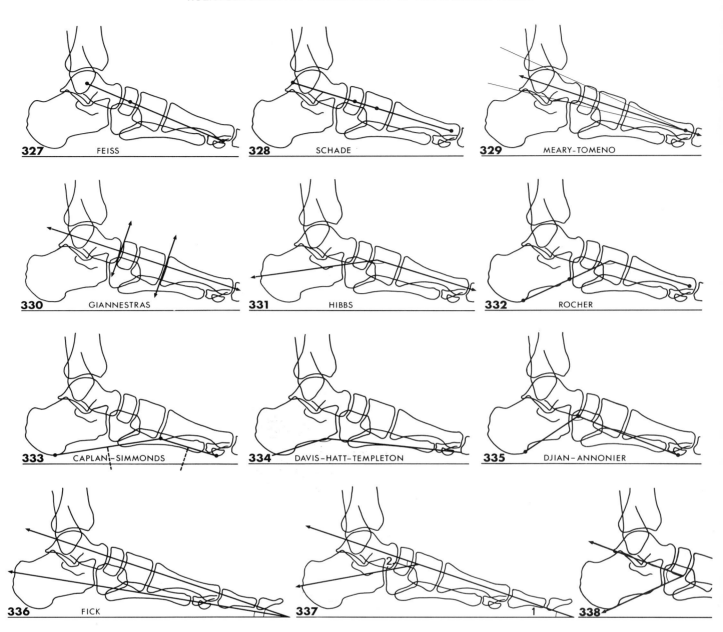

327. Feiss line. In the normal foot, this line extends from the center of the navicular bone and the trochlea of the talus to the lowest point of the first metatarsal head. Generally, the center of the trochlea of the talus is projected on a level with the anterior tubercule of the medial malleolus.

328. Schade line. In the normal foot, this line extends from the lower margin of the posterior aspect of the talo-trochlea to the center of the navicular, the medial cuneiform, and the first metatarsal head which are in a straight line.

329. Meary line. Usually, the axis of the neck of the talus is continuous with the axis of the first metatarsal shaft.

To be more precise, Tomeno uses the following marks :

— the midtalar axis is the bisecting line of the angle formed by the lines tangential to the superior and inferior aspects of the talus ;

— the first metatarsal midshaft axis is a line parallel to its superior margin, drawn through the center of its head ;

— usually, these two axes coincide (Meary axis).

330. Medial series of bones of the foot, after Giannestras : the articular surfaces of the talonavicular and cuneiform-first metatarsal joints are parallel and at right angles to the Meary line.

331. Hibbs angle or angle of planus : usually, the mid-calcaneal line and the axis of the first metatarsal shaft form an angle of 130°.

332. Rocher angle : the line extended from the lowest point of the posterior tuberosity of the calcaneus to the lowest point of the calcaneocuboidal joint and the axis of the first metatarsal shaft form a normal angle of 140°.

333. Caplan and Simmonds angle : the line extended from the lowest contour of the medial sesamoid bone to the lowest point of the first metatarsal base and a second line extended from this point to the lowest point of the posterior calcaneal tuberosity form a normal angle of 150°. The authors prefer the complementary angle (30°).

334. Davis-Hatt and Templeton angle : an obtuse angle is usually formed by the line passing through the inferior cortex of the calcaneus and the inferior cortex of the fifth metatarsal. An acute angle is pathologic.

335. Djian-Annonier angle : the line drawn from the inferior contour of the medial sesamoid through the lowest point of the talonavicular joint forms an angle, usually 120-125°, with the line drawn from this last point to the lowest point of the calcaneus.

336. Fick angle : the axis of the first metatarsal shaft and the horizontal plane make an angle of approximately 18-25° ; this angle decreases to 5° for the fifth metatarsal.

337. Talar pitch (1) : the midtalar line forms, usually with the horizontal plane, an angle of 25°. Angle of talocalcaneal divergency (2) : the axes of the talus and the calcaneus form an angle of 20-35°.

338. Angle of talocalcaneal convergency : the tangents to the inferior margins of the talus and calcaneus form a normal angle of 25-35°.

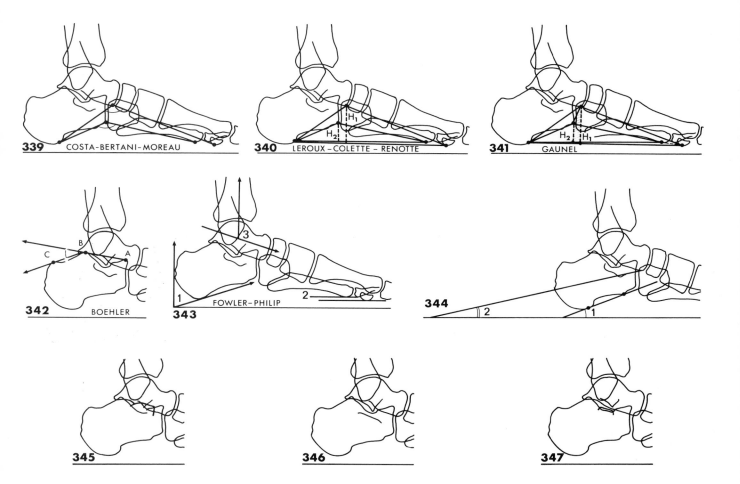

339 COSTA-BERTANI-MOREAU 340 LEROUX-COLETTE-RENOTTE 341 GAUNEL

342 BOEHLER 343 FOWLER-PHILIP 344

345 346 347

339. Costa - Bertani and Moreau angles. The angle of the medial arch is formed by the line extended from the lower contour of the medial sesamoid to the lowest point of the head of the talus and a second line extended from this last point to the lowest point of the posterior tuberosity of the calcaneus. Normal value : 115⁰. The angle of the lateral arch is formed by the line extended from the lowest point of the 5th metatarsal head to the lowest point of the calcaneocuboid joint and a second line extended from this last point to the lowest point of the posterior tuberosity of the calcaneus. Normal value : 145⁰.

340. Leroux, Colette and Renotte triangles. With the above well-defined points, it is possible to draw a triangle inscribed in the medial or lateral arch. The proportion between altitude and base in named « rise » of the external or lateral arch.

341. Gaunel prismatic volume. The inscribed triangles of the medial and lateral arch form Gaunel's prismatic volume. In the lateral radiograph, the vertex and the altitudes of the Leroux, Colette and Renotte triangles form a quadrangle, which is the frontal section of the prismatic volume. The distortions of this quadrangle allow Gaunel to figure the abnormalities of the static foot.

342. Boehler critical angle : the line drawn form the postero-superior margin of the talocalcaneal joint through the postero-superior margin of the calcaneus makes an angle of usually 28-40⁰ with a second line drawn from the postero-superior margin of the talocalcaneal joint to the superior articular margin of the calcaneocuboid.

343. Fowler and Philip angle (1) : angle formed by the tangent to the posterior aspect of the tuber calcanei and a second line extended from the lowest weight-bearing point of the calcaneus to the inferior part of the calcaneocuboid joint. Normal value : 44-70⁰. This angle is wider than 70⁰ in the anatomical calcaneal variant called « Haglund disease ».

If the pressure of the first metatarsal head on the ground is inadequate (2) : the height between the horizontal tangents to the fifth metatarsal head and to the sesamoid bone of the great toe usually does not exceed 5 mm.

Tibiotalar angle (3) : the axis of the shaft of the tibia and the midtalar line form an angle of usually 90-105⁰.

344. Calcaneal pitch (1) : inferior aspect of the calcaneus and the horizontal plane form a normal angle of 15⁰.

Angle of the calcaneal pitch (2) : the midcalcaneal line usually forms an angle of 20⁰ with the horizontal plane.

345, 346, 347. Radiographic appearance of the frontal relationships of the posterior tarsus with the leg in a lateral radiograph.
345. Normal radiograph of the sustentaculum tali ; **346.** Appearance of the sustentaculum tali in a case of calcanean varus ; **347.** Radiographic appearance of the sustentaculum tali in a case of calcanean valgus.

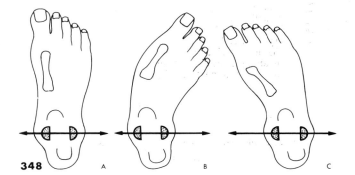

348 A B C

348. Changes in the radiographic image of the foot in the lateral projection, according to the pathological deviation of the forefoot. Diagram of the foot seen from above, the ankle being exactly in lateral position.

A) No deviation : the medial arch of the foot is parallel to the plane of the X-ray plate. So, axes and angles are projected without any distortion.

Forefoot valgus (B) and forefoot varus (C) : the medial arch is not more parallel to the plane of the plate. The projection of the axes and angles is distorted.

SAGITTAL PLANE

FRONTAL RADIOGRAPHY OF THE WEIGHT-BEARING ANKLE

The frontal radiograph of the ankle of a patient in upright position shows the axial relationships of the leg and the heel. The outline of the calcaneus is best shown with the heel raised (3-4 cm) by a cork block. The frontal plane passes through both malleoli, it is parallel to the plane of the vertical film and it is visualized by a lead wire : Meary's technique (351-352), or metallic marks (Djian's technique, 352). Xeroradiography (357) gives a better radiographic appearance even with the shoe on (358).

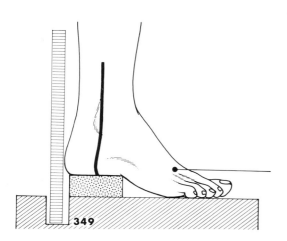 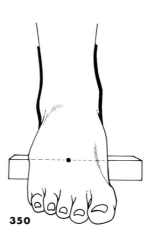 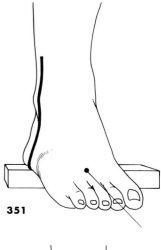

349 → 352. Schemas of the incidence.
Position : patient standing on both feet, medial aspects of feet brought together, heels raised by a cork block* (349).

350, 351. Meary's method : Both malleoli are encircled by a lead wire passing under the heel.

352. Djian's method : metallic marks are placed in contact with the skin of the heel, on both sides of the calcaneus, plumb with the malleoli.
Center : midway between the dorsal aspect of the feet with the horizontal X-ray beam.**

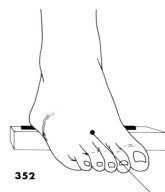

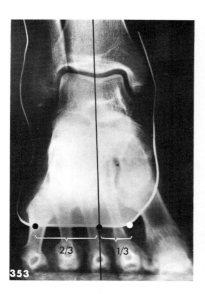 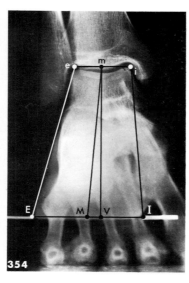

353. Radiograph of the weight-bearing ankle in the anteroposterior projection with the Meary lead wire. The axis of the tibial shaft usually passes through the junction between the inner and the outer two-thirds of the straight under-calcaneal lead wire portion.
If the tibial axis passes inside this crossing point, there is a calcaneal valgus; outside, there is a calcaneal varus.

354. Radiograph of the weight-bearing ankle (bearing the full weight of the body), in the anteroposterior projection, with Djian's metallic marks. Points e and i are the inner and outer extremities of the superior margin of the talar trochlea surface.
Points E and I are the inner and outer extremities of the cutaneous weight-bearing calcaneal surface, visualized by metallic marks.
E-I-e-i is the hindfoot weight-bearing quadrangle, usually asymmetrical.
The line passing through the midpoint of the bases of this quadrangle and the vertical weight-bearing line of the lower limb form an angle of 8[0] (physiological calcaneal valgus).

---

* Strictly frontal radiograph of the ankle is not compulsory, for the axial relationships between the heel and the leg are estimated according to the following references : the axis of the tibial shaft, the weight-bearing plane of the heel, and the superior margin of the talar trochlea surface.
** For the same reason, as*, it is unnecessary to obtain a radiograph with a horizontal X-ray beam tangential to the weight-bearing plane of the calcaneus. By all means, one must use a radiographic projection which could be repeated in the operating-room.

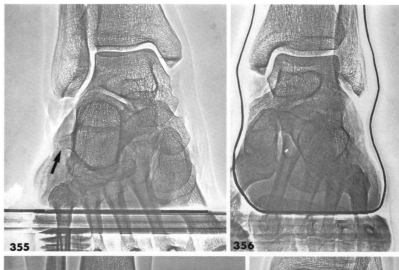

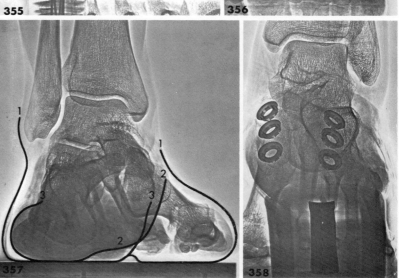

355 → 358. Frontal xeroradiographs of the ankle.

355. With the heel raised and Djian's metallic marks. Note the large trochlear process (→) of the os calcis (peroneal process).

356. With Meary's lead wire.

357. With the heel flat, without marks. On the xeroradiograph, the tangential lines to the skin are clearly defined, 1 : tangency to the weight-bearing plane of the metatarsal heads : 2 : tangency to the apex of the plantar arch ; 3 : tangency to the weight-bearing point of the heel.

358. With the shoe on.

AXIAL RADIOGRAPHY OF THE WEIGHT-BEARING SESAMOIDS

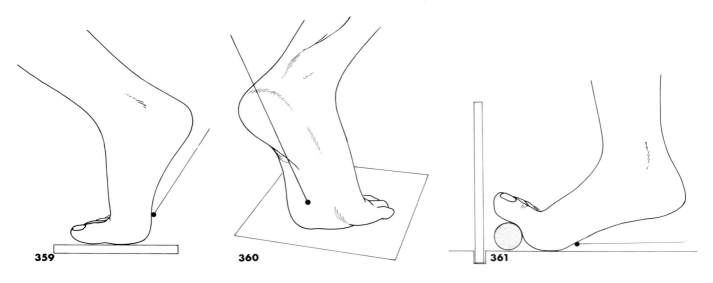

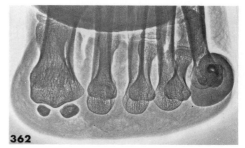

359 → 361. Schemas of the incidences.

359, 360. *Position :* the patient is in starting sprint position ; the knee flexed and the heel raised, with the toes pressed against the horizontal film.
Center : to the first metatarsal head with the angled X-ray tube.

361. *Position :* the patient is in upright position, the hell slightly raised, the plantar aspect of the toes pressing against a cork roller.
Center : to the first metatarsal head with the central ray at a right angle to the film, supported vertically against the toes.

362. Axial xeroradiograph of the sesamoids.

WEIGHT-SUPPORTING FRONTAL RADIOGRAPH OF THE FOREFOOT

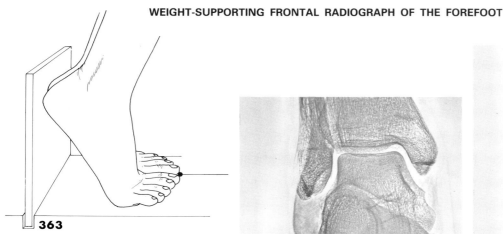

363. Schema of the incidence.
Position : the patient is standing, with the heels elevated.
Center : to the toes with the central beam horizontal, and the plate vertical.

364. Xeroradiograph of the weight-bearing forefoot in the frontal projection (half tiptoe) : the metatarsal heads and the sesamoid bones are usually in a straight line.

365. Xeroradiograph of the weight-bearing forefoot in the frontal projection (tiptoe) : the metatarsal heads and the sesamoid bones are still in a straight line. (1 - 2 - 3) medial, intermediate and lateral cuneiforms; (4) cuboid - fifth metatarsal joint ; (5) medial cuneiform - navicular joint ; (6) cuneo-first metatarsal joint ; (7) pyramidal process of the first metatarsal base.

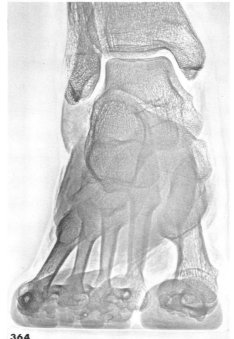

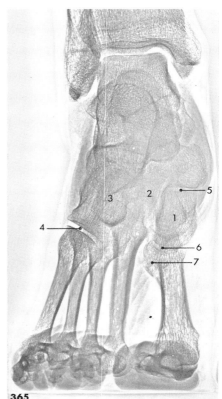

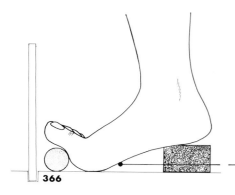

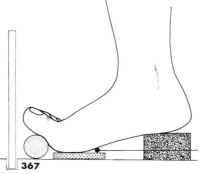

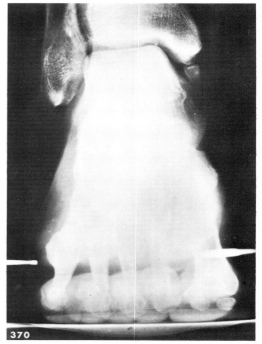

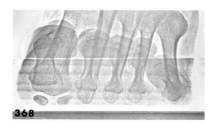

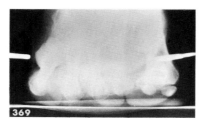

366, 367. Schemas of the incidences (metatarsal heads).

366. Ch. Rocher and Wangermez procedure.
Position : the patient is standing, with the heels elevated by a 4-cm cork-block, the plantar aspect of the toes pressing against a cork roller.
Center : on the metatarsal heads with the X-ray tube horizontal.

367. H. Rocher procedure. Position, centering and direction of the central X-ray are identical with the above procedure (**366**) but a 18-mm-thick rubber sponge is placed between the forefoot and the supporting surface. This technique shows the weight-bearing planes of the toes and of the metatarsal heads.

368. Xeroradiograph with Ch. Rocher and Wangermez technique : on *a hard plane,* all the metatarsal heads are on a same straight line.

369. Radiograph with Ch. Rocher procedure. Usually, the five metatarsal heads are on the same horizontal straight line. Bottomed forefoot with hyperpressure of the fourth and fifth metatarsal heads, and hammer-toe deformities.

370. Radiograph with the technique of Ch. Rocher, modified by J. Moutounet.
The author uses Djian's metallic marks and makes a double exposure, one for the ankle and one for the forefoot. Finally, we see on the same radiograph ankle joint, the weight-bearing surfaces of the heel and of the metatarsal heads. Note on this radiograph the rocker deformity of the forefoot and the os subtibiale.

WEIGHT-SUPPORTING AXIAL VIEW OF THE CALCANEUS

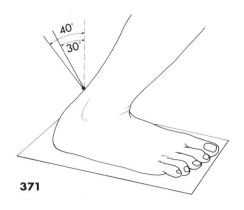

371

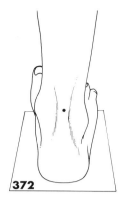

372

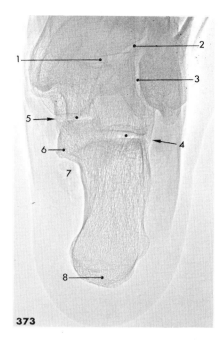

373

371, 372. Schemas of the incidence.

Position : the patient stands with the foot on the horizontal film, the body leaning forward with the knee flexed.
Center : to the heel with the tube angled 30⁰ to 40⁰ from the vertical (often bilateral projection).

373. Axial xeroradiograph of the calcaneus.

1 : ankle joint ; 2 : cuneocuboid joint ; 3 : distal tibiofibular joint ; 4 : posterior talocalcanean joint ; 5 : anterior talocalcanean joint ; 6 : sustentaculum tali ; 7 : calcaneal groove ; 8 : tuber calcanei.

WEIGHT-SUPPORTING VIEW OF THE SUBTALAR JOINT

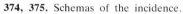

374, 375. Schemas of the incidence.

Position : the patient stands with both feet together on a small 15⁰ angle block. This wedge places the lower ankle in valgus and the upper one in varus **(374)**.
Center : between the feet at the level of the dorsal aspect of the foot, with the tube directed slightly downward (10⁰), the film being placed vertically behind the heels.

A second reverse radiograph is necessary with a wedge angled oppositely **(375)**.

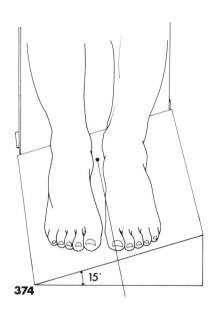

374

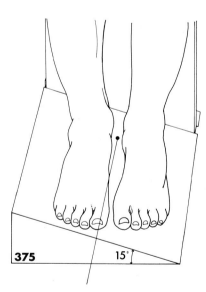

375

376, 377. Xeroradiograph of the right ankle in varus-valgus position with the above technique.

The articular margins of the subtalar joint are parallel. The slipping of the talus on the calcaneus is usually smaller than 5 mm.

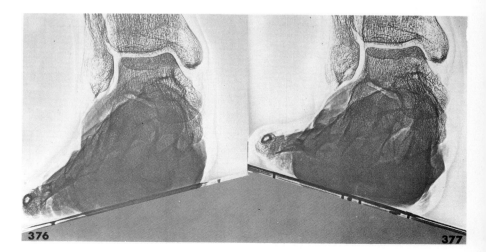

376

377

STATIC DISORDERS
DEVIATIONS IN THE HORIZONTAL PLANE

The axial relationships of the foot are measured on the anteroposterior weight-bearing radiograph

INTERPHALANGEAL CLINODACTYLY OF THE GREAT TOE IN VALGUS

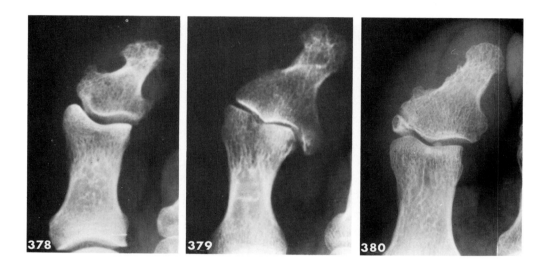

378, 379. Lateral deviation (40⁰) of the distal phalanx due to a medial prominence of the head of the proximal phalanx.

380. Lateral deviation (35⁰) caused by a medial hypertrophy of the base of the distal phalanx, with a separate ossification center.

METATARSOPHALANGEAL CLINODACTYLY OF THE GREAT TOE
IN VALGUS (HALLUX VALGUS)

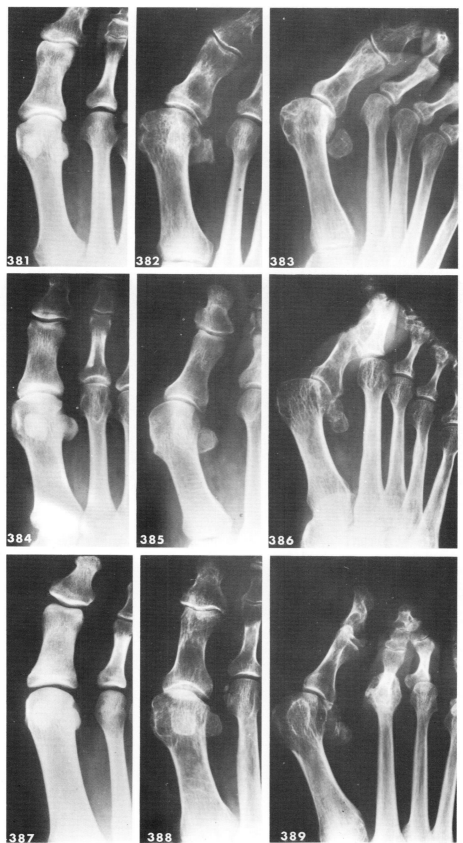

381 → **383.** Measurement of the lateral deviation of the great toe.

381. Angulation 20⁰.

382. Angulation 45⁰.

383. Angulation 60⁰.

384 → **386.** The three stages of sesamoid displacement.

384. Lateral sesamoid projecting on the lateral cortex of the first metatarsal head.

385. Lateral sesamoid projecting on the intermetatarsal area.

386. Dislocation of the two sesamoids in the intermetatarsal area. See axial views on the following page.

387 → **389.** Measurement of the metatarsus varus.

387, 388. Angulation 20⁰.

389. Angulation 50⁰.

In hallux valgus, to a variable extent, the hallux pronates or everts at the metatarsophalangeal joint. Because of the laterally deviated great toe, the weight-bearing bony point supporting the maximum pressure is the second metatarsal head. This stress produces degenerative changes in the second metatarsophalangeal joint and dorsal luxation of the proximal phalanx.

METATARSOPHALANGEAL CLINODACTYLY OF THE GREAT TOE
IN VALGUS (HALLUX VALGUS)

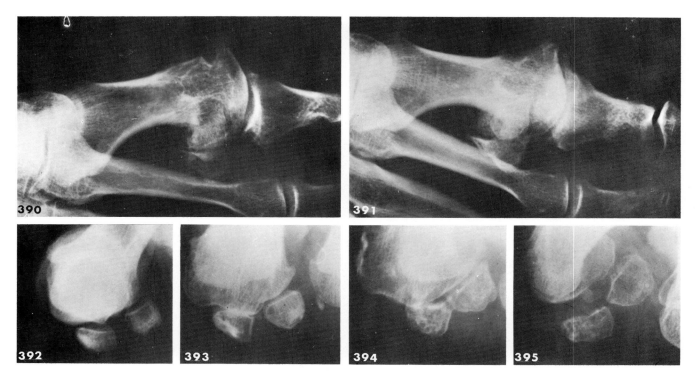

390, 391. Hallux valgus. Dorsiplantar oblique projection : superomedial erosion of the first metatarsal head caused by bursitis. Degenerative changes of the metatarsosesamoid joint.

392→395. Various stages of sesamoid displacement into the intermetatarsal space (axial views).

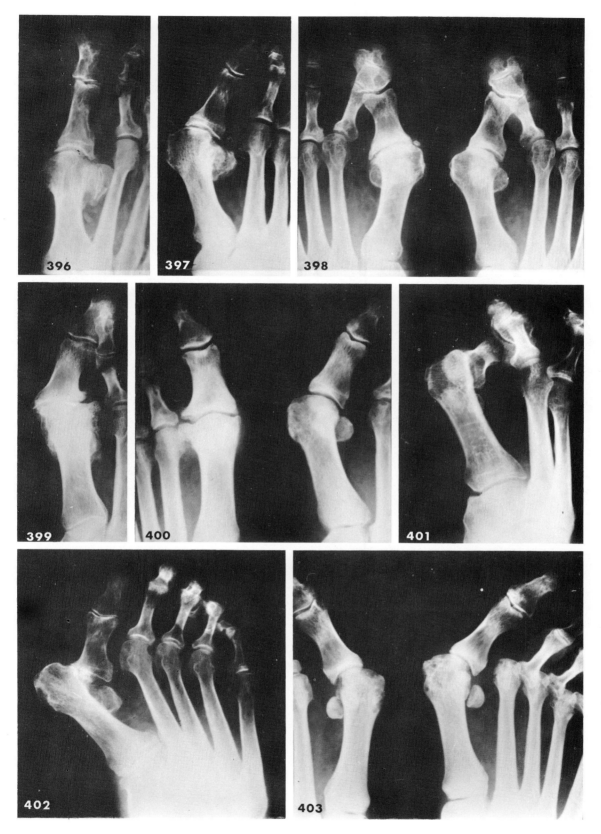

396. Hallux valgus. Dorsiplantar oblique projection. Degenerative changes of the metatarsosesamoid joint. Calcification of the distal arteries (diabetes).

397. Hallux valgus. Osteoarthritis of the metatarsosesamoid joint.

398. Hallux valgus. Arthrosis of both metatarsophalangeal joints and overriding or underriding of the second toes.

399. Marked degenerative changes of the first metatarsophalangeal joint (hallux rigidus) with lateral deviation of the great toe simulating an hallux valgus with arthrosis.

400. Same patient : right foot, hallux valgus, characterized by lateral deviation of the great toe, sesamoid displacement and metatarsus varus. Left foot, hallux rigidus, characterized by narrowness of the metatarsophalangeal joint with osteophytes, without phalangeal angulation, metatarsus varus, sub or luxation of the sesamoids.

In hallux valgus, the osteoarthritis is secondary, late, with a slow course, and produces lateral osteophytes.

In hallux rigidus, the arthrosis is primary, early, has a quick course, with dorsal exhuberant osteophytosis.

401. Hallux valgus due to an agenesis of two median rays.

402. Severe luxation into valgus of the great toe after marked destruction of the first metatarsophalangeal joint during a chondrocalcinosis. Note that such a localization is exceptional in this disease.

403. Luxation into valgus of the great toe after metatarsophalangeal joint destruction in rheumatoid arthritis. Arthritis and lateral dislocations of all the metatarsophalangeal joints : « peroneal blast ».

Compare with the static luxation of the second metatarsophalangeal joint (**389**).

METATARSOPHALANGEAL CLINODACTYLY OF THE GREAT TOE
IN VARUS (HALLUX VARUS)

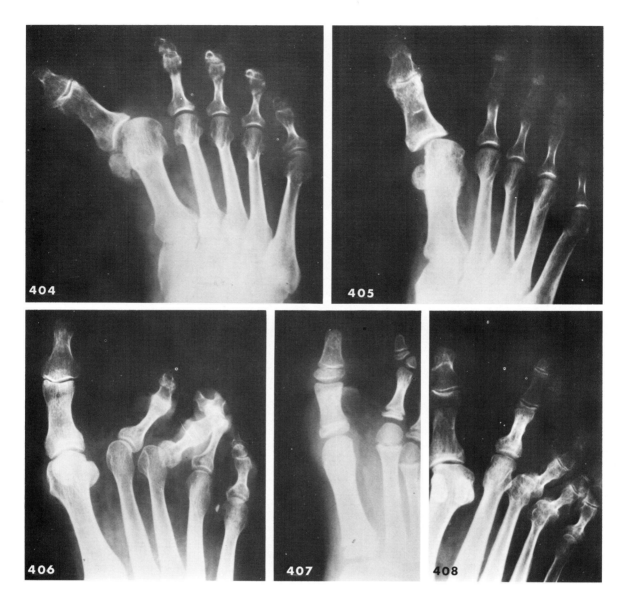

404. Hallux varus unfortunately due to overcorrection of a hallux valgus treated by Smith-Petersen procedure.

405. Hallux varus untoward result due to overcorrection of a hallux valgus after surgery (McBride procedure).

406. Deceptive appearance of hallux varus due to clinodactyly of the toes.

407. False hallux varus due to the divergency of the first two toes in Down syndrome : plantar cutaneous furrow continuous with the interdigital commissure. Note the second toe : the conical-shaped epiphysis of the proximal phalanx and the triangular distal phalanx.

408. Hallux varus.

CLINODACTYLY OF THE FIFTH TOE

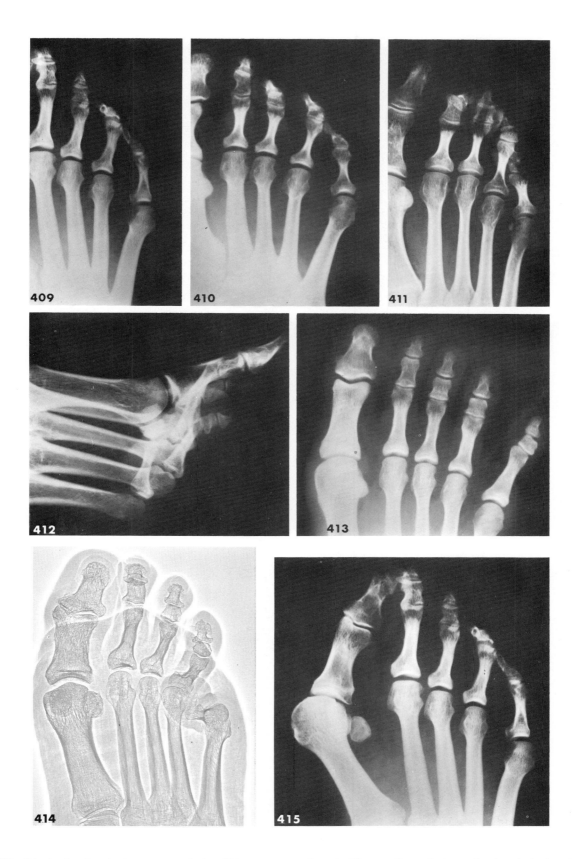

409. Distal clinodactyly into varus of the fifth toe : congenital quintus varus of the fifth metatarsal without associated valgus.

410. Quintus varus with metatarsus valgus of the fifth digit.

411. Quintus varus and swan-neck clawing of the second toe (frequent association).

412. Quintus varus and overriding, same case as **414**. The lateral oblique radiograph shows the dorsal clawing, but not the varus.

413. Distal clinodactyly into valgus of the fifth toe : congenital quintus valgus.

414. Quintus varus and overriding fifth toe.

415. Quintus varus and hallux valgus forming a characteristic triangular forefoot.

CLINODACTYLY OF THE MEDIAN TOES

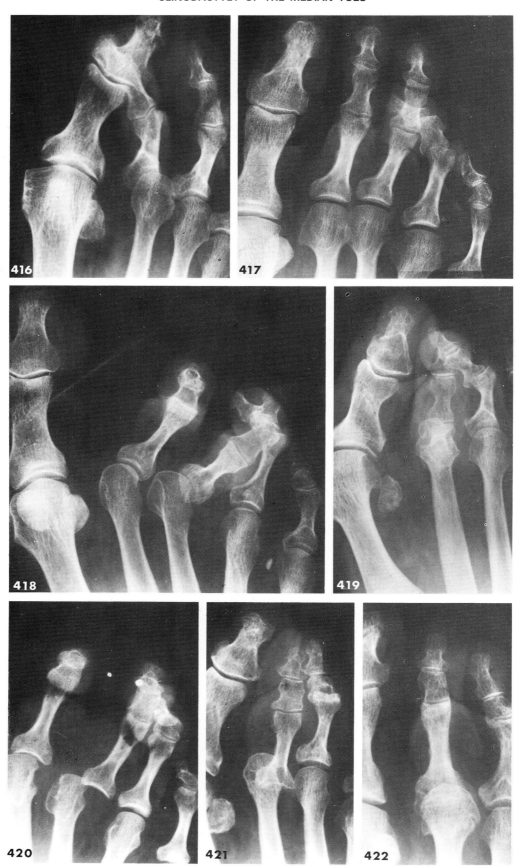

416 → 419. Clinodactylies.

416. Clinodactyly of the second toe.

417. Clinodactyly of the fourth toe.

418. Clinodactyly of the second and third toes.

419. Clinodactyly of the third toe. Note the clawing of the second toe, forming a swan-neck with a vanishing view of the proximal phalanx. Hallux valgus with shortening of the first metatarsal.

420 → 422. Dislocations.

420. Traumatic lateral dislocation of the second toe.

421. Static dorsal dislocation of the second toe.

422. Isolated static dorsal dislocation of the second toe with degenerative changes of the metatarsophalangeal joint.

TALOCALCANEAN DIVERGENCY

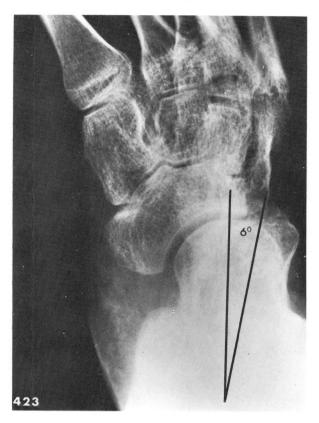

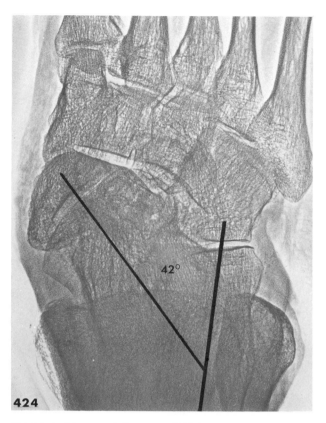

423. No divergency in an equinocavus varus foot deformity. Note the osteonecrosis of the lateral aspect of the navicular.

424. Marked increased divergency (42⁰) in a pes planovalgus, with osteonecrosis of the lateral part of the navicular.

MIDTARSAL DEVIATION

The abduction of the forefoot (metatarsus valgus) is one element of deformity in the static valgus flat foot.

This midtarsal deviation only appears on the weight-bearing dorsoplantar radiograph. It is measured by the angulation between the longitudinal axes of the talus and the second metatarsal.

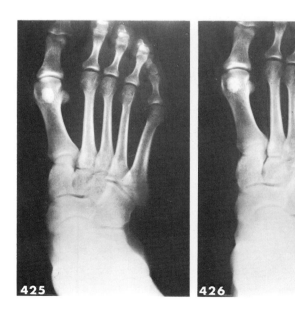

425, 426. Static valgus flat foot deformity
425. Weight-bearing.
426. Non weight-bearing.

STATIC DISORDERS
SAGITTAL DEVIATIONS

FLAT FOOT

The static pes planovalgus is characterized by a fourfold deformity : supination and abduction of the forefoot ; pronation and equinism of the hindfoot.

The weight-bearing dorsoplantar view of the foot shows the abduction of the forefoot, but the metatarsus valgus is absent in the simple flat foot.

The increased size of the talocalcaneal angle and of the second metatarsal-talar angle is a good indication of the valgus tilt of the forefoot (G. Lang) (**425**). The talar sliding forward and inward (talo-calcanean olisthesis of Viladot and Escarpenter) pushes the medial malleolus posteriorly (**431**), producing a rotation of the bimalleolar axis. The torsion of this axis is absent in the isolated heel valgus very frequent in childhood (**430**).

The weight-bearing lateral view of the foot shows the collapse of the medial longitudinal arch of which the roentgenographic measurement is exact only for the simple flat foot. In the pes planovalgus, the abducted forefoot and the heel valgus produce an apparent decrease in the height of the medial longitudinal arch as the size of the projected angles is greater than the true angle (**348**).

So, it is more advisable to measure the flatfootedness at the level of the first metatarsal (B. Tomeno) (**432**). The stress films in plantar and dorsiflexion demonstrate the equinus tilt (**613, 614**).

The frontal radiograph of the weight-bearing ankle shows the heel valgus (**456**).

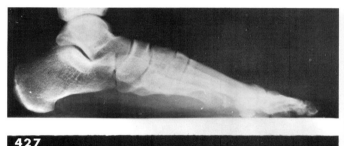 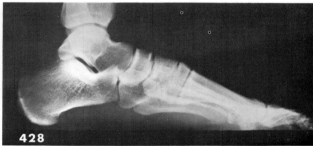

427, 428. Static valgus flat foot deformity : the flatfootedness appears on the lateral radiograph only in the standing position.
427. Weight-bearing.

428. Not weight-bearing.

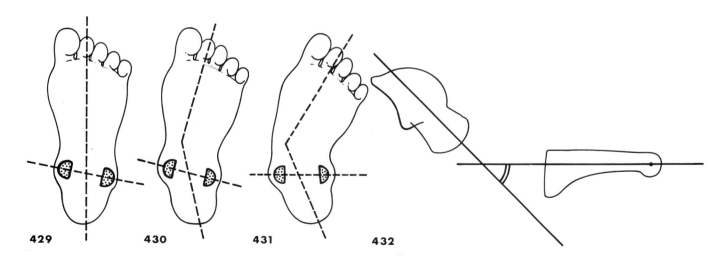

429. Normal foot.
430. Isolated heel valgus.

431. Pes planovalgus.
432. Angular measurement of the flatfootedness (Tomeno).

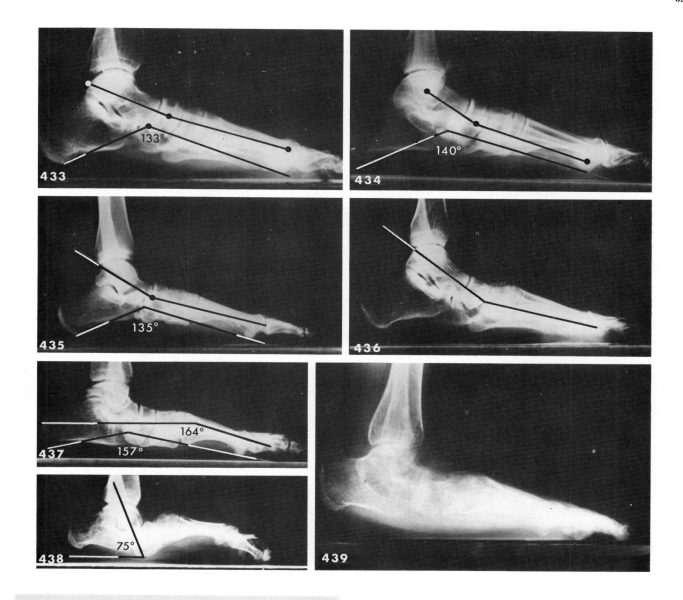

CHIEF TYPES OF FLAT FOOT

Congenital flat foot (page 102)

    Convex pes valgus with talonavicular subluxation

    Dysostosis or osteochondrodysplasia with joint hypermobility

    Severe flat foot with vertical talus without talonavicular subluxation.

    With tarsal coalition

Infective flat foot (osteitis) or inflammatory flat foot (rheumatoid arthritis)

Paralytic flat foot

Static flat foot (page 96)

    Counterbalancing flat foot : genu valgum, abnormal rotation of the skeletal leg, increased torsion angle of femur

    Flat foot with neuromyotendinous abnormalities
    — congenital or spastic short Achilles tendon
    — peroneus tertius and tibialis anterior muscles inserted too far anterior

    Flexible pes planovalgus in childhood

    Stiff pes planovalgus in youth

    Trophostatic flat foot in menopause and obesity

Traumatic flat foot

433. Slight static flat foot (Djian-Annonier angle : 133⁰).

434. More marked static flat foot (Djian-Annonier angle : 140⁰). Medial longitudinal arch flattened at the cuneonavicular joint level.

435. Static flat foot (Djian-Annonier angle : 135⁰). Collapse of the medial longitudinal arch at the talonavicular joint level.

436. Static flat foot. Medial longitudinal arch flattened at the cuneonavicular joint level.

437. Severe static flat foot (Djian-Annonier angle : 157⁰).

438. Poliomyelitic convex flat foot. The talus is in extreme plantar flexion (pitch 75⁰). Talonavicular dislocation with the navicular subluxated over the talar neck. The forefoot dorsiflexes at the midtarsal level.

439. Fallen forefoot and hindfoot equinus.

CAVUS FOOT DEFORMITY

The pes cavus is characterized by the exaggeration of the normal curvature of the plantar arch due to the verticality either of the forefoot (anterior pes cavus), or of the hindfoot (posterior pes cavus), or of both the fore and hindfoot (mixed pes cavus). The cavus is demonstrated radiologically in a standing lateral radiograph, but with the same reservation as in the flat foot deformity for the true value of the angles measured (see **348**). The verticality of the posterior tarsus is defined by the angle formed between the midcalcaneal line or the calcaneal pitch with the weight-bearing surface. The anterior cavus is measured by the angle between the midtalar line and the midaxis of the first metatarsal shaft. The lack of balance associated with cavus depends on the etiology of this foot deformity : the heel may keep its normal posture but, most frequently, the calcaneus deviates into varus (eg Friedreich disease), very rarely into valgus (eg spinal dysraphism). In the sagittal plane, the hindfoot is most often in talus (eg anterior poliomyelitis by paralysis of the triceps surae), sometimes in equinus (eg pes cavus equinovarus in myopathies).

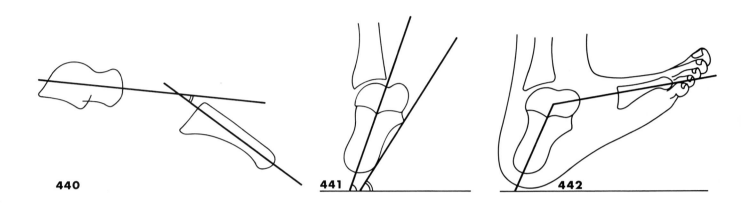

440   441   442

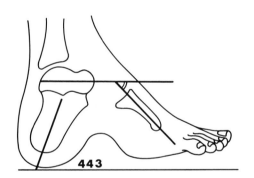

443

440. Cavus angle (Tomeno).

441. Talus angle.

442. Posterior pes cavus. Simple cavus. Pistol-butt-like shape.

443. Pes cavus talus.

444. Pes equinus.

445. Pes equinocavus.

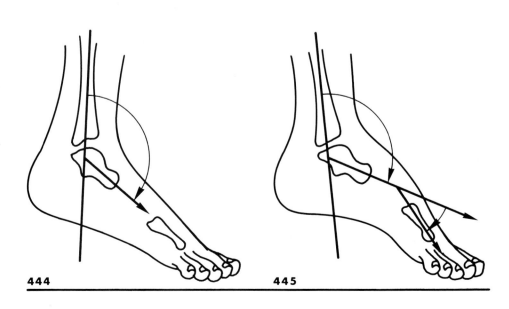

444   445

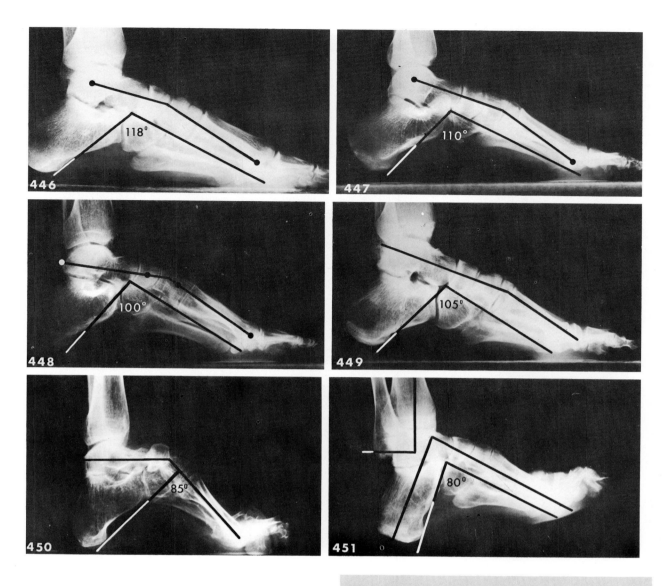

446. Moderate cavus foot deformity : Djian-Annonier angle : 118°

447. Anterior pes cavus : verticality of the forefoot with the medial and lateral longitudinal arches both abnormally high : the first and fifth metatarsal heads are on the same plane and their shafts are parallel. It is a simple anterior pes cavus.

448, 449. Anterior pes cavus : verticality of the forefoot with increased height of the longitudinal medial plantar arch alone, the axis of the fifth metatarsal remaining horizontal.
Often, the first metatarsal head is projected over the fifth metatarsal head, because the forefoot is pronated to avoid the painful pressure of the vertical first metatarsal on the ground.

450. Mixed pes cavus.

451. Posterior pes cavus : talus 80°.

ETIOLOGIC TABLE OF THE PES CAVUS

Extrinsic causes (bridles, burns)

Idiopathic pes cavus, often neurologic

Neuropathic pes cavus

    Conus medullaris disorders : malformations (spinabifida), traumatic sequelae, medullar compression, angioma, tumors, etc.

    Dejerine-Sottas disease.

    Extrapyramidal syndromes : Parkinson disease, Wilson disease.

    Medullar or cerebral acquired extrapyramidal syndromes of tumorigenic, inflammatory, vascular or degenerative origins

    Myopathies : myotonic dystrophy, Govers syndrome, etc.

    Peripheral neuropathies : toxic (lead), inflammatory (gonorrhea), post-traumatic

    Poliomyelitis-Acute idiopathic polyneuritis of Landay-Guillain-Barré

    Spinocerebellar heredodegenerative syndromes : Freidreich disease, Roussy-Levy disease, hereditary cerebellar ataxia, familial spastic paraplegia, Charcot-Marie-Tooth syndrome

Traumatic and post-surgical pes cavus

EQUINUS FOOT DEFORMITY

The heel equinus may be either a straight calcaneus or a varus, or valgus calcaneus.

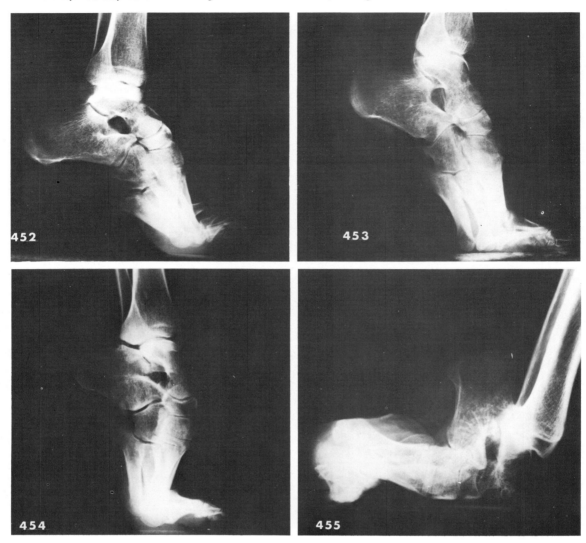

452. Pes equinocavus.

453. Simple pes equinus.

454. Simple pes equinus. Note the abnormal articular surfaces between the talus and the calcaneus.

455. Extreme foot deformity : the patient walks on the dorsal aspect of the foot.

ETIOLOGY
OF PES EQUINUS

Congenital causes

Myopathies

Neurologic causes

   Cauda equina syndrome
   Cerebral palsy
   Contusion and wound of the nerves
   Hemiplegia
   Poliomyelitis
   Polyneuritis (diabetes, alcoholism)
   Polyneuritis in the rheumatoid arthritis
   Radiculalgia
   Root sciatica
   Spinocerebellar heredodegenerative syndromes (Frei-
     dreich disease, Charcot-Marie-Tooth syndrome, etc.)

Rheumatoid causes

   Juvenile rheumatoid arthritis
   Rheumatoid arthritis in a bedridden patient
   Sympathetic reflex algodystrophy

Traumatic causes

   Retracted Achilles tendon
   Sequelae of the marginal fracture of the tibia or
     bimalleolar fracture of the ankle

Vascular causes

STATIC DISORDERS
FRONTAL DEVIATIONS

HINDFOOT

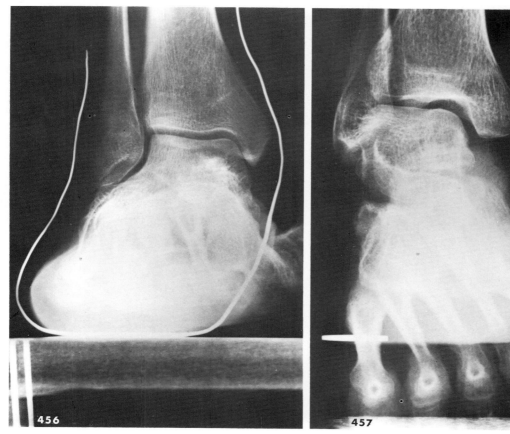

456. Heel valgus.

457. Heel varus

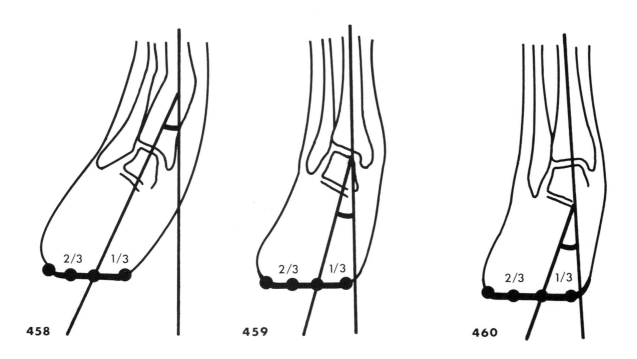

458, 459, 460. Pattern of the hind foot axial deviations in the frontal plane, according to Meary and Tomeno. The axial relationship must be measured from the starting-point of the deviation, as the surgical treatment will be applied there.

TOES

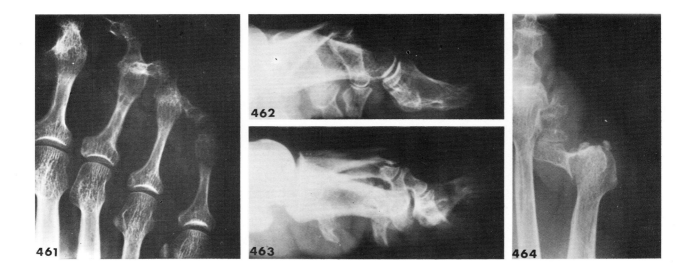

461. Distal clawing : flexion at the distal interphalangeal joint.

462. Proximal clawing : flexion at the proximal interphalangeal joint (swarn-neck deformity).

463. Complete and reverse clawing : flexion at the proximal interphalangeal joint and extension at the distal interphalangeal joint (swan-neck deformity).

464. Clawing of the fifth toe.

METATARSAL ALIGNMENT

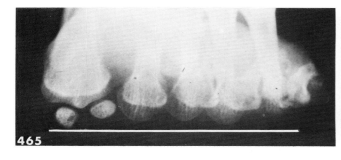

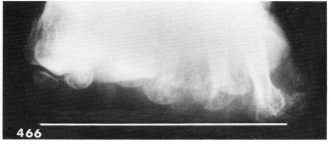

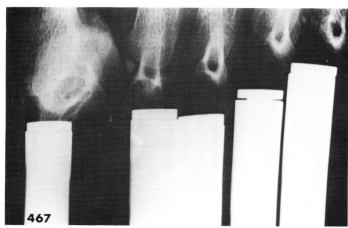

465. Weight-bearing metatarsal alignment. The horizontal plane is tangential to the sesamoids and to the metatarsal heads. Lack of pressure on the fifth metatarsal head.

466. Weight-bearing metatarsal alignment : marked pressure on the fifth metatarsal head. No pressure of the medial part on the forefoot.

467. Study of the frontal weight-bearing alignment of the metatarsal heads with the Baropodometer of J. Martorell-Martorell. This apparatus uses five cylinders, the pistons of which, connected together, sink in proportion with the transmission of the pressure of the body weight through each metatarsal head.

STATICS OF THE FOOT
WITH THE SHOE ON

STUDY OF THE CURVATURE OF THE PLANTAR ARCH
IN THE SAME PATIENT STANDING IN VARIOUS POSITIONS

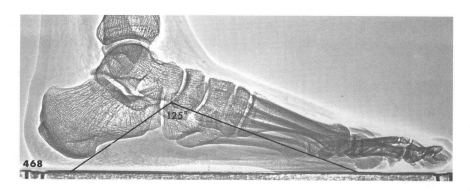

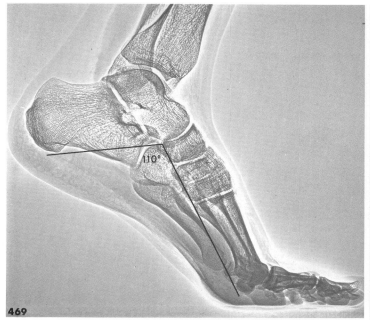

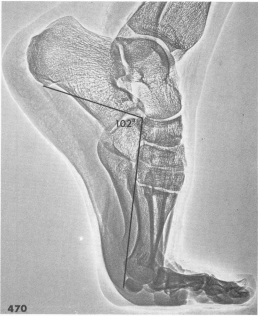

468. Barefoot.
469. Barefoot and on half tip toe.

470. Barefoot and on tip toe. The Djian-Annonier angle decreases as the patient rises on the tip of his toes, because of the increased tonicity of the tensor muscles of the plantar arch.

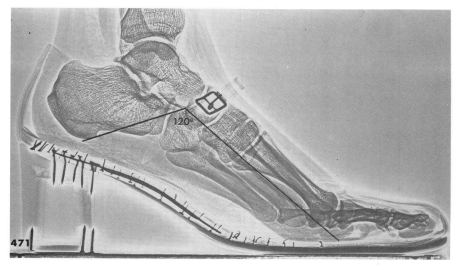

471. Foot in a shoe. A heel of 4 cm only slightly changes the curvature of the plantar arch : light straining of the muscles.

STUDY OF A CORRECTIVE ORTHESIS

Xeroradiograph of the bare foot, and wearing a shoe with or without a corrective insole.

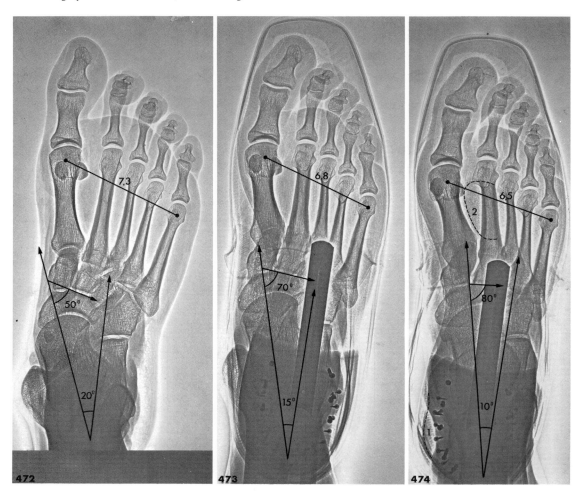

472 → 474. Roentgenoradiographic measurements on the antero-posterior view.

472. Barefoot : pes planovalgus.

473. Shoewear with a heel 4 cm high : the talocalcanean divergency decreases by 5 degrees. Squeezed foot.

474. The orthesis increases the metatarsal squeezing and again decreases the talocalcanean divergency. 1 : valgus heel wedge ; 2 : metatarsal bar.

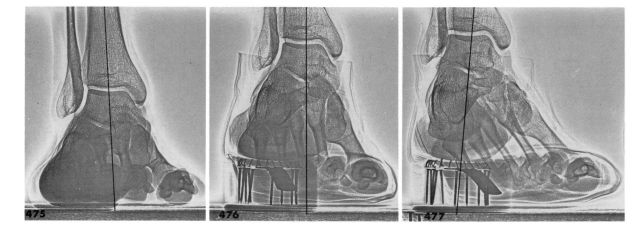

475 → 477. Radiographic measurements on the frontal view.

475. Barefoot : calcaneal valgus.

476. Shoewear with a heel of 4 cm : the valgus decreases because of the tonicity of the triceps surae.

477. Hypercorrective orthosis with calcaneal varus.

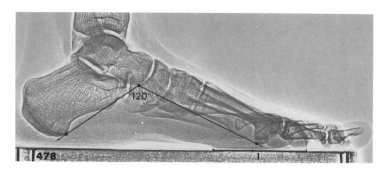

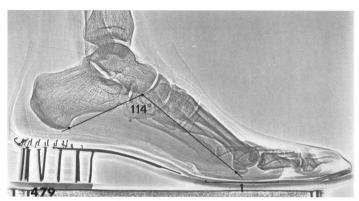

478 → 480. Roentgenographic measurements on the lateral view.

478. Barefoot : pes planovalgus.

479. The shoe with a heel 4 cm high produces a moderate equinus foot, with a slight increase of the curvature of the plantar arch and a decrease of 1 cm in length of the supporting surface of the forefoot (1).

480. Shoewear and corrective insole including a wedge of the metatarsal bar type, placed behind the metatarsal heads (2) in conjunction with a valgus heel wedge (3). This orthesis decreases for the second time the size of the Djian-Annonier angle. The supporting surface of the forefoot (1) increases by 3 cm in length, according to the width of the metatarsal bar (2).

**CONTRASTS
CHINESEFOOT**

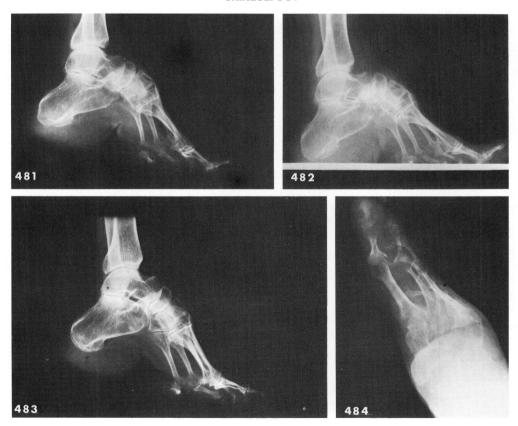

481 → 484. Double mutilation of the chinesefoot :

— squeezing of the forefoot by plantar flexion of the toes which tuck under the sole of the foot and by folding of the four last metatarsals around the first one (**484**) ;

— shortening of the foot by extreme exaggeration of the curvature of the plantar arch due to a break at the anterior tarsus level (**481, 483**).

Statics of a Chinese acquired pes cavus equinovarus in upright position : vertical calcaneus which represents the single bony point supporting body weight, the distal phalanx of the great toe being a very accessory supporting surface (**482**).

**CONTRASTS
BALLET DANCER'S FOOT**

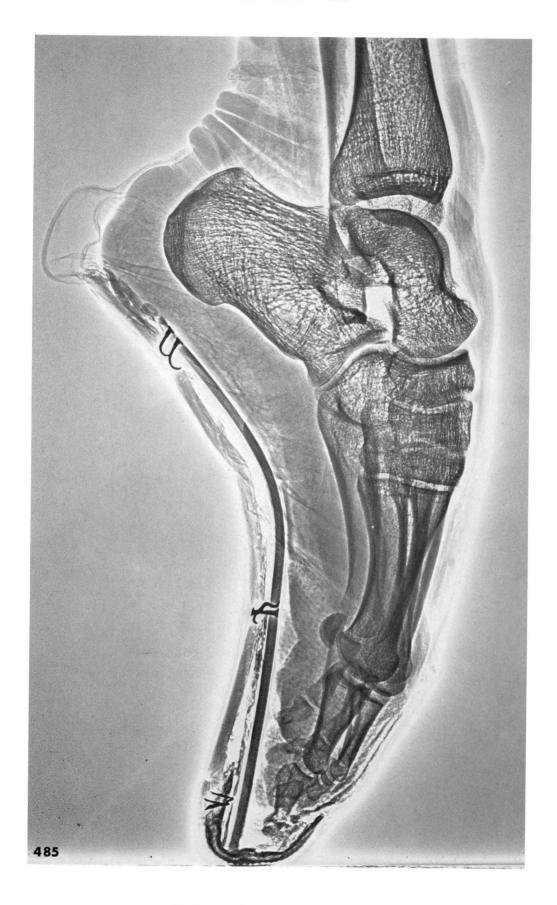

485. Foot on tip toe in sandal : flying off.

3

THE FOOT IN CHILDHOOD

BONE GROWTH

NORMAL APPEARANCES

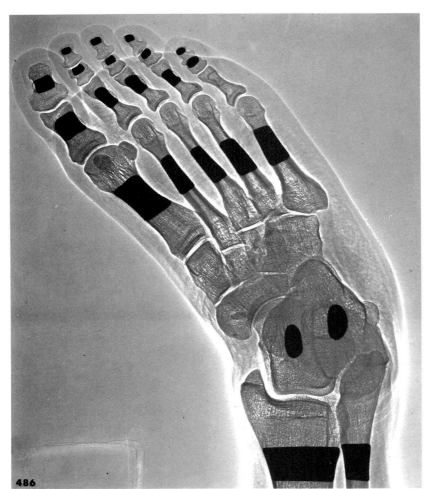

OSSIFICATION CENTERS

486. Xeroradiograph of an adult foot : ossification centers visible at birth are indicated in black.

Normal ranges of ages at epiphyseal fusion
Tibia : 16-19 years
Fibula : 18-22 years
Calcaneus : 16-20 years
Phalanges : 13-20 years. In chronological order, the distal phalanx, the middle phalanx, the proximal phalanx.

486

Ossification centers	Mean age of ossification onset at centers		Normal range of ossification onset at secondary centers	
	Boys	*Girls*	*Boys*	*Girls*
Cuboid	25 days	18 days	Birth to 3 m 1/2	Birth to 2 m
Lateral cuneiform	5 m 1/2	3 m	20 days to 1 year 7 m	Birth to 15 m
Epiphysis 2d Ph. great toe	14 m 1/2	9 m	9 m to 2 years 1 m	4 m 1/2 to 20 m
Epiphysis 2d Ph. 4th toe	14 m 1/2	11 m	5 m to 2 years 11 m	4 m 1/2 to 3 years
Epiphysis 1 st Ph. 3d toe	18 m	1 year 15 days	11 m to 2 years 6 m	6 m to 23 m
Epiphysis 1st Ph. 4th toe	20 m	15 m	11 m to 2 years 8 m	7 m 1/2 to 2 years 7 m
Epiphysis 1st Ph. 2d toe	21 m	14 m	11 m 1/2 to 2 years 8 m	7 m 1/2 to 2 years 1 m
Epiphysis 2d Ph. 2d toe	2 years	14 m	11 m to 4 years	6 m to 2 years 3 m
Medial cuneiform	2 years 2 m	17 m	11 m to 3 years 9 m	6 m to 2 years 10 m
Epiphysis 1st Ph. great toe	2 years 4 m	19 m	17 m to 3 years 4 m	10 m 1/2 to 2 years 6 m
Epiphysis 1st Ph. 5th toe	2 years 5 m	21 m	18 m to 3 years 8 m	11 m 1/2 to 2 years 8 m
Intermediate cuneiform	2 years 8 m	22 m	14 m to 4 years 3 m	9 m 1/2 to 3 years
Second metatarsal epiphysis	2 years 10 m	2 years 1 m	23 m to 4 years 4 m	1 year 3 m to 3 years 5 m
Navicular	3 years	23 m	13 m 1/2 to 5 years 5 m	9 m to 3 years 7 m
Third metatarsal epiphysis	3 years 6 m	2 years 6 m	2 years 4 m to 5 years	2 years 6 m to 3 years 8 m
Epiphysis 3d Ph. 5th toe	3 years 11 m	2 years 4 m	2 years 4 m to 6 years 4 m	2 years 4 m to 4 years 1 m
Fourth metatarsal epiphysis	4 years	2 years 10 m	2 years 11 m to 5 years 9 m	21 m to 4 years 1 m
Epiphysis 3d Ph. 3d toe	4 years 4 m	2 years 9 m	3 years to 6 years 2 m	16 m to 4 years 1 m
Fifth metatarsal epiphysis	4 years 4 m	3 years 3 m	3 years to 6 years 4 m	2 years 1 m to 4 years 11 m
Epiphysis 3d Ph. 4th toe	4 years 5 m	2 years 7 m	2 years 11 m to 6 years 5 m	16 m to 4 years 1 m
Epiphysis 3d Ph. 2d toe	4 years 8 m	2 years 11 m	3 years 3 m to 6 years 9 m	18 m to 4 years 6 m
Calcaneal epiphysis	7 years 7 m	5 years 4 m	5 years 2 m to 9 years 7 m	3 years 6 m to 7 years 4 m

Boy   Girl

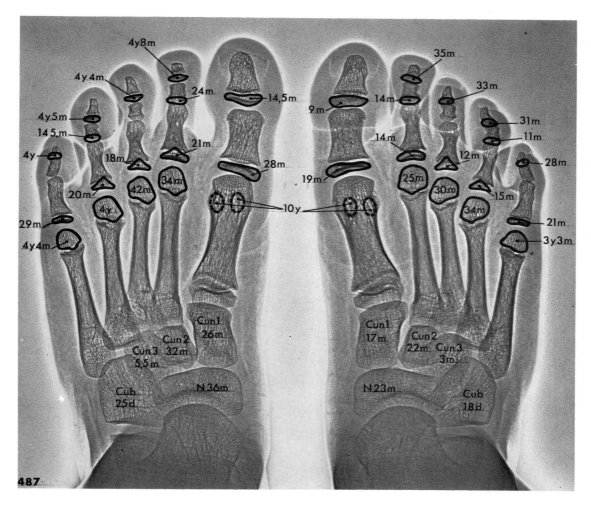

487. Ages at radiographic appearance of foot ossification centers (after Garn, Rohman, Silverman and adapted from A. Coussement).

GENERALIZED ACCELERATED SKELETAL MATURATION

Adrenogenital syndrome (adrenocortical tumor or hyperplasia)
Chondroectodermal dysplasia (Ellis-Van Creveld S.)
Congenital brain defect
Constitutional (congenital tall stature)
Ectopic gonadotropin production (hepatoma, choriocarcinoma, teratoma)
Encephalitis
Excessive androgen or estrogen administration or production (virilizing adrenal tumor or hyperplasia, androgen- or estrogen-secreting gonadal tumor, hypergonadism)
Exogenous obesity with overgrowth and tall stature
Homocystinuria
Hydrocephalus
Hyperthyroidism (maternal or acquired)
Hypothalamic or parahypothalamic neoplasm or inflammation with sexual precocity (eg, craniopharyngioma, tuberculosis)
Idiopathic isosexual precocious puberty
Neurofibromatosis
Pinealoma, primary or ectopic
Pituitary or cerebral gigantism
Polyostotic fibrous dysplasia (esp. Albright S.)
Primary hyperaldosteronism
Total lipodystrophy
Tuberous sclerosis

GENERALIZED RETARDED SKELETAL MATURATION

Addison disease
Anemia, chronic (eg, sickle cell anemia, thalassemia)
Cerebral hypoplasia
Congenital heart disease (esp. cyanotic)
Congenital syndromes of dwarfism or mental retardation
Congenital hyperuricosuria
Constitutional delay of growth and adolescence
Diabetes mellitus, juvenile
Hypogonadism (eg Turner syndrome)
Hypopituitarism with growth hormone deficiency (idiopathic or secondary to craniopharyngioma or other neoplasm)
Hypothyroidism, congenital or acquired
Idiopathic
Intrauterine growth retardation
Malabsorption
Malnutrition
Nephrosis or other renal disease
Oculocerebral-renal syndrome (Kowe)
Phenylketonuria
Rickets, all types
Severe constitutional disease (eg celiac disease, ulcerative colitis)
Steroid therapy ; Cushing syndrome

LOCALIZED RETARDED SKELETAL MATURATION

Enchondromatosis (Ollier disease)
Hypervitaminosis A
Infarction (eg sickle cell anemia)
Neoplasm
Osteomyelitis (eg, bacterial, yaws, smallpox)

Radiation injury
Rickets
Scurvy
Thermal injury
Trauma

BONE AGE

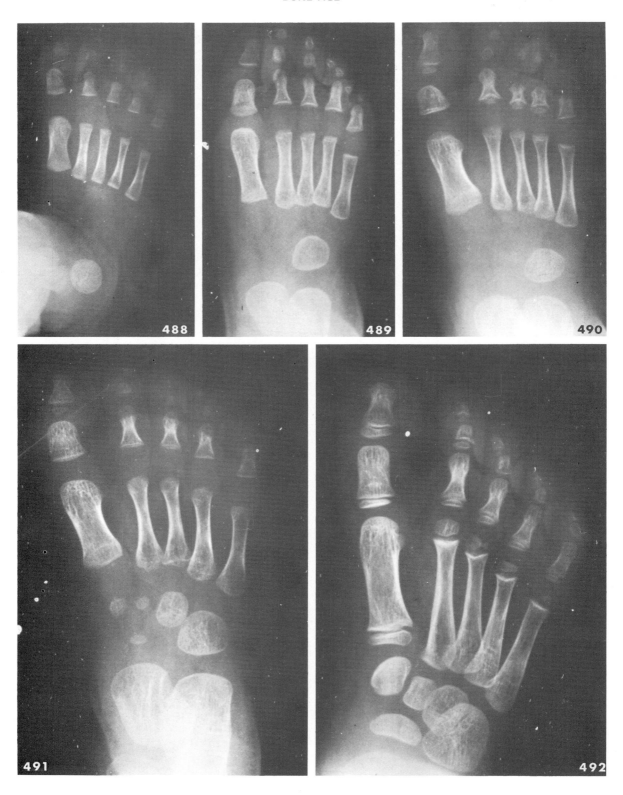

488 → 492. Illustrations of osseous changes in the forefoot according to age in the male child.

488. 15 days.
489. 3 months.   **491.** 2 years.
490. 20 months.   **492.** 3 years.

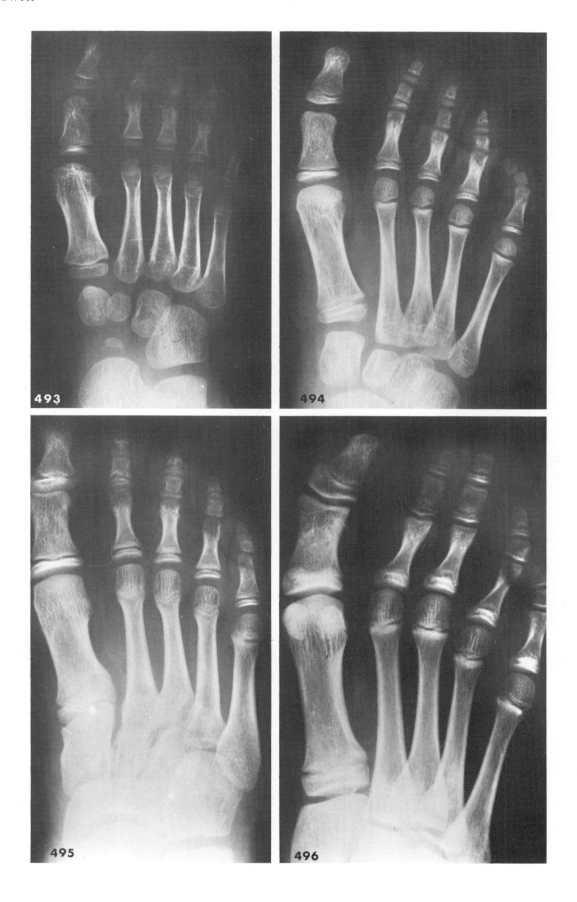

493 → 496. Illustrations of osseous changes in the forefoot according to age in the female child.

493. 6 years.	**495.** 12 years.
494. 9 years.	**496.** 13 years.

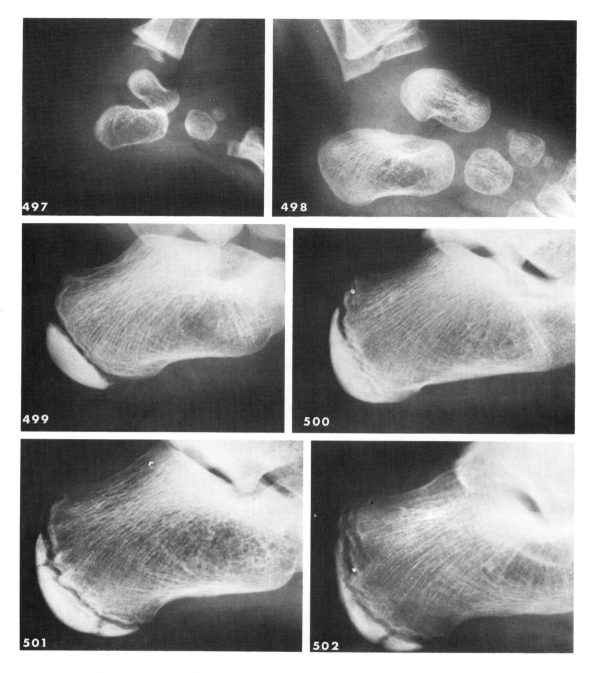

497 → 502. Illustrations of calcaneal changes according to age in the male child.

497. 5 months.	**500.** 10 years.
498. 2 years.	**501.** 12 years.
499. 5 years	**502.** 13 years.

CONE-SHAPED EPIPHYSES

Achondroplasia
Acrocephalosyndactyly (Apert S.)
Asphyxiating thoracic dysplasia
Beckwith-Wiedemann S.
Chondroectodermal dysplasia (Ellis-Van Creveld S.)
Cleidocranial dysplasia
Dactylitis (esp. sickle cell, smallpox)
Epiphyseal dysplasia
Hypervitaminosis A
Idiopathic or normal
Neonatal hyperthyroidism
Orodigitofacial S.
Osteopetrosis
Otopalatodigital S.
Peripheral dysostosis (acrodysostosis)
Phalangeal gigantism
Pseudohypoparathyroidism, pseudo-
    pseudohypoparathyroidism
Rhinotrichophalangeal S.

NORMAL VARIANTS

PHALANGES AND METATARSALS

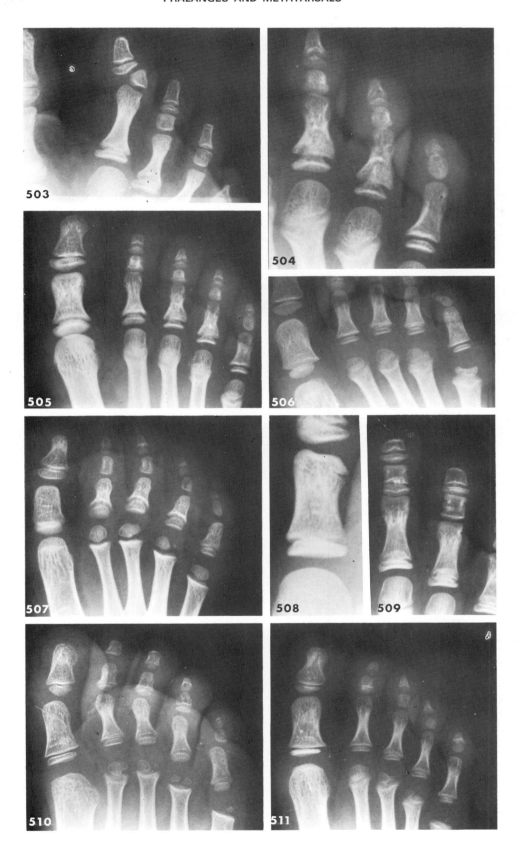

503. Triangular phalanx.

504, 505. Cone-shaped epiphyses.

506, 507. Anatomic variants of the ossification centers of the metatarsal heads.

508, 509. Incomplete developmental fissure in the phalanges simulating a fracture. To be distinguished from the epiphyseal growth-plate which is more proximal.

510. Anatomic variants of the ossification centers of the metatarsal heads.

511. Dense epiphysis of the base of the proximal phalanx of the great toe.

METATARSALS

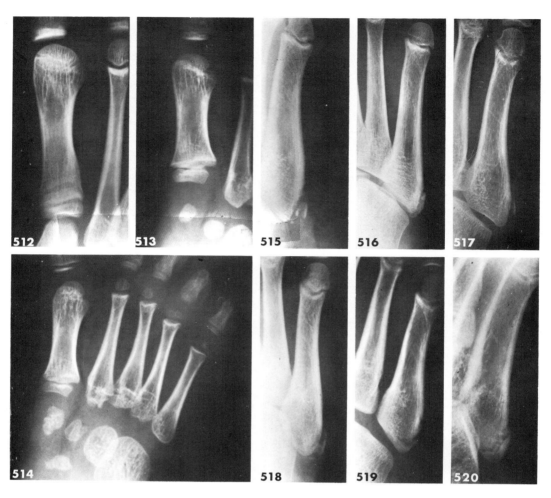

512, 513. Accessory ossification center of the first metatarsal head.

514. Accessory ossification center of the base of the second and third metatarsals and multicentric ossification centers of the cuneiforms.

515 → 520. Styloid tuberosity on the lateral side of the fifth metatarsal base.

515, 516. Accessory ossification center.

517. Avulsion.

518. Accessory ossification center.

519. Fracture.

520. Accessory ossification center.

SUPERNUMERARY EPIPHYSEAL OSSIFICATION CENTERS
Cleidocranial dysplasia Down S. (mongolism) Hand-foot-uterus S. Hypothyroidism Idiopathic Larsen S. Otopalatodigital S. Peripheral dysostosis

IRREGULARITY, FRAGMENTATION, OR STIPPLING OF MULTIPLE EPIPHYSEAL OSSIFICATION CENTERS
Aseptic necrosis ; osteochondrosis Cerebrohepatorenal S. Chondrodysplasia punctata (congenital stippled epiphyses, Conradi disease) Cockayne S. Cretinism Down S (mongolism) Dysplasia epiphysealis hemimelica (Trevor disease) (unilateral knee and ankle) Enchondromatosis (Ollier disease) ; Maffucci S. Hereditary arthro-ophthalmopathy (Stickler S.) Hereditary multiple epiphyseal disturbances (Ribbing) Homocystinuria (stippled physeal plates) Kniest disease Metatrophic dwarfism Mucopolysaccharidosis (eg, Morguio) Multiple epiphyseal dysplasia (Fairbank) Normal (at certain ages) Osteopetrosis Osteopoikilosis ; osteopathia striata Parastremmatic dwarfism Pituitary gigantism Rhinotrichophalangeal S. Smith-Lemli-Opitz S. Spondyloepiphyseal dysplasia (congenital and pseudoachondroplastic types)

« METATARSAL EPIPHYSITIS »

The borderlands of the normal variant picture and early pathologic radiologic appearance are difficult to define : the terms of epiphysitis, apophysitis, epiphysosis, apophysosis, must be used only for syndromes with preponderant clinical signs.

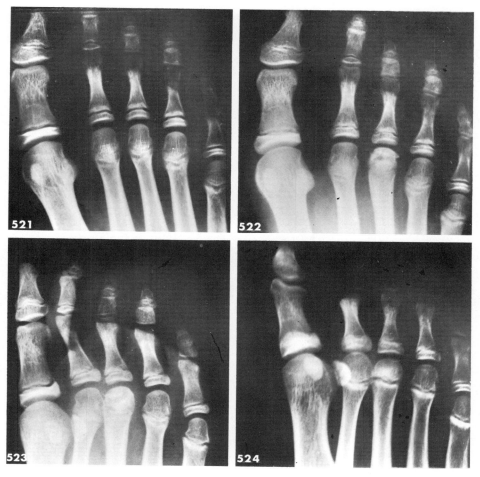

521 → 524. Same patient.

521. 12-year-old girl. Pain for month at the third metatarsophalangeal joint. At this time, there is no radiographic abnormality. Note the normally dense epiphysis at the base of the proximal phalanx of the great toe.

522, 523. 6 months later, evident osteochondrosis : focal aseptic osteonecrosis of the third metatarsal head. An isolated fragment of bone is set in an island of rarefaction surrounded by a zone of sclerosis.

524. In 6 months, complete bony replacement of the necrotic area, without any deformation of the metatarsal head (see Freidberg disease) has occurred. During that time, the patient lived a busy life, wearing a plantar orthosis with a rocker bar, set just behind the metatarsal head to relieve it from the full body weight.

« ASEPTIC NECROSIS » OF THE TARSAL NAVICULAR

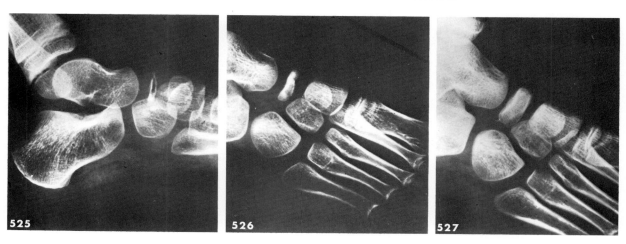

525 → 527. Course of Kohler-Mouchet disease ending in complete healing.

525. First radiograph.

526. Seven months later.

527. Two years after onset.

NAVICULAR-CALCANEUS

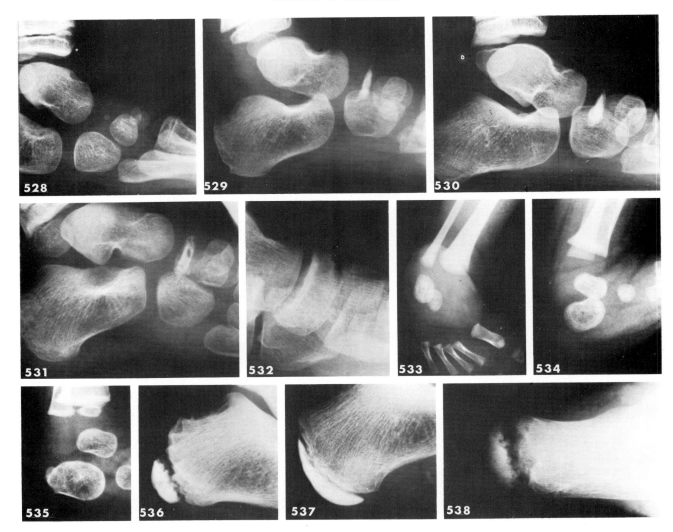

528 → 532. Navicular.

528. Double ossification center of the navicular bone in a 6-year-old boy.

529 → 531. Sclerotic, compressed, fragmented, irregular ossification center of the navicular bone. If these radiographic appearances coexist with symptoms of pain, this clinical entity is called the Kohler-Mouchet disease.

532. Stair-like aspect simulating an avulsion or a fracture.

533 → 538. Calcaneus.

533, 534. Physiologic concentric rings of calcification in the ossification center of the calcaneus ; **533.** 3-day-old female ; **534.** 4-month-old male.

535. Double ossification center for the body of the calcaneus. Note the transient calcaneal spur (always disappears before 1 year of age) which is directed posteriorly, opposite in direction to the degenerative calcaneal spur.

536 → 538. The density and fragmentation of the calcaneal secondary ossification center are all normal manifestations of growth. In case of focal pain, the term calcaneitis is applied (Server disease).

> « BONE WITHIN
> BONE » APPEARANCE
>
> Delay of growth (eg, due to disease, stress, chemotherapy)
> Hypervitaminosis D
> Normal neonate
> Osteopetrosis
> Paget disease
> Phosphorus ingestion
> Sickle cell anemia
> Thorotrast

DYSOSTOSES (malformations *)

Dysostosis is the malformation of individual bones, single or in combination with other bone abnormalities.

ADACTYLY - APHALANGY

The toes or phalanges may be lacking, in part or as a whole. The aplasia may be transversal (eg absence of all the phalanges) or longitudinal metameric topography (eg middle metatarsals missing).

The aplasia may be associated with other malformations, eg, the aglossia-adactylia syndrome.

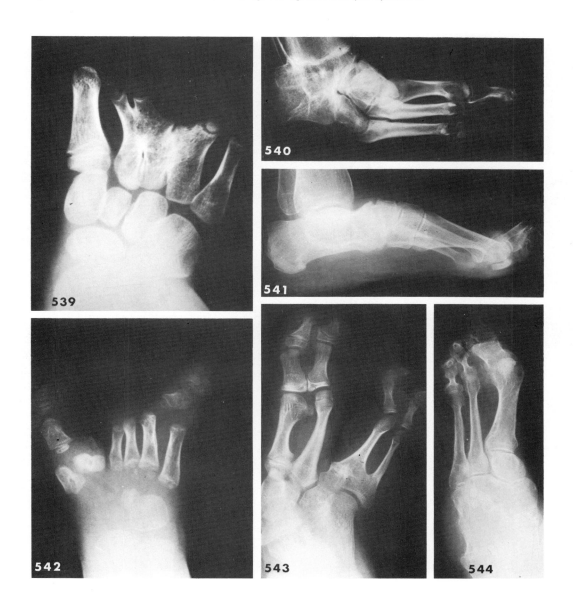

539. Total aphalangy and metatarsal synostoses.

540, 541. Incomplete aphalangy (third and fourth metatarsals) and tarsal coalition.

542. Partial aphalangy and first toe duplication.

543. Partial adactyly (middle metatarsal missing) lobster-claw-like aspect. Syndactyly of the first and second toes.

544. Partial adactyly (third and fourth metatarsals).

* See also chapter 4.

POLYDACTYLY

Polydactylism is a congenital abnormality characterized by supernumerary toes, often with malformations. The polydactyly may be due to a supernumerary or a duplicated toe (bifid toe). The duplication may take place on the phalanx or on the metatarsal. Diplopodia is rare (557, 558).

Polydactyly is often associated with other dysostoses (syndactyly-hyperphalangy). It may be only one component of a more complex deformity. eg Werner syndrome (see page 89), acrofacial dysosto-sis (Weyer), Ulrich-Feichtiger syndrome. Laurence - Moon - Bardet - Biedl syndrome which includes retinitis, obesity, hypogonadism, mental retardation (552), orodigitofacial syndrome (Papillon-Leage) (649).

Polydactyly may be associated with osteochondrodysplasia, eg, chondroectodermal dysplasia (Ellis - Van Creveld) it includes micromelia, abnormalities of nails and teeth, heart malformation (550).

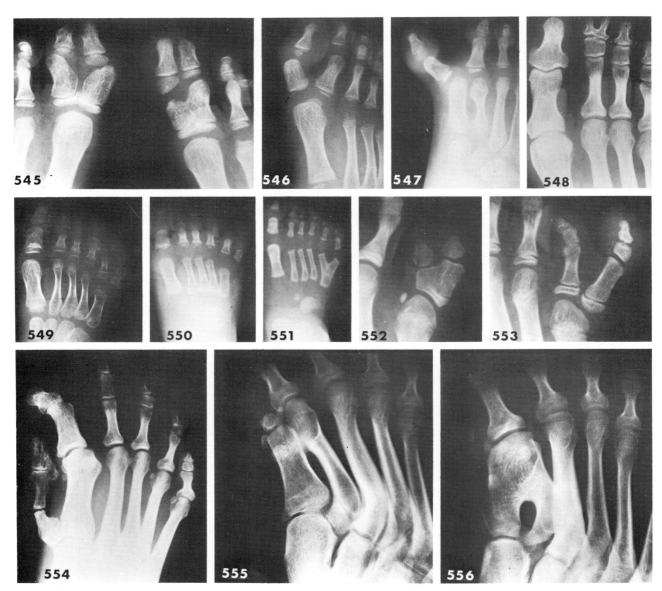

545. Bifid bilateral great toe : the two phalanges are developed from a single epiphyseal disk. Right syndactyly.

546. Duplication of the great toe : each phalanx is developed from a specific growth plate.

547. Supernumerary bone between first and second metatarsal with hallux varus.

548. Double distal phalanx of the second toe.

549 → 553. Polydactyly by duplication of the fifth toe. Supernumerary phalanges (549, 550, 553). Doubling of the metatarsal shaft (551). Doubling, distal aplasia and syndactyly (552).

554. Supernumerary great toe : pre-hallux.

555. Complete duplication of the great toe.

556. Incomplete duplication of the great toe.

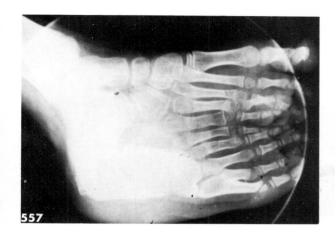 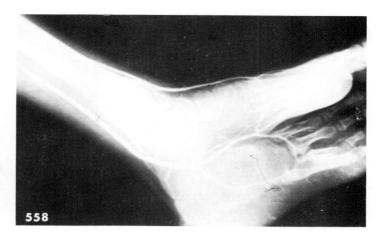

557, 558. Distal schizomelia : rare complete double of the foot.

557. Radiograph.

558. Arteriography : the vascularization of the double foot is mostly supplied by the posterior tibial artery and a branch of the peroneal artery.

POLYDACTYLY

Acrocephalopolysyndactyly (Carpenter S.)
Acrofacial dysostosis
Asphyxiating thoracic dysplasia
Biemond S.
Blakfan-Diamond anemia
Bloom S.
Brachydactyly B
Chondrodysplasia punctata (Conradi disease)
Chondroectodermal dysplasia (Ellis-Van Creveld S.)
Ectodermal dysplasia, Robinson type
Fanconi S. (pancytopenia-dysmelia S.)
Focal dermal hypoplasia (Goltz S.)
Holt-Oram S.
Isolated anomaly
Laurence-Moon-Biedl S.
Mesomelic dwarfism variant
Orodigitofacial S. I and II
Polydactyly-syndactyly S.
Rubinstein-Taybi S.
Short-rib polysyndactyly S.
Smith-Lemli-Opitz S.
Trisomy 13 S.
Ulnar dimelia

SYNOSTOSIS - SYNDACTYLY

We have described in chapter 1 « Normal variants » (pp. 24, 25), individual (namely between only two bones) and isolated (viz not combined with skeletal abnormalities) synostosis.

But some coalitions are only one element of a more intricate dysostosis or affect many bones, such as acrospondylopectoral dysplasia, carpal and tarsal fusion, or multiple synostosis disease, etc.

The incomplete and isolated syndactyly of the second and third toes is rather common. Syndactyly may be associated with other dysostoses, eg acrocephalosyndactylia (Apert syndrome), etc.

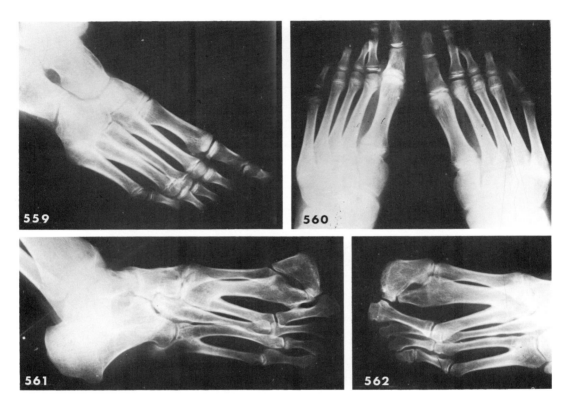

559, 560. Multiple synostoses disease : tarsal coalition and symphalangism.

561, 562. Apert syndrome : tarsal and metatarsal synostoses with syndactyly.

SYNDACTYLY (CUTANEOUS OR OSSEOUS)

Aarskog-Scott S. (shawl scrotum S.)	Mandible hypoplasia (Pierre Robin S.)
Acrocephalopolysyndactyly (Carpenter S.)	Neurofibromatosis
Acrocephalosyndactyly (Apert S.)	Oculodentodigital S.
Aminopterin-induced S.	Orodigitofacial S.
Bloom S.	Otopalatodigital S.
Brachydactyly B	Pectoral aplasia syndactyly S. (Poland S.)
Chondrodysplasia punctata (Conradi disease)	Polydactyly-syndactyly S.
Cornelia de Lange S.	Popliteal pterygium S.
Down S. (mongolism) (toes)	Prader-Willi S.
Ectodermal dysplasia, Robinson type	Pseudohypoparathyroidism
Fanconi S.	Russell-Silver S.
Focal dermal hypoplasia (Goltz S.)	Smith-Lemli-Opitz S.
Hallerman-Streiff S.	Thrombocytopenia
Incontinentia pigmenti S.	Trisomy 13 S.
Laurence-Moon-Biedl S.	Trisomy 18 S.

LONGITUDINAL HEMIAPLASIA

Longitudinal hemiaplasia is the congenital absence of the tibia or fibula. Aplasia or hypoplasia of the fibula is far more frequent than tibial aplasia. Commonly aplasia is associated with a reduction of the digits of the foot or other dysostosis, eg Werner syndrome : tibia and thumb aplasia, polydactyly of the foot.

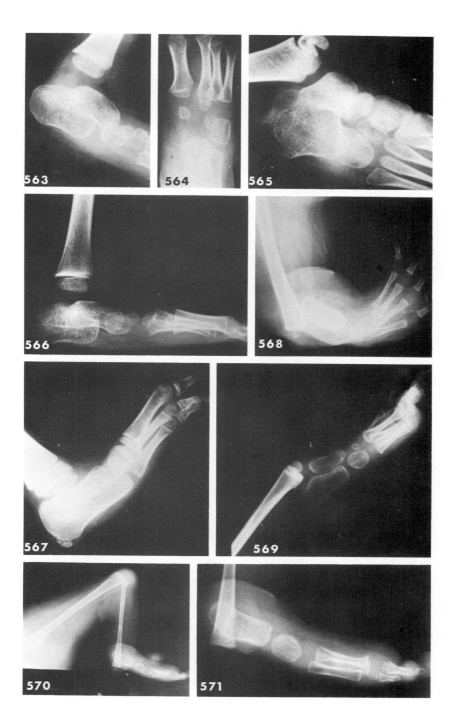

563. Fibula aplasia and talocalcaneal fusion.

564. Fibula aplasia and reduction of the fifth digit of the foot.

565. Single aplasia of the fibula.

566. Fibula aplasia and posterior tarsal coalition with flatfoot (standing patient).

567. Fibula aplasia and absence of the fourth and fifth digits of the foot.

568. Tibial aplasia and absence of the first digit with clubfoot.

569. Isolated aplasia of the tibia.

570. Bilateral tibial aplasia : general view of a lower limb.

571. Same case : tibial aplasia with absence of the second and third digits.

MALPOSITIONS AND DEFORMITIES

CONGENITAL TALIPES EQUINOVARUS

This deformity occurs in approximately 1 per 1.000 live births. It is three times as common in males as in females, and is bilateral in 52 % of cases. When unilateral, it usually effects the left foot.

Abnormal posture results from the combination of varus and equinus.

Varus is produced by two elementary distorsions : adduction or the inward placement of the forefoot, and supination or the turning inward of the sole of the foot. Equinus is an irreducible plantar flexion of the foot, often hidden, and which appears only if adduction and supination are reduced.

The adduction of the foot takes place :

— between the hindfoot and the leg ;

— in the subtalar joint where the calcaneus moves inward (it heaves*) ;

— between the hindfoot and the forefoot, in the transverse midtarsal joint. In the newborn, the skeleton of the leg is in medial rotation, the ankle turns in and this movement increases.

The supination of the foot takes place in the subtalar joint where the calcaneus is tucked upward on its medial side (it rolls*).

The equinus occurs in the ankle (the talus approaches the vertical) and the subtalar joint (the calcaneus pitches*).

The radiographic examination of the congenital talipes equinovarus is difficult, because the deformity is complex. The exact measurement of one abnormal posture is possible only after correction of the other ones ; but the capsular, ligamentous and muscular retractions often make the deformities irreducible. Nevertheless, the foot must be X-rayed in the optimal position, taking into account that adduction takes place essentially between hind and forefoot (frontal radiograph), supination is localized, especially in the subtalar joint (because of the tilted calcaneus) (lateral radiograph), and the equinus has its seat particularly in the ankle joint (because the talus is tilted downward) (lateral radiograph).

Frontal radiograph

— Adduction between fore and hindfoot : the midtalar line passes outside of the first ray and the cuboid is not in front of the calcaneus.

— Adduction of the calcaneus superimposes it on the talar radiographic appearance.

— Supinated calcaneus : the talocalcaneal angle is null.

— Supinated forefoot : the metatarsal bases overshadow each other.

Lateral radiographs

— Equinus : measurement of the tibiotalar angle.

— Subtalar joint mobility : comparative view with the foot brought in plantar and dorsal flexion.

— Supinated calcaneus : measurement of the talocalcaneal angle : tarsal sinus obliterated.

— Supination of the forefoot : metatarsal outspread.

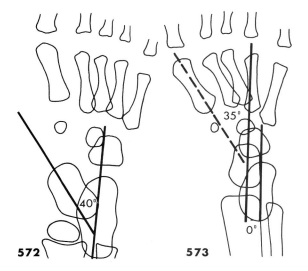

572, 573. Diagram of the deformities and their measurement (frontal view).

572. Normal foot. Anteroposterior view : the angle between the midtalar and midcalcaneal lines is 40⁰. The cuboid is in front of the calcaneus. A line drawn through the long axis of the talus should pass inside the first metatarsal.

573. Congenital talipes equinovarus. Anteroposterior view : supination and adduction of the calcaneus : the talocalcaneal angle is zero. Adduction of the metatarsus : the line drawn through the long axis of the talus should pass outside the first metatarsal and the cuboid is not in front of the calcaneus.

* After Farabeuf.

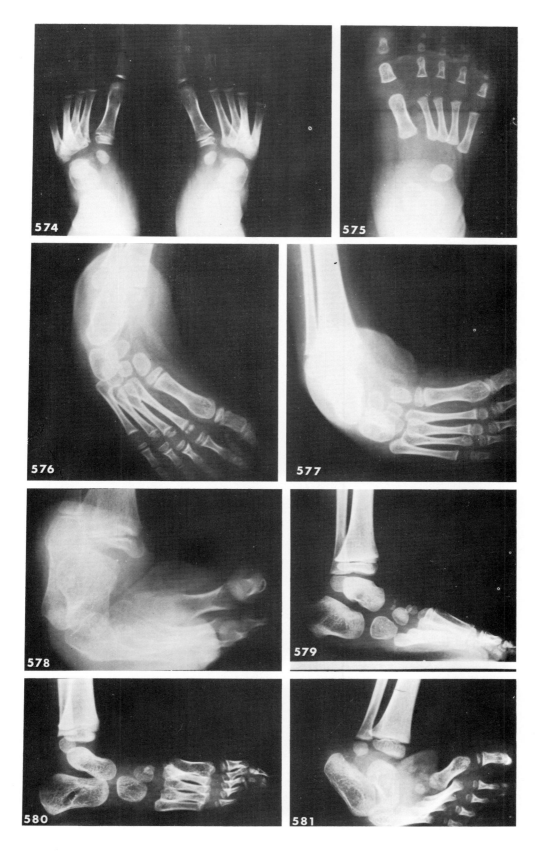

574. Bilateral congenital talipes equinovarus : 5-year-old boy. The adduction of the metatarsus and supination of the foot are irreducible.

575. Congenital talipes equinovarus : 8-month-old boy. The suppleness of this foot makes it possible to reduce the adduction and supination of the foot : normal radiographic appearance.

576, 577. Bilateral congenital talipes equinovarus (Arthrogryposis).

578. Congenital talipes equinovarus (patient standing). Irreducible adduction and supination of the forefoot : skin furrow digging into the medial side of the foot. The calcaneus and the talus are vertical and project one on the other.

579. Congenital talipes equinovarus : lateral radiograph in the static position : 10-year-old boy. The midtalar and midcalcaneal lines are parallel. Tarsal sinus obliterated. Slight supination.

580. Congenital talipes equinovarus : irreducible supination.

581. Congenital talipes equinovarus : extreme abnormal posture : « rocker » deformity : 4-year-old girl. Spinal dysraphism of the fourth lumbar vertebra with meningomyelocele.

CONGENITAL TALIPES EQUINOVARUS

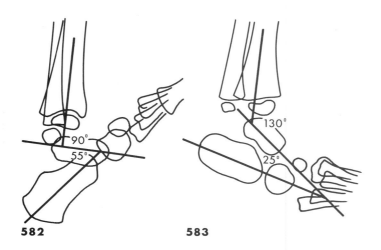

582   **583**

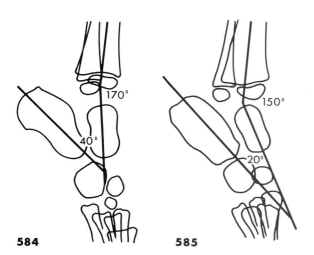

584   **585**

582 → 585. Pattern of deformities and their measurement (lateral view).

582. Normal foot, in maximal dorsal flexion : tibiotalar angle 90°. Talocalcaneal angle 55°. The tarsal sinus is clearly visible.

583. Congenital talipes equinovarus brought in maximal dorsi-flexion. The tibiotalar angle is wider than 90° (equinus). The talocalcaneal angle decreases to 25°. Midtalar and midcalcaneal lines approach parallelism. The calcaneus has a potato-like aspect (from Boppe) and the tarsal sinus disappears by supination of the calcaneus.

584. Normal foot brought in maximal plantar flexion : the tibiotalar angle increases to 60° or more (normal range of mobility of the ankle). The talocalcaneal angle decreases of 5-10°.

585. Congenital talipes equinovarus : foot brought in maximal plantar flexion (lateral view). The range of movement of the ankle decreases.

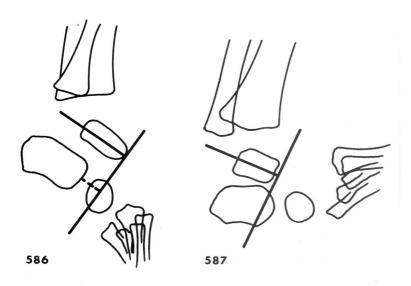

586   **587**

586, 587. Congenital talipes equinovarus. The range of movement of the subtalar joint is analyzed in the lateral view by the comparative relationship of the talar and calcaneus, according to the position (flexed or extended) of the foot.

586. Maximal plantar flexion : on a lateral view, the anterior aspect of the calcaneus is at the rear of the projection of the talar anterior aspect.

587. Maximal dorsal flexion : the calcaneus moves forward : the subtalar joint is not stiffened.

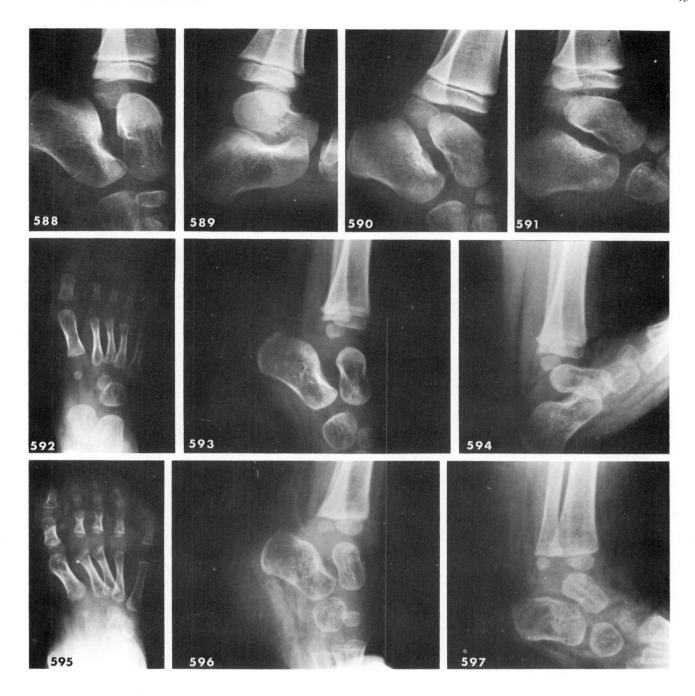

588 → 591. Clubfoot : stress film of the ankle, with maximum plantar or dorsal flexion of the foot.

588, 589. Normal foot. Plantar and dorsal flexion. 5-year-old boy.

590, 591. Congenital talipes equinovarus. Plantar and dorsal flexion. 5-year-old boy.

592 → 597. Congenital talipes equinovarus. Routine radiographs. Frontal radiograph and lateral projection (plantar and dorsal flexion of the foot).

592 → 594. Normal foot in a 2-year-old girl.

595 → 597. Congenital talipes equinovarus in a 2-year-old boy.

CONGENITAL TALIPES EQUINOVARUS

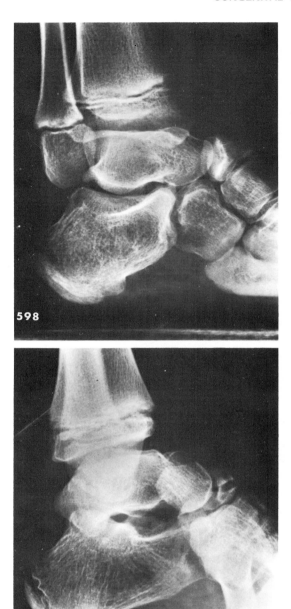

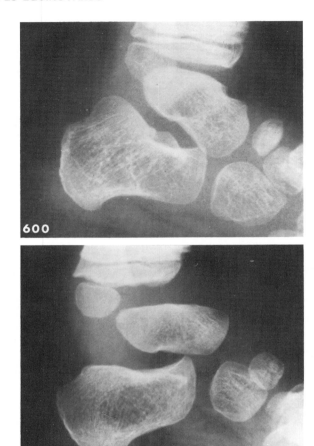

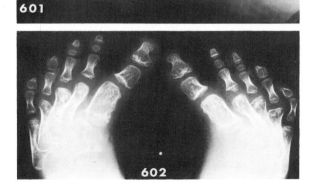

598 → 602. Particular radiological aspects of the clubfoot : The bones of the posterior tarsus, particularly the talus, may show peculiar radiological shapes, generally non-pathologic, for they are due only to the radiographic projection. In that aspect, R. Seringe insists on the necessity of including in the radiographic examination of a clubfoot, a *strictly* lateral projection of the ankle.

598. Routine lateral view of the foot : the lateral malleolus is projected rearward, the tarsal sinus is obscured, and the talar trochlea looks flattened.

599. Strict lateral view of the ankle, with the leg and the clubfoot medially rotated : normal view of the lateral malleolus. The tarsal

sinus and the talar dome reappear. Note the vanishing view of the forefoot, with a falsely vertical first metatarsal.

600. Standard lateral radiograph of the foot : apparent hypertrophic tuber calcanei.

601. Standard lateral radiograph of the foot : apparent flattening of the talus due to orthopedic maneuvers.

602. Bilateral congenital clubfoot and dwarfism (Maroteaux). This recessive, autosomic hereditary skeletal dysplasia consists also of micromelia and evolutive scoliosis. Likewise the ovoid aspect of the first metatarsal shaft is typical.

METATARSUS VARUS

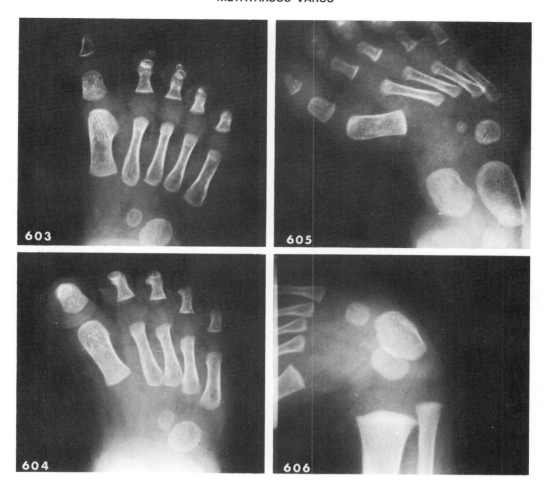

603. Normal foot in frontal projection.

604. Congenital metatarsus varus. Slight adduction of the metatarsals.

605. Congenital metatarsus varus in a 9-month-old child. The radiograph shows that the metatarsals are adducted relative to the midtarsus (pes adductus). The cuboid is in front of the calcaneus.

606. Clubfoot : the metatarsus adductus is associated with the adduction of the cuboid which slipped inside of the calcaneal tuberosity.

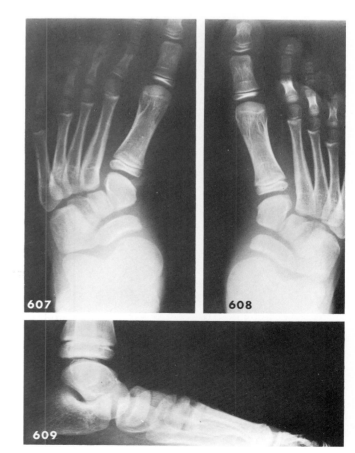

607 → 609. Metatarsus varus and flat foot : 8-year-old boy.

607, 608. Frontal radiographs : adduction of all metatarsals.

609. Lateral radiograph : flattening of plantar arch.

STATIC FLAT FOOT*

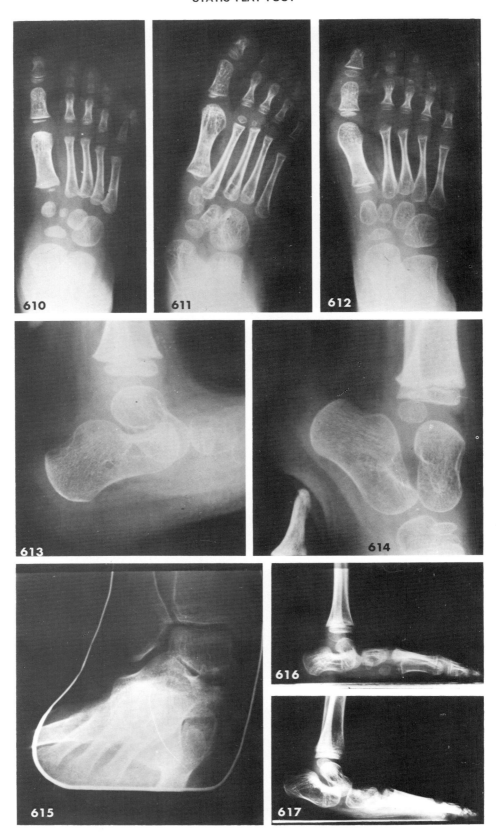

610. Flexible flat foot of the child. Valgus of the calcaneus (increased talocalcaneal angle).

611. Flexible flat foot of the child with metatarsus valgus.

612. Flexible flat foot of the child : calcaneus valgus.

613, 614. Flat foot : lateral radiographs with plantar and dorsiflexion for the equinus.

615. Pes planovalgus in a weight-bearing frontal radiograph of the ankle.

616. Hypotonic flat foot.

617. Hypotonic flat foot with shrinking of the Achille tendon.

See pages 65 and 102.

FLAT FOOT

The static pes planovalgus of the adolescent has been studied in the chapter « The Foot in Standing ». The supple flat foot of the child is more common and asymptomatic but in some cases, it has particular etiologies : paralysis, synostosis.

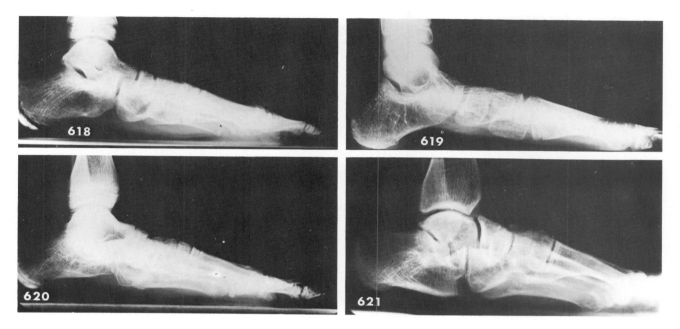

618. Paralytic flat foot : poliomyelitis.

619. Hypotonic flat foot : Marfan syndrome (congenital hypotonia) : vertical position of the talus, elongation of bones, fibrillar osteoporosis with coarsening of trabeculae.

620. Flat foot with tarsal coalition : a single stiff painful flat foot must lead to studies for possible synostosis.

621. Flat foot associated with tarsal dysostosis.

CONGENITAL CONVEX PES VALGUS

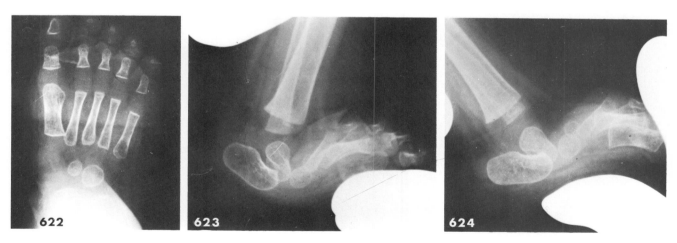

622 → 624. Same patient, 1-year-old boy.

622. Frontal radiograph : increased talocalcaneal angle. Outspread metatarsals (valgus).

623. Lateral radiograph with the foot brought in dorsiflexion : irreducible vertical talus, with the navicular subluxated on the talar neck.

624. Lateral radiograph with the foot in plantar flexion. Residual talus position of the forefoot. Overshadowing of the metatarsals (valgus).

TALIPES CALCANEUS

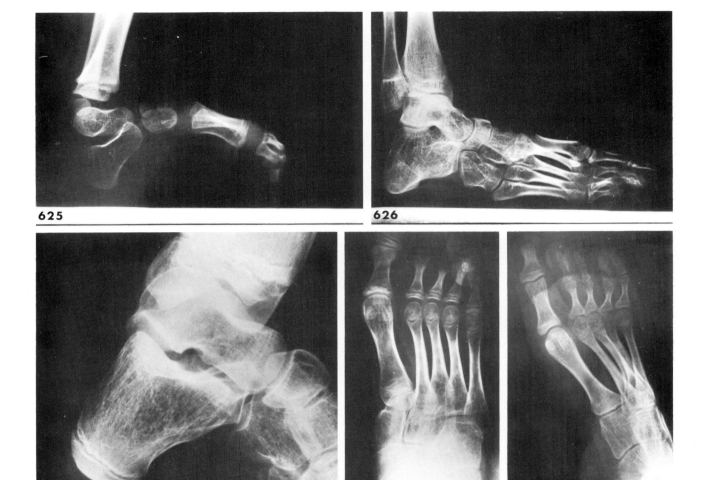

625. Pes talus valgus cavus : paraplegia out of medullary ischemia : (lateral view) ; vertical position of the calcaneus ; exaggeration of the medial longitudinal normal arch of the foot ; superimposed projection of the metatarsals (valgus).

626. Pes talus varus : poliomyelitis (lateral view) vertical position of the calcaneus. Separate projection of the metarsals (varus).

627. Pes talus valgus : poliomyelitis (lateral view) vertical position of the calcaneus. Apparent subtalar joint (valgus).

628. Same case as **627** (frontal view). Distinctly projected metatarsals on the radiograph (valgus).

629. Same case as **626** (frontal view). The metatarsals are adducted (varus) and overshadow each other (supination).

PES CAVUS*

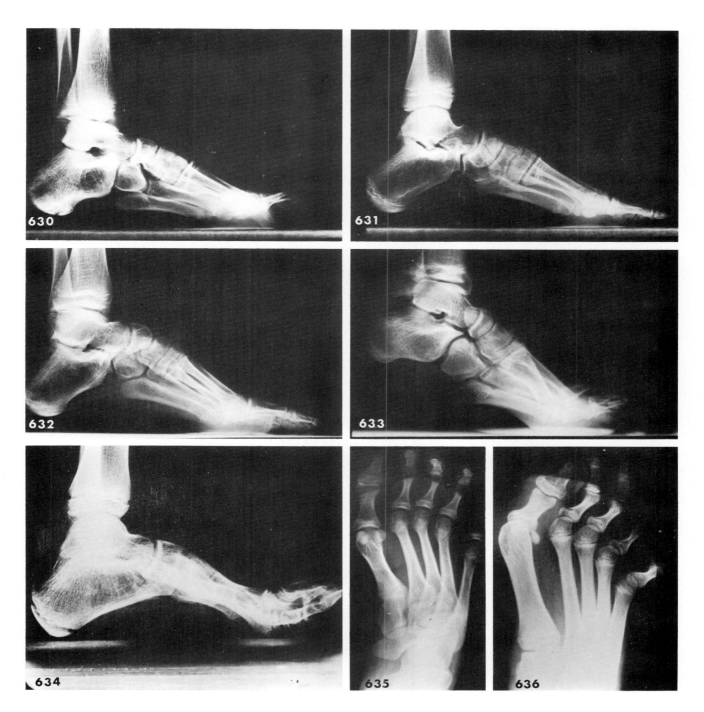

630. Anterior pes cavus with high medial longitudinal arch. Djian-Annonier angle 110^0, Meary line broken at a level with the cuneonavicular joint.

631. Anterior pes cavus with high medial and lateral arches. Djian-Annonier angle 110^0, Meary line broken at a level with the talonavicular joint.

632. Posterior pes cavus : talus value 96^0.

633. Talipes equinovarus and cavus. Compare with **643**.

634. Apert disease. 6-year-old girl. Synostoses and cavus.

635. Talipes equinovarus and cavus.

636. Pes cavus : clawing of the toes.

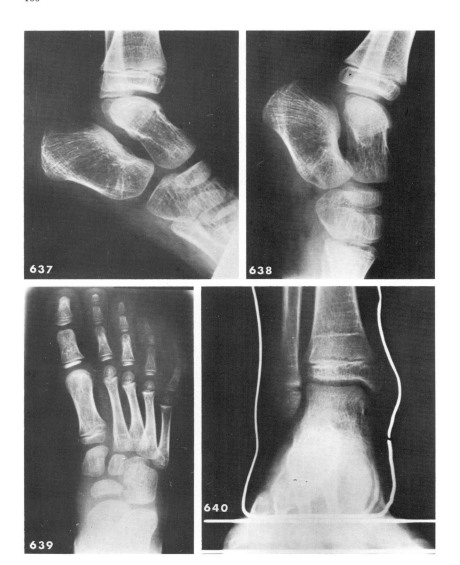

PES EQUINUS*

637 → 640. Talipes equinus.
637. Dorsiflexion.
638. Plantar flexion.
639. Horizontal plane : normal axes.
640. Vertical plane : normal axes.

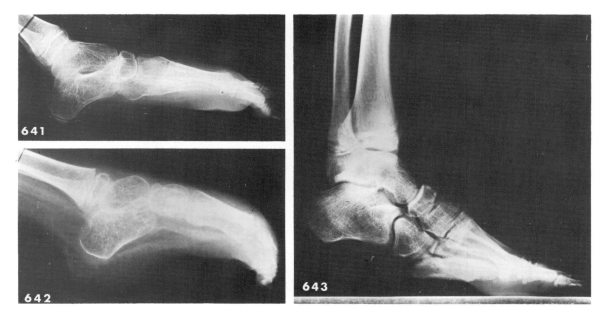

641, 642. Talipes equinus in arthrogryposis.

643. Talipes equinus : lateral view. Absent cavus, compare to **634.**

* See page **68.**

MAJOR DEFORMATION

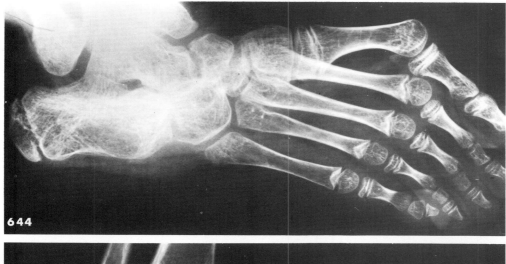

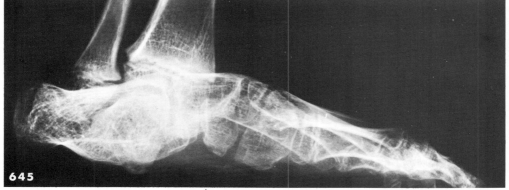

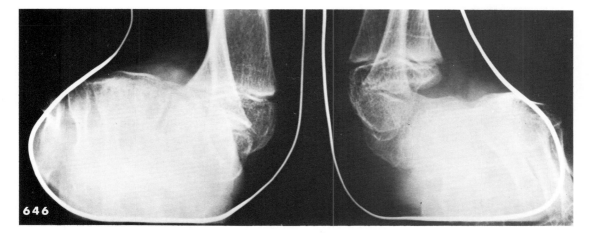

644 → 646. Larsen syndrome : congenital generalized joint hyperlaxity with multiple dislocations and osseous anomalies, including flattened facies and cleft palate.

644. *Anteroposterior* radiograph with weight-bearing foot.

645. *Lateral* radiograph with weight-bearing foot.

646. Frontal radiograph of the ankles with the patient standing erect.

CONGENITAL SYNDROMES WITH JOINT HYPERMOBILTY

Bird headed dwarfism (Seckel S.)
Down S. (mongolism)
Ehlers-Danlos S.
Focal dermal hypoplasia (Goltz S.)
Geroderma osteodysplastica
Hereditary arthro-ophthalmopathy (Stickler S.)
Marfan S.
Metaphyseal chondrodysplasia (McKusick)
Morquio S.
Oculocerebral-renal S.
Osteogenesis imperfecta
Pseudoachondroplastic dysplasia

ETIOLOGY OF STRUCTURAL DEFORMITIES OF THE FOOT

I - CONGENITAL MALPOSITIONS AND DEFORMITIES

Deformities likely due to neurologic intrauterine disorders :
— congenital talipes equinovarus (clubfoot)
— arthrogryposis
— congenital convex pes valgus

Deformities due to malposition in utero :
— congenital vertical talus
— congenital metatarsus adductus and varus
— congenital talipes calcaneovalgus

Chromosom aberrations :

— sex chromosomes : X X X X Y syndrome ; X X X X X syndrome
— autosomes : trisomy 13 (clubfoot) ; trisomy 18 (clubfoot) ; trisomy 8 (clubfoot) ; deletion of the long arm of chromosome 18 ; deletion of the short arm of chhromosome 4 (Wolf-Hirschorn syndrome)

Disorders of muscles and ligaments : Myotonic dystrophy of Steinert (clubfoot), Larsen syndrome (clubfoot), Ehlers-Danlos disease (flat foot)

Pharmacotoses (Recklinghausen)

Inherent disorders of bone growth :

— overgrowth of bone : Marfan disease (flat foot) ; hemihypertrophy (clubfoot)
— small stature : with mental retardation : Smith-Lemli-Opitz syndrome (varus-metatarsus varus) ; Coffin syndrome (flat foot) ; Cornelia de Lange syndrome
without mental retardation : Freeman-Sheldon syndrome (clubfoot), Bloom syndrome (equinus), otopalatodigital syndrome

Metabolic abnormalities : Morquio disease (flat foot) and other mucopolysaccharidoses (flat foot or cavus), Refsum-Thiebaut disease, aminopterin (varus), homocystinuria (flat foot or cavus)

Dysostoses : Moebius syndrome (clubfoot), cerebrohepatorenal syndrome of Zellweger (clubfoot, metatarsus varus), acrosyndactyly (clubfoot), onychodysostosis (clubfoot), tibial aplasia (clubfoot), peroneal aplasia, congenital coalitions.

Osteochondrodysplasia : chondrodysplasia punctata (clubfoot), Kniest disease (flat foot), diaphyseal dysplasia of Camurati-Engelmann (flat foot), Pyle disease (flat foot), dysplasia epiphysealis hemimelica (flat foot), spondyloepiphyseal dysplasia (clubfoot), diastrophic dwarfism (clubfoot), chondroectodermal dysplasia of Ellis-van Creveld (valgus).

II - ACQUIRED MALPOSITIONS AND DEFORMITIES

Static disorders without paralysis
— counterbalancing (knee - hip)
— idiopathic (flat foot - pes cavus)

Paralyses

— cerebral cause : encephalopathies ; meningitides ; hemiplegia
— medullar cause : poliomyelitis (pes talus, pes cavus, flat foot) ; Werdning-Hoffmann disease (flat foot) ; paraplegia ; tetraplegia ; spinocerebellar heredodegenerative syndromes (Freidreich disease, Charcot-Marie disease, etc.) (pes cavus) ; spina-bifida

— peripheral nerves : diabetic and alcoholic polyneurites ; neurites ; wound of the nerves (common fibular nerve)

Bone trauma

Infectious and inflammatory diseases

Vascular disorders.

4

BONE AND JOINT ANOMALIES OF SHAPE AND SIZE

ETIOLOGIC CLASSIFICATION OF THE FOLLOWING RADIOGRAPHS

DYSOSTOSES (MALFORMATIONS)
— Brachydactyly : brachyphalanges or brachymetatarsals ; single or in combination : oral-facial-digital syndrome.
— Macrodactyly.

OSTEOCHONDRODYSPLASIA
— With disturbances of growth :
  - Marked dwarfism : achondroplasia ; chondrodysplasia punctata ; metatropic dwarfism.
  - Dwarfism in combination : cleidocranial dysplasia.
  - Small stature : metaphyseal chondrodysplasia Schmid-type ; spondyloepiphyseal dysplasia ; epiphysometaphyseal dysplasia : pseudoachondraplasia, acrodysplasia.
— With disorganized development of cartilage : dysplasia epiphysealis hemimelica.

BONE GROWTH SECONDARY ABNORMALITIES
— Essential disorders :
  - Small stature : Rubinstein-Taybi syndrome.
  - Osseous overgrowth : Marfan disease ; hemihypertrophy ; Klippel-Trenaunay syndrome ; gigantism.
  - Hormonal disturbances : hypothyroidism ; acromegaly.
  - Metabolic abnormalities : Hunter disease ; Morquio disease ; Refsum disease.
— Miscellaneous diseases : poliomyelitis ; phacomatoses ; osteoid osteoma ; myositis ossificans progressiva ; burns.

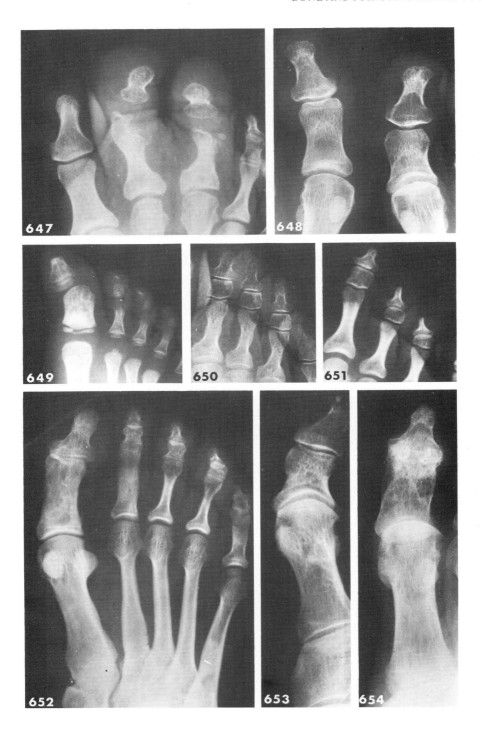

647. Macrodactyly of second and third toes with phalangeal maldevelopment.

648. Idiopathic short proximal phalanx of the right big toe.

649. Massive first phalanx of the big toe (with small radiolucent areas of osteoporosis) and medial deviation of the distal phalanx : typical radiographic findings of orodigito-facial syndrome (Papillon-Leage and Psaume). This one is characterized by facial and buccal maldevelopment associated with various anomalies of the feet and hands (eg brachydactyly, polydactyly, syndactyly).

650. Normal variant : square middle phalanges.

651. Normal variant : pointed distal phalanges.

652. Enlarged phalanges : altered trabecular architecture with pseudocystic radiolucent areas of rarefaction : fibrous dysplasia.

653. Idiopathic short proximal phalanx of the great toe.

654. Hypertrophic great toe with enlarged proximal phalanx, osteoporosis, thinning of the cortex. Patient, aged 75 years, with tabetic neurogenic arthropathies of the hindfoot and other regions. Is this condition « Alajouanine's tabetic big toe » ?

CONGENITAL SYNDROMES WITH SHORT PHALANGES

Acrocephalopolysyndactyly (Carpenter S.)
Acrocephalosyndactyly (Apert S.)
Asphyxiating thoracic dysplasia
Basal cell nevus S. (Gorlin)
Cleidocranial dysplasia
Cornelia de Lange S.
Diastrophic dwarfism
Dilantin therapy to mother
Familial brachydactylies
Fanconi S. (pancytopenia-dysmelia S.)
Holt-Oram S.
Myositis (fibrodysplasia) ossificans progressiva
Otopalatodigital S.
Poland S.
Rhinotrichophalangeal S.
Rubinstein-Taybi S.
Trisomy 13 S.
Trisomy 18 S.

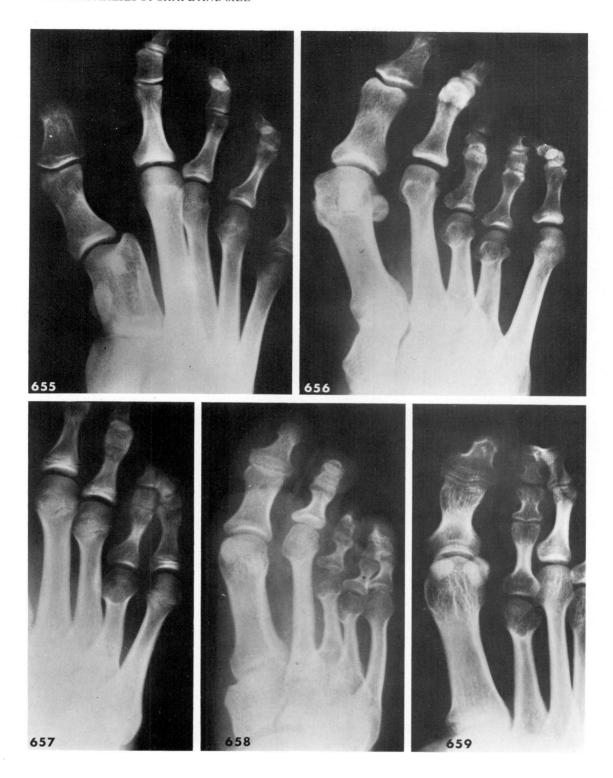

655 → 659. Shortening of the metatarsals*.

655. Short great toe and hypertrophic second metatarsal.

656. Short third and fourth metatarsals in Turner syndrome.

657. Short fourth metatarsal.

658. Short third and fourth metatarsals.

659. Short second metatarsal.

See page 116.

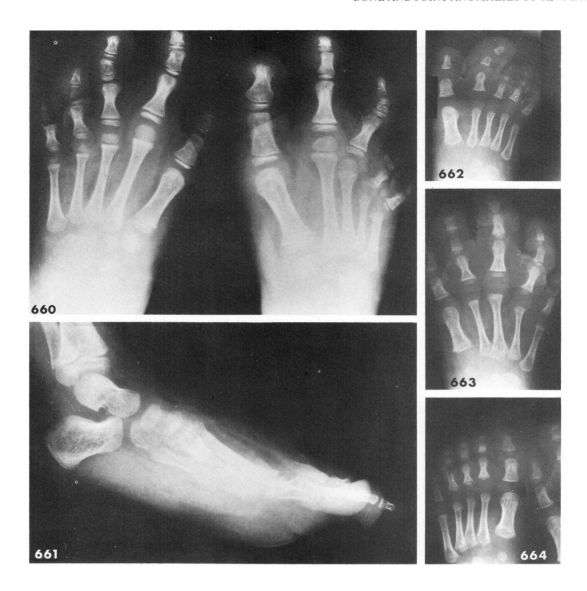

660, 661. Klippel-Trenaunay-Weber syndrome : segmental hypertrophy of skeleton and soft tissues caused by congenital venous anomalies which delay blood returning.

662. Localized hypertrophy of the soft tissues and phalanges of the second toe : phacomatosis in a 20-month-old boy.

663. Idiopathic hypertrophic right foot in a 2-year-old girl.

664. Same case : left foot.

GENERALIZED OR WIDESPREAD ELONGATION OF BONE

Cerebral gigantism (hypothalamic)
Hemihypertrophy
Homocystinuria
Hyperpituitarism
Klinefelter S.
Marfan S.
Total lipodystrophy

LOCALIZED ELONGATION OR OVERGROWTH OF BONE

Arteriovenous fistula
Chronic arthritis (eg, tuberculous, juvenile rheumatoid)
Chronic osteomyelitis (eg, tuberculous, tropical ulcer)
Dysplasia epiphysialis hemimelica (Trevor disease)
Healing fracture
Hemangioma, lymphangioma
Hemihypertrophy
Hemophilic hemarthrosis
Hyperemia, any cause
Idiopathic
Macrodystrophia lipomatosa ; congenital macro dactyly
Neurofibromatosis

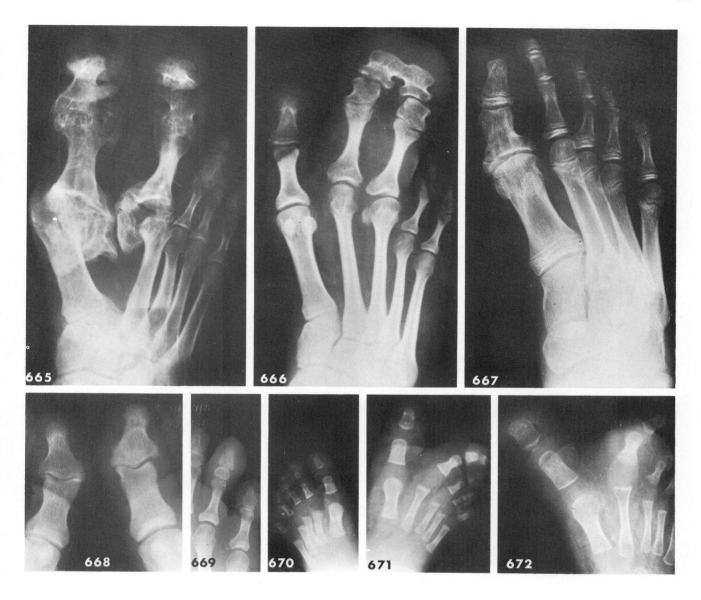

665. First and second hypertrophic toes, sequela of burns in childhood.

666. Idiopathic hypertrophy of the second and third toes associated with osseous and cutaneous syndactyly.

667. Total symmetrical increase of the bony foot with hypertrophic epiphyses, altered trabecular architecture of the first metatarsophalangeal joints. *This 11-year-old girl* has enlargement of the epiphyses of all the bones and multiple painful epiphysial aseptic necroses.

668. Hypertrophic great toe caused by chronic eczema.

669. Hypertrophic fourth toe caused by an osteoid osteoma of the distal phalanx.

670, 671. Right idiopathic macropodia with syndactyly. Radiograph at birth.

672. Same case, 2 years later.

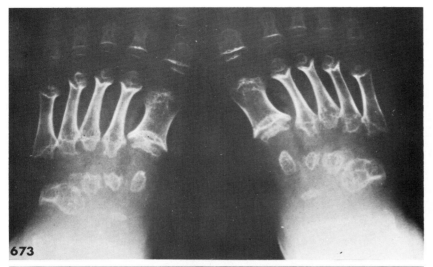

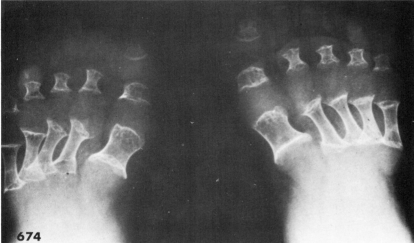

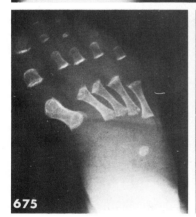

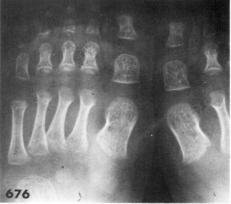

CONGENITAL SYNDROMES WITH SHORT FEET

Aarskog-Scott S. (shawl scrotum S.)
Achondroplasia
Chondroectodermal dysplasia (Ellis-Van Creveld S.)
Cockayne S.
Diastrophic dwarfism
Enchondromatosis (Ollier disease)
Hypochondroplasia
Metaphyseal chondrodysplasia
Metatrophic dwarfism
Mucopolysaccharidosis (eg, Hurler, Hunter, Morquio)
Multiple cartilaginous exostoses
Multiple epiphyseal dysplasia (Fairbank)
Noonan S.
Orodigitofacial S.
Peripheral dysostosis
Prader-Will S.
Progeria
Pseudohypoparathyroidism, pseudopseudohypoparathyroidism
Rhinotrichophalangeal S.
Smith-Lemil-Opitz S.
Spondyloepiphyseal dysplasia, pseudoachondroplastic type
Spondylometaphyseal dysplasia
Thanatophoric dwarfism
Weill-Marchesani S.

ACQUIRED DISEASES CAUSING SHORT FEET

Acro-osteolysis (see page 171)
Leprosy
Lipoid dermatoarthritis
Osteomyelitis, severe (eg, bacterial, yaws, smallpox)
Rheumatoid arthritis, arthritis mutilans

673. Pseudo-achondroplasia : epiphysometaphyseal dysplasia characterized by the same micromelia as in achondroplasia, but without facial dysmorphia and with more marked shortening of the hands and the feet. Radiolucent, broadened and flaring metaphyses. Irregular and frayed epiphyseal plates with side hooks or spurs.

674. Metatrophic dwarfism (viz variable) : the micromelia prevails at birth, then it is oblitered during childhood by an evolutive kyphoscoliosis. Pudgy foot with shortened and diabolo-like bones.

675. Metatrophic dwarfism : in this case, the metatarsals are longer, and they show increased density of the metaphyseal margin.

676. Achondroplasia : the foot bones are short and squat but less so than in the pseudoachondroplasia (**673**).

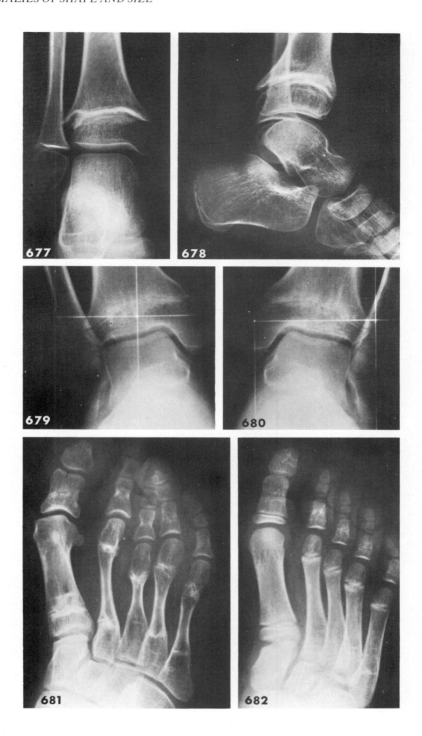

677, 678. Metaphyseal chondrodysplasia (Schmid dominant type) : characterized by a moderate micromelia where the skull, the spine, the hands and the feet are spared. However, in the recessive type (McKusick) the hands and the feet are affected and hair is light-colored, fine and sparse, (cartilage-hair hypoplasia). Differential diagnosis includes metaphyseal alterations of pancreatic insufficiency (with or without neutropenia) and thymoaplasia with lymphopenia. Metaphyseal cupping. Irregular transverse radiolucent bands alternating with transverse zones of increased density in the metaphysis. However the growth, the shape and the structure of the epiphyseal centers are normal.

679, 680. Achondroplasia (in an adolescent) : discrepancy in epiphyseal growth ; oblique ankle joint - metaphyseal cupping.

681. Cleidocranial dysostosis : the Pierre-Marie-Sainton disease is characterized by clavicular aplasia, cranio-facial dysmorphia and delayed osseous development. In addition to these classic findings, the following are sometimes noted at the foot : shortening of the talus and calcaneus, spindle-shaped, short metatarsals and phalanges, pseudoepiphyses.

682. Cleidocranial dysostosis : small decrease in length of the phalanges.

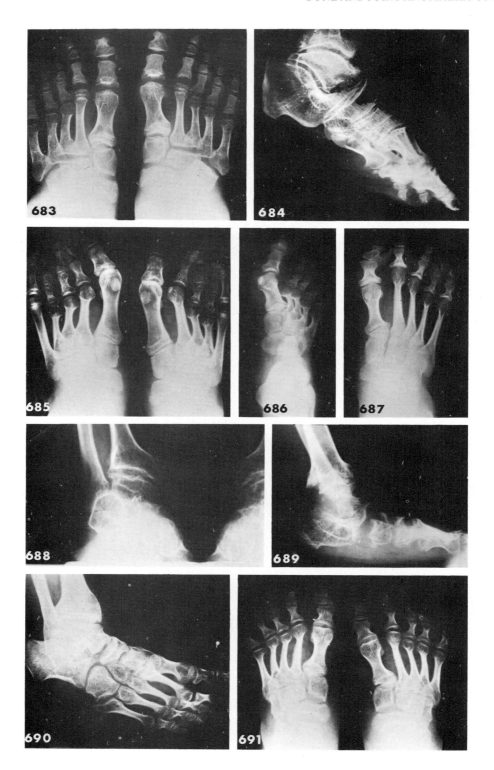

683. Polyepiphyseal dysplasia (16-year-old boy) : broadened epiphyses ; thickened metatarsal bases.

684. Polyepiphyseal dysplasia (43-year-old male) : thickened and widened foot bones caused by underdevelopment of the epiphyses.

685. Spondyloepiphyseal dysplasia (17-year-old boy) : broadened epiphyses ; short metatarsals.

686. Acrodysostosis : congenital syndrome characterized by marked shortening of the hands and the feet associated with facial dysmorphia, fatness, and mental retardation (16-year-old girl). Very short metatarsals.

687. Polyepiphyseal dysplasia : less important manifestations.

688, 689. Same case. Spondyloepiphyseal dysplasia (10-year-old boy) : no ossification of the dysplastic epiphyseal centers.

690, 691. Same patient. Polyepiphyseal dysplasia (14-year-old boy).

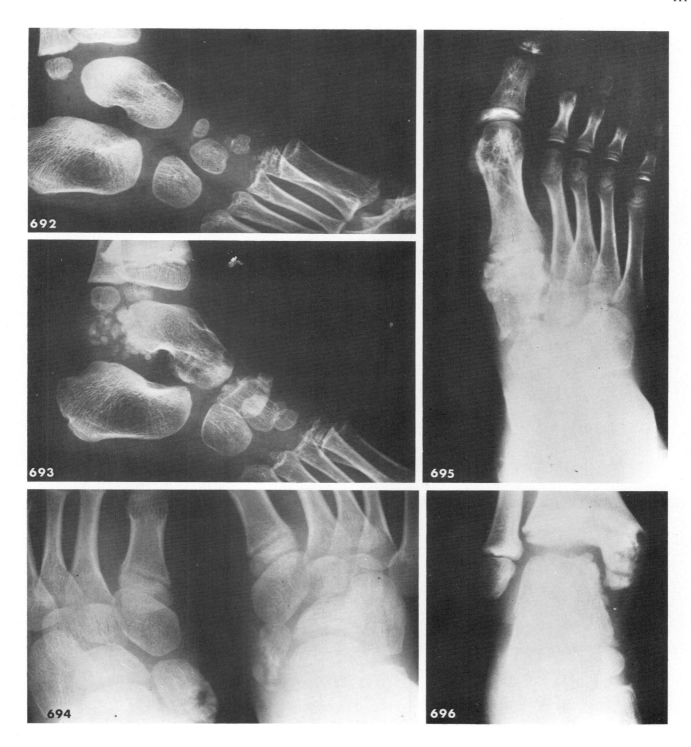

692, 693. Hemimelia epiphysealis dysplasia (tarsomegaly of Mouchet-Belot or tarso-epiphyseal aclasia of Trevor and Fairbank) : disorganized development of the epiphyseal cartilages and the tarsal ossification centers, localized to only one lower limb and generally to the medial side.

692. Normal foot.

693. Tarsal changes : overdevelopment of the talus and navicular with multiple ossification centers.

694. Bilateral hypertrophic os tibiale externum or bipartite navicular.

695, 696. Tarsomegaly : epiphyseal changes of the first metatarsal and the ankle.

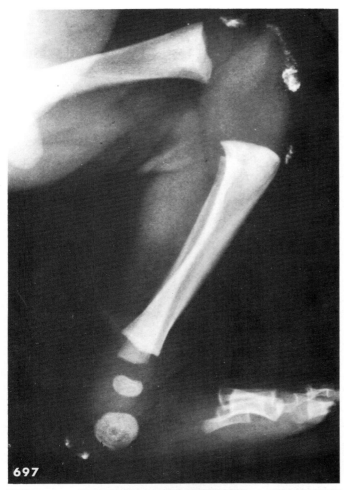

697

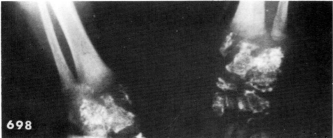

698

697, 698. Chondrodysplasia punctata (Conradi-Hünermann disease). Congenital entity, twice more frequent in the girl : characterized by cutaneous lesions, cataract, heart anomalies and variable morphologic changes : adactyly, syndactyly, clubfoot, micromelic dwarfism, shortening of long bones, kyphoscoliosis, facial dysmorphia, stippled epiphyses. Radiologically, the calcifications are localized in the epiphyses and in the periarticular soft tissues ; all bones can be affected. These punctate areas of calcification are variable in size and shape. Mosekilde describe three radiographic appearances :

— patchy sclerotic foci, of variable size, surrounding the ossification center ;
— regular, dense, circumscribed sclerotic areas, simulating an ossification center ;
— cloud-like opacity, instead of cartilaginous tissues.

The significance of the radiographic findings is proportionate to the limb deformities.

These calcifications decrease progressively and disappear before the fourth year of age, by resorption or incorporation in the ossification center. These pathologic calcifications may be mistaken for the normal variations in appearance of the bone ossification centers, eg particularly the cuboid bone.

STIPPLED EPIPHYSES AND APOPHYSES

Anencephaly
Down syndrome
Isolated stippled calcaneus
Sequelae of the arthritides
Trisomy 18 syndrome
Zellweger syndrome (Cerebrohepatorenal
    syndrome)

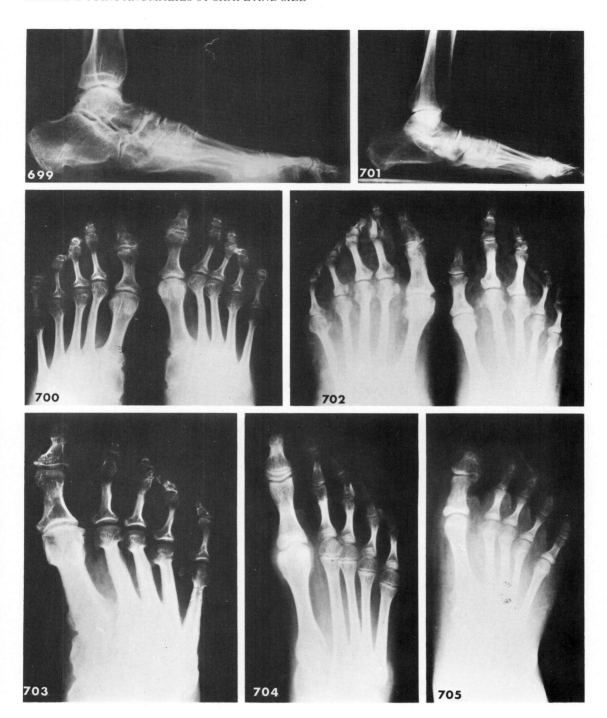

699, 700. Gigantism : large size shoe, size of the foot 39 cm. Compare to normal foot **701.**

701. Normal foot (same scale).

702. Klippel-Trenaunay syndrome : localized hypertrophy of the lower limb involving skeleton and soft tissues and due to hereditary vascular abnormalities blocking the venous return.

703. Acromegaly : the metatarsal and phalangeal shafts are markedly thickened. Enlargment of the articular space due to articular cartilage hypertrophy.

704. Arachnodactylia (Marfan disease) : hereditary, congenital growth disturbance characterized by funnel-shaped thorax, scoliosis, cardiovascular malformations (aneurysm), dislocation of the ocular lens, hypermobile muscles, tendons and ligaments with articular dislocation (frequent flat foot) and excessive growth and elongation of the bones. Eleven - year-old girl : tapered and markedly elongated metatarsals and phalanges, with respect to cortex, metaphysis and epiphysis of bone.

705. Rubinstein-Taybi syndrome : dwarfism with mental retardation, facial dysmorphia (thin and beaked nose, prominent forehead) and typical abnormalities of the hands and feet which are broad and short (particularly the thumb and the great toe) - triangular hypertrophic distal phalanx (sometimes bifid or duplicated) showing a slight change in the osseous trabecula.

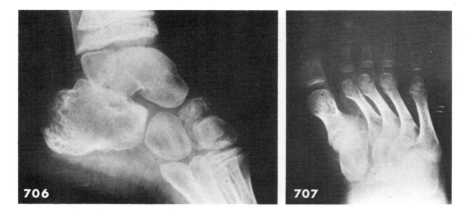

706, 707. Infantile hypothyroidism : the congenital myxedema produces a delayed osseous development and epiphyseal abnormalities.

This is an 18-year-old girl with a bone age of 10 years and a mental age of 2 years. Irregular appearance of the navicular ossification center and calcaneal posterior apophysis. Sometimes, an osteosclerosis exists simulating Albers-Schönberg disease.

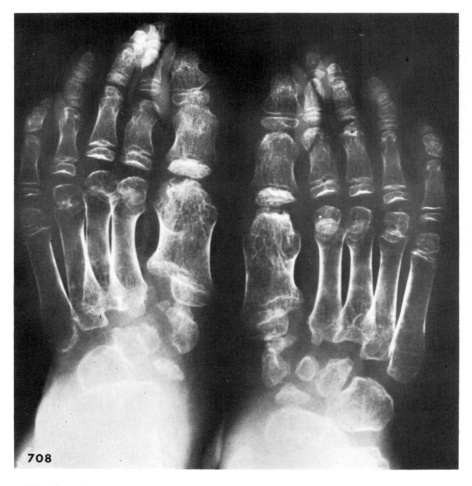

708. Morquio disease : congenital spondyloepiphysometaphyseal dysplasia due to an error of mucopolysaccharide metabolism (type IV) and characterized by dwarfism, facial dysmorphia with backward flexion of the head, knock-knee and flat foot. The evolution of the epiphyseal defects is typical of Morquio disease : hardly visible in the child, these osseous abnormalities increase during growth and lead to marked osteoporosis, platyspondyly, coxa valga, etc. Morquio disease : conical metacarpal ends — but normal modeling contrary to other types of mucopolysaccharidoses. At the foot, anomalies in length of the metatarsals and dysplastic epiphyses.

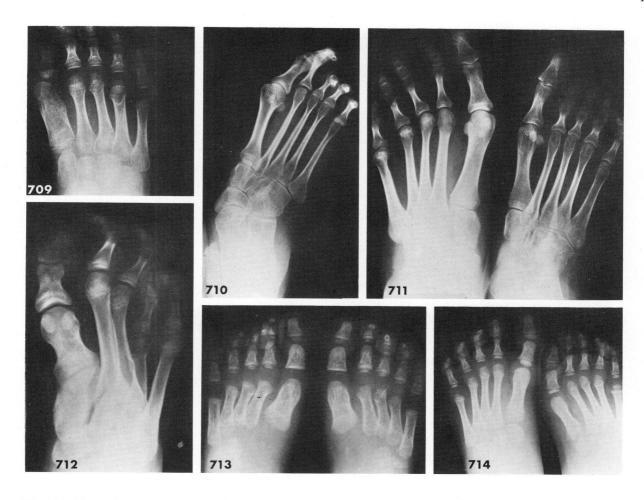

709. Myositis ossificans progressiva : rare disease, unknown etiology. The changes in the hands and feet make diagnosis possible early in the disease, long before the ossifications appear in the connective tissues and muscles. First metatarsal, short and thick, of which the narrow head is curved in varus, or even separated from the shaft. Same defects at the thumb. Short phalanges and symphalangism may be associated.

710. Neonatal meningitis : long and slender metatarsals.

711. Poliomyelitis (at the right side), long and slim metatarsals.

712. Refsum-Thiebaut disease : heritable autosomal neuropathy characterized by hypertrophy of Schwann's sheath as in Dejerine-Sottas disease, but more over associated to encephalic and cerebellar disorders, and due to congenital enzymatic deficiency : incomplete metabolism of the phytol in decarboxylic acid by hereditary absence of phytanate and oxydase. Phytanic acid accumulation in myelin, serum, urine and miscellaneous tissues is responsible for ocular. cardiac, cutaneous and osseous lesions (elbow, knee, foot).

15-year-old boy : polyneuritis of the lower limbs - bilateral foot dysplasia with shorteness of the first and fourth toes.

713. Hunter disease : mucopolysaccharidosis type III (see above), very similar to Hurler disease, type I, characterized by kyphosis, facial dysmorphia (gargol-like facies), limitation of joint motion, mental retardation. In type I, abnormalities of modeling of the metatarsal and metacarpal metaphyses. In type II, more severe skeletal changes. In a 3-1/2-year-old child, thickened metatarsal and first phalanx of the great toe.

714. Right clubfoot in a 4-1/2 year-old child operated at 11 months of age.

BRACHYDACTYLY

Acro-osteolysis (eg, congenital, leprosy) (see page 171)
Arthritis
Basal cell nevus S. (Gorlin)
Cone-shaped epiphyses (see page 80)
Congenital syndromes with short hands and feet (esp. chondrodysplasias, mucopolysaccharidoses) (see page 108)
Congenital syndromes with short metacarpals or metatarsals (see opposite gamut)
Congenital syndromes with short phalanges (see page 104)
Enchondromatosis (Ollier disease)
Familial brachydactylia
Idiopathic
Kaschin-Beck disease (in Manchuria, Russia)
Myositis (fibrodysplasia) ossificans progressiva
Oculodentodigital S.
Orodigitofacial S.
Osteomyelitis (eg, bacterial, yaws, smallpox)
Pseudohypoparathyroidism, pseudopseudohypoparathyroidism
Sickle cell anemia (hand-foot syndrome)
Smith-Lemli-Opitz S.
Trauma (eg, thermal, electrical, epiphyseal cartilage injury, fracture)
Turner S.
Weill-Marchesani S.

SHORT METATARSALS AND METACARPALS (EXCLUDING GENERALIZED SHORTENING)

Basal cell nevus S. (Gorlin)
Beckwith-Wiedemann visceromegaly S.
Biemond S.
Brachydactylia, familial
Chondrodysplasia punctata (Conradi disease)
Cockayne S.
Cornelia de Lange S.
Cri du chat S.
Diastrophic dwarfism
Dyschondrosteosis
Epiphyseal dysplasia
Fanconi S. (pancytopenia-dysmelia S.)
Hand-foot-uterus S.
Holt-Oram S.
Idiopathic (isolated anomaly)
Klinefelter S.
Larsen S.
Leri pleonosteosis
Long arm 18 deletion S.
Multiple hereditary osteocartilaginous exostoses
Myositis (fibrodysplasia) ossificans progressiva
Neonatal hyperthyroidism
Orodigitofacial S.
Osteomyelitis (eg, bacterial, yaws, smallpox)
Peripheral dysostosis
Post-infarction (eg, sickle cell anemia)
Pseudohypoparathyroidism, pseudopseudohypoparathyroidism
Radial hypoplasia
Radiation or radium injury
Rhinotrichophalangeal S.
Rubinstein-Taybi S.
Russel-Silver S.
Trauma (eg, thermal, electrica, epiphyseal cartilage injury, fracture)
Turner S.

5

SOLITARY OR MULTIPLE OSTEOSCLEROTIC BONE LESIONS

OSTEOCHONDRODYSPLASIA WITH SCLEROTIC CHANGES

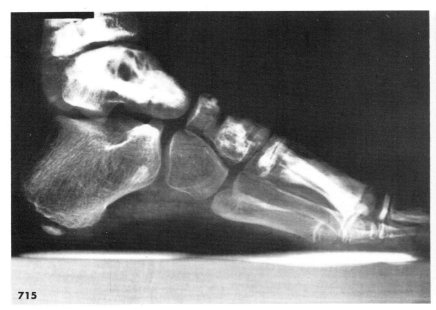

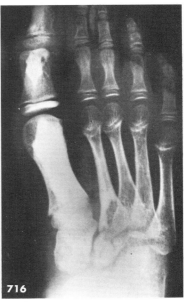

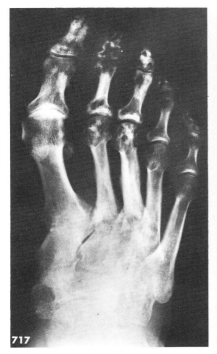

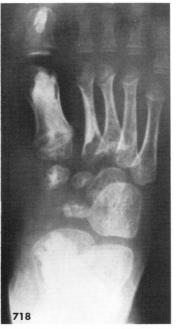

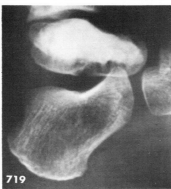

715 → 719. Melorheostosis : usually affects a unilateral group of bones - characterized by patchy sclerotic foci or tape-like osseous condensations extending all along the medial or lateral side of a limb and resembling a drop of wax flowing from a candle. This disease often reveals itself only at the adult age, but may be seen at a younger age, producing discrepancy in length of a limb and walking disorders.

The melorheostosis may be associated with osteopoikilosis or localized scleroderma (Maroteaux).

715, 716. Melorheostosis : child-medial unilateral sclerosis (tibia, talus, first rayon) and second metatarsal shaft, pes cavus.

717. Melorheostosis : osteosclerosis flowing inside and outside the marrow, especially at the second and third rays level.

718, 719. Melorheostosis : monomelic osteosclerotic changes and deformed ossification centers of the navicular and medial cuneiform in a child.

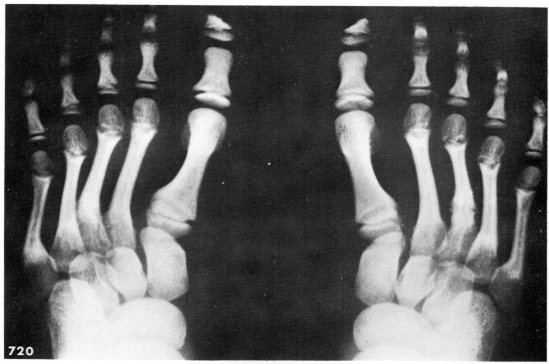

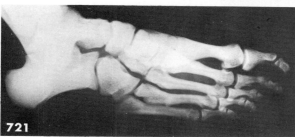

720, 721. Pyknodysostosis (pyknos = compact) : a recessive autosomal hereditary condition. This entity has been classified in the dysplasia group by Lamy and Maroteaux.

It is characterized by short stature, prominence of frontal bossae, generalized osteosclerosis and osseous fragility. Diffuse sclerosis with narrow medullary cavities.

No band-like or streak-like bone condensations are present as in Albers-Schönberg disease. At the hands and feet, progressive resorption of the distal phalanges is seen (see **1040**).

720. Pyknodysostosis in a child : fracture of the third metatarsal shaft.

721. Pyknodysostosis in an adult : oblique view showing the fracture of the fourth metatarsal shaft.

TRANSVERSE LINES OR ZONES OF INCREASED DENSITY IN THE METAPHYSES

Aminopterin-induced syndrome
Cretinism, hypothyroidism
Estrogen in high doses or heavy metal therapy to mother during pregnancy
Heavy metal or chemical absorption (eg, bismuth, arsenic, phosphorus, fluoride, mercury, lithium, radium)
Hypervitaminosis D
Idiopathic hypercalcemia
Lead poisoning
Leukemia, treated
Metaphyseal chondrodysplasia (Schmid)
Methotrexate therapy
Normal variant (esp. in the neonate)
Osteopetrosis
Oxalosis
Parathormone therapy
Protracted anemia (eg, sicklemia, thalassemia)
Radiation from bone seeking isotopes (Sr^{90}, Y^{90}, P^{32})
Rickets, renal osteodystrophy (healing)
Scurvy, healing
Steroids (in high doses)
Systemic illness or stress in infancy (growth lines)
Transplacental infection (eg, toxoplasmosis, rubella, cytomegalic inclusion disease, herpes, syphilis)

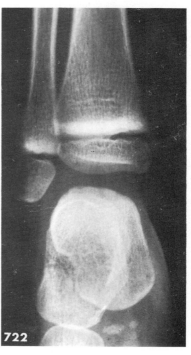

722. Oxalosis : metabolic heritable disorder characterized by a widespread deposition of calcium oxalate crystals, especially in the kidney's. 5-year-old child. Homogeneous sclerotic metaphyseal band of the tibia.

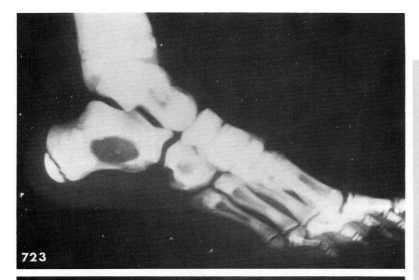

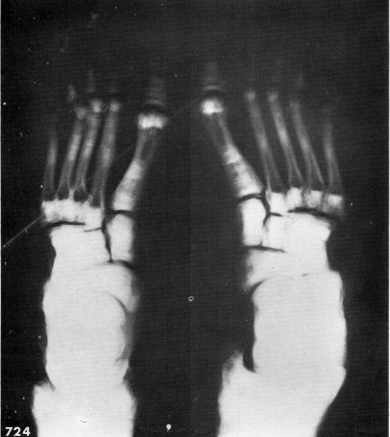

723, 724. Osteopetrosis (Albers-Schönberg disease, marble-bone disease) : Congenital recessive autosomal dysplasia with anemia, hepato and splenomegaly, and nervous system disorders (compression of the central nervous system at the base of the skull. The skeletal manifestations are an osseous fragility and a generalized, symmetrical osseous condensation. This osteosclerosis is diffuse or streak-like, and leads to obliteration of narrow spaces.

723. Lateral view. Severe osteosclerosis : homogeneous or with a radiolucent center, or rosette-like with alternate dense and lucent rings.

724. Anteroposterior view. The condensation is located particularly at the metatarsal epiphyses. Abnormalities of metaphyseal modeling of the tibia and the first metatarsal base. Longitudinal or transverse sclerotic streaks, fracture of the left second and third metatarsal shafts.

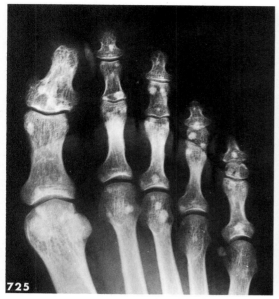

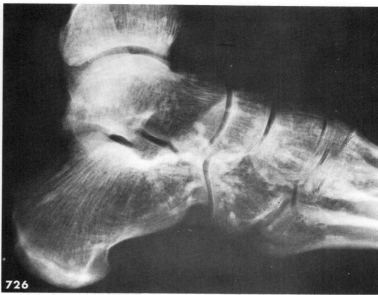

725, 726. Osteopoikilosis : hereditary dysplasia, radiologically characterized by multiple, dense, pea-sized islands of compact bone, symmetrically located in the epiphyses and metaphyses (« spotted » bones from G. Ledoux-Lebard). They may also be seen as prolate oval sclerotic foci or with a radiolucent central portion. Usually asymptomatic, this disease is twice more frequent in males than in females and it may be associated with melorheostosis and scleroderma (P. Maroteaux) or skin changes (dermatosis lenticularis disseminata of Buschke-Ollendorff and Curth, or keratoderma palmaris et plantaris). At the foot, the great number of sclerotic patches and the presence of other speckled bones make the differential diagnosis possible, with benign bone islands, single or in small numbers, often observed in the calcaneus and the talus (see **734** and **768**).

727. Osteopathia striata (Voorhoeve disease) : dysplasia characterized radiologically by band-like bone condensations in metaphyses, running parallel to the bone axis. The condition is frequently associated with morphologic abnormalities (polydactyly, syndactyly) or skin changes (localized dermatofibrosis lenticularis from Goltz).

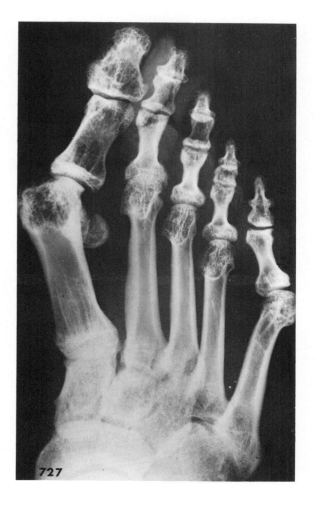

BONE ISLANDS

Benign, distinctly circumscribed sclerotic areas of compact bone located in a normal spongiosa in epiphyses as well as in metaphyses. They are shaped like a round or a long oval island, measuring 5 to 15 mm.

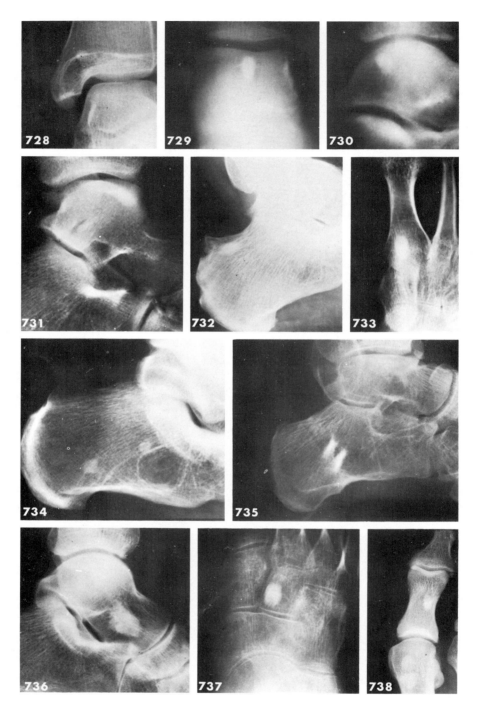

728. Tibial bone island.

729, 730. Talar bone island (tomograms).

731. Avulsion of the tip of the lateral malleolus (**140**).

732. Calcanean bone island. Note the rheumatoid cortical erosion.

733. Bone island of the first metatarsal base.

734. Two calcanean bone islands. Note the simulated calcanean cyst (see page 155)

735. Calcanean osteotomy from Dwyer and bone grafting procedure.

736. Large bone island ; the term osteoma is inappropriate.

737. Intermediate cuneal bone island.

738. Bone island of the proximal phalanx of the great toe.

MISCELLANEOUS OSTEOSCLEROSES

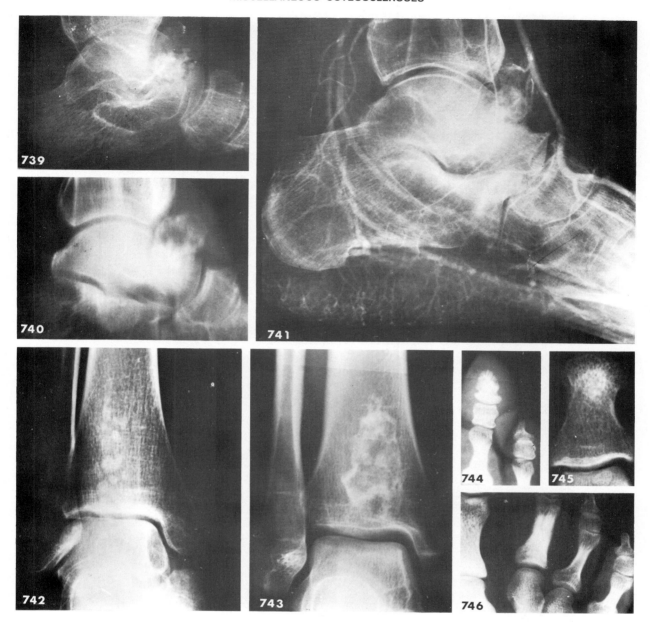

739 → 741. Osteoid osteoma : solitary benign formation of osteoid tissue affecting adolescents or young adults, more frequently males than females. Its course follows a slow run. Radiologically, it is a small, isolated, well delineated, radiolucency (nidus) measuring at the outside 1 cm., usually full in the middle of a dense osteosclerotic zone. But atypical changes are frequent, according to the site of the nidus : nidus with a central sclerotic focus, considerable thick sclerotic area obscuring the nidus, eccentric or outside nidus, sclerosis extending in the soft tissues, hypertrophy of the soft tissues (toe and nail).

739, 740. Osteoid osteoma of the talar neck : outside nidus in the soft tissues (lateral radiograph and tomogram).

741. Advantage of angiography : opacification of the highly vascularized nidus.

742. Calcification in an Achilles tendon (see lateral view, 1423).

743. Bone infarct : idiopathic type, no clinical significance, detection usually by radiography. Typical osteosclerotic change in the spongiosa of the metaphysis : heterogeneous irregular cloud-like patchy osseous condensation.

744. Osteoid osteoma of the distal phalanx of the fourth toe with edema of the tissues.

745. Dorsal exostosis of the distal phalanx of the great toe (see lateral radiograph 1400).

746. Osteoid osteoma of the proximal phalanx of the second toe.

SOLITARY OSTEOSCLEROTIC BONE LESION

Avascular necrosis
Bone infarct
Bone island
Bone sarcoma (eg, osteosarcoma, chondrosarcoma, Ewing)
Callus (healed or healing fracture)
Chondroid lesion (eg, enchondroma, osteochondroma)
Fibrous dysplasia ; ossifying fibroma
Healed or healing benign bone lesion (eg, bone cyst, nonossifying fibroma, fibrous cortical defect, brown tumor)
Lymphoma ; reticulum cell sarcoma
Mastocytosis
Osteoblastic metastasis (see page 126)
Osteoblastoma
Osteoid osteoma
Osteoma, endosteoma
Paget disease
Sclerosing osteomyelitis (eg, Garre ; Brodie abscess ; granuloma)
Syphilis ; yaws

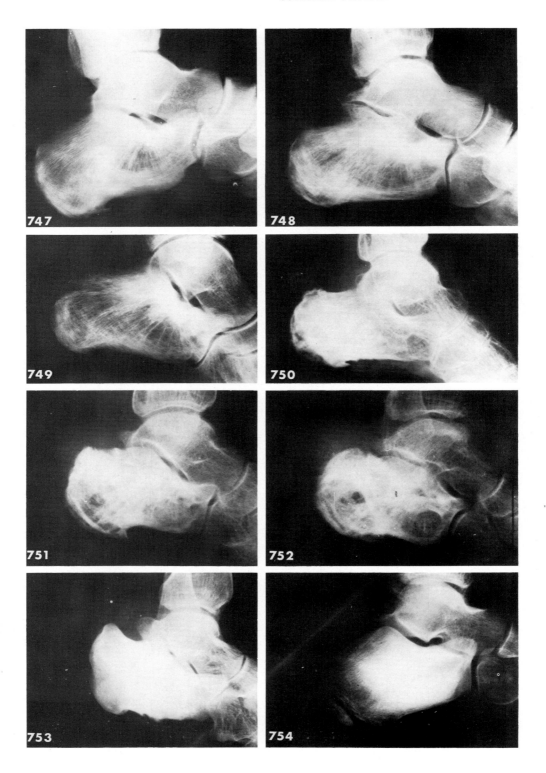

747 → 749. Paget disease. Uncommon localization at the foot, 1 % of cases.

747. Mottled wooly trabecular architecture.

748. Broad, coarse trabecular architecture and some sclerotic bone patches. Note degenerative changes of the posterior talocalcanean joint with beak-like spur formations which have also a remodeled osseous structure.

749. Calcaneal coarsely reticulated architecture.

750. Calcaneal condensans osteitis by heel scab.

751. Condensing tuberculous osteitis with cyst-like area of radiolucency and edematous soft tissues.

752. Tuberculous osteitis : same radiographic picture.

753. Massive osteosclerosis and deformity : chronic osteomyelitis.

754. Uniform sclerosis with preserved osseous architecture : osteomyelitis.

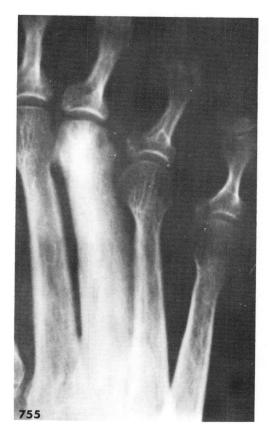

755. Paget disease : widened, thickened osteosclerotic shaft of the third metatarsal with undifferentiated cortical and spongiosa structures.

756, 757. Mycetoma. Mycotic tumor originating in the teguments and the soft tissues. Then, on an average of 2 years after the inoculation, it expands in the osseous tissues. This chronic infection, involving usually the foot (Madura foot) is caused by two principal groups of microorganisms : Actinomycetes (including several species of *Streptomyces)* and true fungi (including miscellaneous strains of *Madurella).* The mycotic tumefactions are characterized by multiple sinuses from which exudate drains - this exudate contains granules of variable color and size, which permit identification of each species. *Streptomyces pelletieri* (red granules) has the strongest affinity for osseous tissues ; it is the most destructive and the most quickly progressive.

In the late mycetoma, the radiographic findings are mixed osteolytic and osteosclerotic changes.

Radiologically, in a few cases, it is possible to determine the specific responsible fungus for, on the X-ray film, the size of the lytic bone defect is in proportion with the size of the granules which it contains. The importance of osteosclerosis is also conditioned by each pathogenic strain.

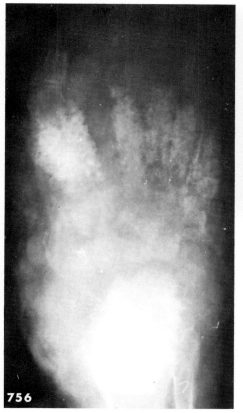

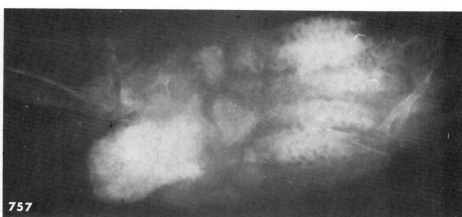

756, 757. Madura foot : 28-year-old male, 3 years after inoculation by scrub thorns.

— Swelled mamelonated soft tissues with numerous draining sinuses.

— Intense demineralization of the foot and the ankle.

— Admixture of sclerosis and lysis (but predominant sclerosis changes with *Streptomyces pelletieri*) : effacement of the bony contours of the cuneiforms and cuboid with widening of the anterior tarsal joints ; complete osteolyses, no sequestra ; multiple cystlike lesions, 1-2 mm. of diameter (red granules), pitting the metatarsals. Because of the dense, massive bone condensation, the weight of the metatarsal shafts is doubled ; their mass is also doubled by the marked periosteal thickening. « Ivory » calcaneus. The talus is often normal.

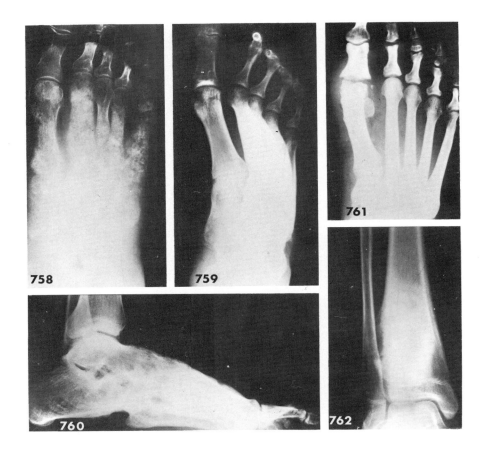

758. Metastases from a breast carcinoma : mixed osteolytic and osteosclerotic radiographic findings.

759, 760. Anterotarsal ankylosis and osteosclerotic metatarsals after healing of a pneumococcal arthritis.

761. Osteosclerotic first ray after arthroplasty.

762. Tibial osteosclerosing sarcoma : classical metaphyseal localization, extension into the cortex and periosteal reaction on the posterior aspect of the tibia ; however, the epiphysis is still protected by its cartilaginous growth plate.

OSTEOBLASTIC METASTASES

Breast carcinoma
Carcinoid
Cerebellar medulloblastoma or sarcoma
Lymphoma
Meningiosarcoma
Other carcinoma (esp. carcinoma of lung, colon, pancreas, urinary bladder, ureter)
Prostate carcinoma

MULTIPLE OSTEOSCLEROTIC BONE LESIONS

Avascular necroses
Bone infarcts
Bone islands
Callus (eg, healed rib fractures)
Chondrodysplasia, punctata (congenital stippled epiphyses, Conradi disease)
Enchondromatosis (Ollier disease)
Fibrous dysplasia
Lymphoma
Mastocytosis
Multiple enchondromas, osteochondromas
Multiple healed or healing benign bone lesions (eg, nonossifying fibromas, fibrous cortical defects, brown tumors, bone cysts, Gaucher disease)
Multiple myeloma
Multiple osteocartilaginous exostoses
Osteoblastic metastases
Osteomas (eg, Gardner syndrome)
Osteomyelitis, chronic or healed (eg, tuberculous, fungal)
Osteopathia striata
Osteopoikilosis
Osteosarcomatosis
Paget disease
Plasma cell granulomas
Syphilis ; yaws
Transversales osteosclerotic metaphyseal bands (see page 119)
Tuberous sclerosis

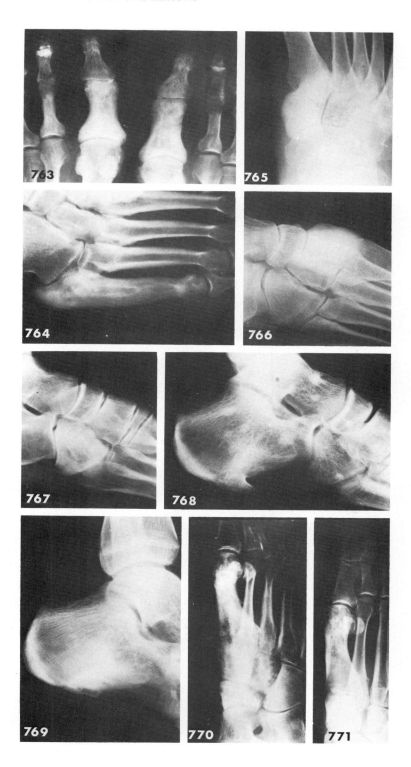

763. Paget disease : remodeling of the trabecular architecture of the proximal phalanx of both great toes : admixture of osteolytic and osteosclerotic changes.

764. Paget disease of the fifth metatarsal : thickened shaft, with undifferentiated cortical and spongiosa structures.

765, 766. Paget disease : osteosclerotic type : dense medial cuneiform.

767. Paget disease of the cuboid : coarsened trabecular.

768. Numerous bone islands.

769. Osteitis by perforating ulcer under the heel.

770. Osteitis of the first metatarsal and the cuneiforms with multiple small cyst-like areas of osteolysis.

771. Osteoarthritis of the intercuneiform joints : reactive bone sclerosis on both sides of the joint.

FATIGUE FRACTURES

Fracture that occurs in a normal bone after repeated or unusual endogenous stress ; for instance, at the level of a metatarsal in people unaccustomed to long hikes (whence the term march fracture suggested by Deutschlander in 1965).

Initially, there are no radiological findings although the lesion produces a severe stabbing pain. Kroening depicts five types of fatigue fracture :

— fissured type (linear) : fine cleft interrupting the bone cortex (**167, 168, 809**) ;
— periosteal type : dense, thick cortical spindle with fracture cleft not always demonstrable ;
— transverse type, observed only on the metatarsal shafts, simulating a fragmentary fracture but with a fusiform heterogenic swelling callus, often hypertrophic (**805, 807, 808**) ;
— condensing type, noticeably typical on the calcaneus ;
— mixed type.

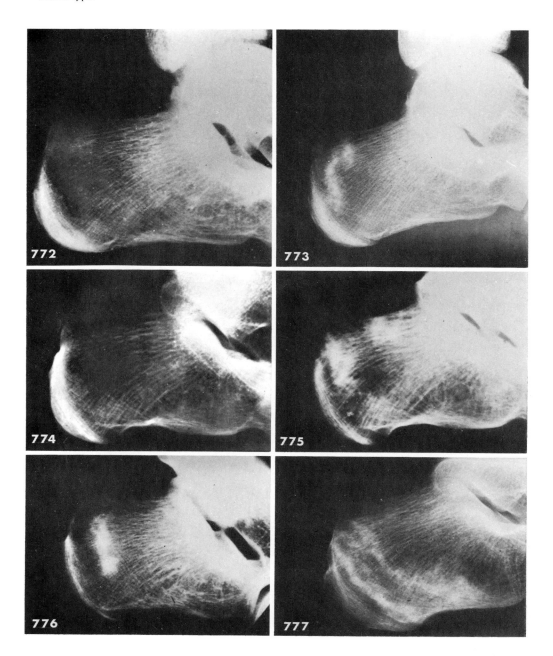

772 → 777. Calcaneal march fracture : the radiographic findings are bandlike bone condensations traversing the spongy bone structures and revealing the impacted lines of the trabecular architecture. The hematoma raises the periosteum and periosteal appositions are later included in the callus.

772, 773. Same patients. 772. Radiograph at the onset of the clinical painful syndrome. 773. Radiograph 15 days later : osteosclerotic band at the calcaneal posterior apophysis level.

774, 775. Same patients. 774. Radiograph at the beginning of the painful clinical syndrome. 775. Radiograph 4 months later : osteosclerosis, proof of the fracture.

776. Fatigue fracture. The radiological picture was identical on both calcanei.

777. Fatigue fracture : radiograph one month after the onset of the clinically painful syndrome.

6

HYPEROSTOSIS AND PERIOSTEAL REACTIONS

CLASSIFICATION OF HYPEROSTOSIS AND PERIOSTEAL REACTIONS

ETIOLOGICAL CLASSIFICATION OF THE PERIOSTEAL REACTIONS

Chronic stimulation of the adjoining periosteum :

— osteoarticular inflammatory lesions,
— hypervascularization of the soft tissues by various disorders (varices, arteriovenous aneurysms and fistulae).

Periosteal detachment :

— in the subperiosteal exudate or granuloma (osteomyelitis, syphilis, leukemia),
— in the subperiosteal hemorrhages (scurvy, trauma, hemophilia).

Awakening of the osteogenic function of the periosteum :

— in trauma (eg callus of a fracture),
— in the osteogenic tumors (eg osteosarcoma).

Unknown or contested etiology :

— pachydermoperiostosis,
— hypertrophic pulmonary osteoarthropathy of Pierre Marie and Bamberger,
— infantile cortical hyperostosis of Caffey-Silverman.

ENDOSTEAL AND SUBPERIOSTEAL HYPEROSTOSIS

The cortex of the shaft may be thickened either from outside to inside, by endosteal osteogenesis at the expense of the medullary spongiosa which narrows, or from inside to outside by coating of periosteal new bone, by a mixed process.

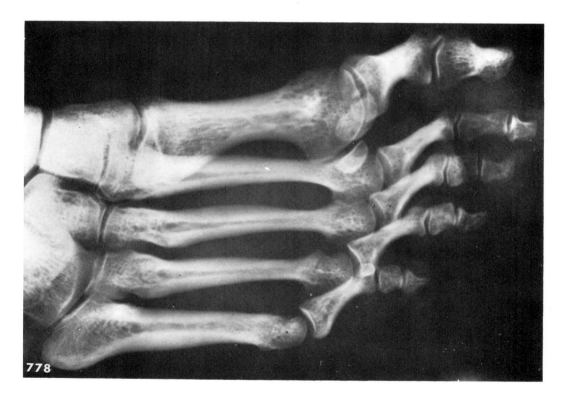

778. Generalized cortical hyperostosis : osteochondro-dysplasia, including a dominant type (Worth) usually clinically asymptomatic (sometimes torus palatinus) characterized by a regular thickening of the diaphysial cortex (endosteal hyperostosis), and a recessive type (Van Buchem), more severe, with mandibular enlarge-

ment and extensive bone condensation which squeezes the cranial nerves.

In this case obliteration of the medullary spaces of the metatarsal shafts.

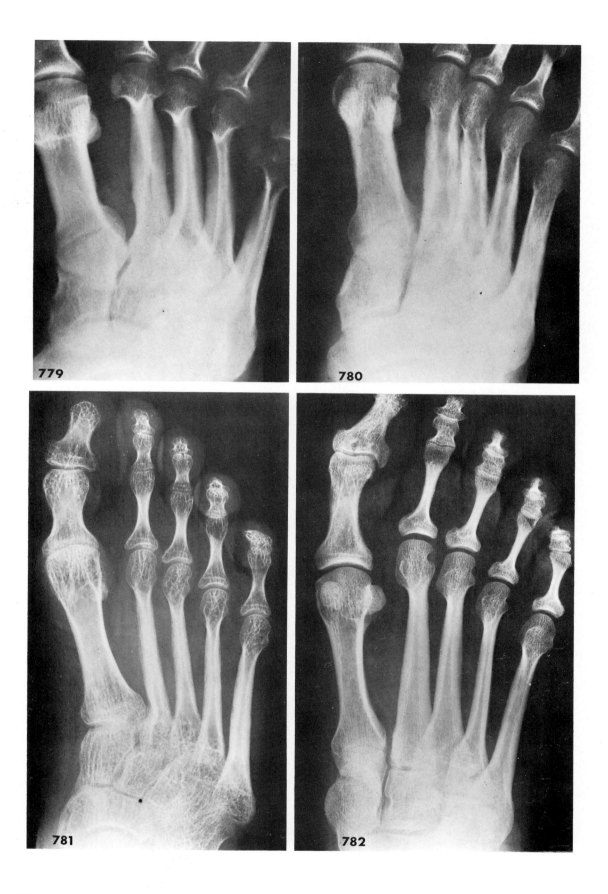

779. Acromegaly : enlargement of the metatarsal shafts without structural osseous abnormalities.

780. Tuberous sclerosis (Bourneville disease) : phaco-matosis characterized by cerebral lesions with mental retardation and seizures, sebaceous adenomas, and skin lesions (white macules) ; irregular periosteal reaction of the metatarsal shafts.

Phacomatosis is a generic term for a group of hereditary diseases characterized by cerebral and verte-bral lesions and small cutaneous and nervous tumors (phacos = lentil) ; including tuberous sclerosis of Bour-neville, neurofibromatosis (Recklinghausen), Sturge-Weber syndrome, Von Hippel-Lindau disease.

781. Lobstein disease : generalized diffuse deminerali-zation of the skeleton with, at the metatarsals, admixture of rarefied osseous structure and, paradoxically, endos-teal hyperostosis.

782. Normal variant : slender aspect of the metatarsal shafts, of which the cortex looks thickened.

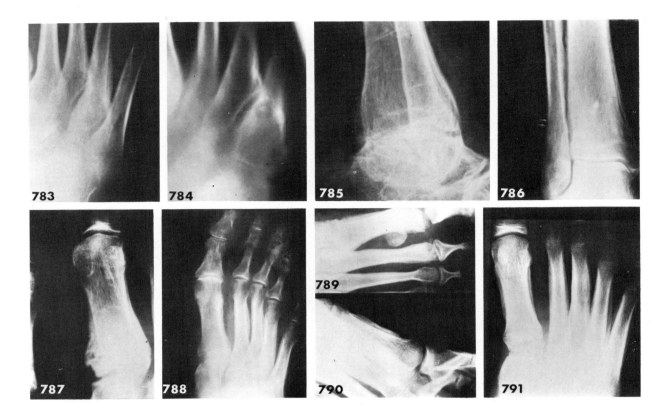

783, 784. Osteoid osteoma. 783. Shell-like periostal appositions of the fourth metatarsal proximal end with a small intraosseous osteolytic area.

784. Tomogram showing the nidus.

785. Varices : laminated periostal appositions of the anterior aspect of the tibia. Linear and reticulated lace-like venous calcifications in the soft tissues. Demineralization of the bony architecture with transverse, irregular, confused sclerotic metaphyseal lines (not like the transverse regular lines of Harris).

786. Hypertrophic pulmonary osteoarthropathy (Pierre-Marie and Bamberger disease) : long parallel layers,

periosteal appositions at the tibial level, rough appositions at the interosseous membrane level.

787. Fatigue fracture of the first metatarsal. Diaphyseal periosteal apposition : regular and laminated at the medial side, rougher and irregular at the lateral side.

788. Hypertrophic pulmonary osteoarthropathy.

789. Sequelae of an arthroplasty of the first metatarsophalangeal joint with perforating trophic ulcer of the sole. Markedly sclerotic metatarsal shaft and periostosis.

790, 791. Hypertrophic pulmonary osteoarthropathy, lamined periosteal new bone appositions at the metatarsals shafts, which are separated from the cortex by a light zone (797).

HYPERTROPHIC OSTEOARTHROPATHY

Benign lung tumor (eg, bronchial adenoma)
Carcinoma of lung
Celiac disease
Chronic liver disease, cirrhosis
Chronic pulmonary infection (eg, tuberculosis, fungus disease, bronchiectasis, empyema)
Chronic ulcerate colitis
Cyanotic congenital heart disease
Familial
Gastrointestinal malignancy
Idiopathic
Lung abcess
Mesothelioma of pleura
Nasopharyngeal carcinoma (Schmincke tumor)
Pachydermoperiostosis
Polyarteritis nodosa
Pulmonary arteriovenous fistula
Pulmonary emphysema
Pulmonary metastases (esp. from osteosarcoma)
Thyroid acropachy

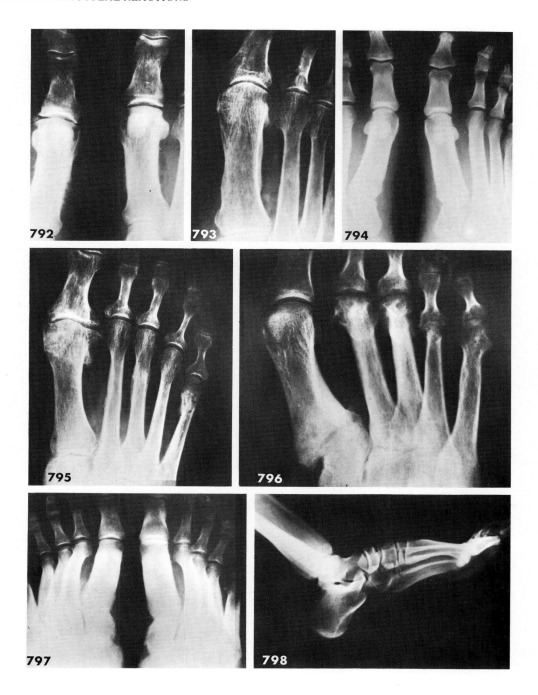

792. Thyroid acropachy. Hypertrophic osteopathy characterized by an elephantiac aspect of the extremities occuring in 1-3 ‰ of hyperthyroid patients during or after specific therapy. It could be due to peripheral action of an hypophyseal hormone, LATS (Long Action Thyroid Stimulator), which also causes exopthalmos and pretibial myxedema. Periosteal reaction in the form of perpendicular spicules on the first metatarsal.

793. Thyroid osteosis. Demineralization by osseous hypermetabolism occurring in 3 % of hyperthyroid individuals. Fatigue fracture of the first metatarsal shaft with periosteal apposition.

794. Thyroid acropachy : tubular-like metatarsals with thickened cortex.

795. Thyroid osteosis : fatigue fracture of the third and fifth metatarsals with periosteal apposition.

796. Diabetes : endosteal hyperostosis of the three first metatarsals. Diabetic arthropathy of the first cuneometatarsal joint and the metatarsophalangeal joints.

797. Pachydermoperiostosis : (Touraine-Solante-Gole disease) characterized by pachydermic coarsening of the facial features with thickening ; furrowing of the skin of the face, scalp and extremities ; and generalized osteosclerosis sparing the skull, the vertebral column, and the pelvic girdle. Thickened hands and feet with clubbing of the digits. Dense sclerosis with smooth bones and post-shaped diaphyses. The periosteal reaction forms one body with the bone cortical, whereas in the hypertrophic pulmonary osteoarthropathy, there are laminated shell-like appositions (De Sèze) (compare to **790, 791**).

798. Thyroid acropachy : large, dense, thickened, cylindrical, tibial, post-like shaft.

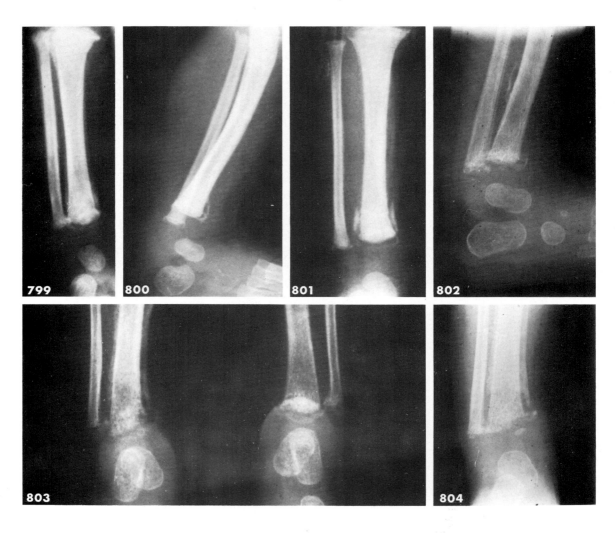

799 → 802. Battered child syndrome (Silverman). Traumatic subperiosteal hemorrhages surrounding the metaphyses and epiphyses.

803, 804. Scurvy : subperiosteal hematomas and osteoporosis.

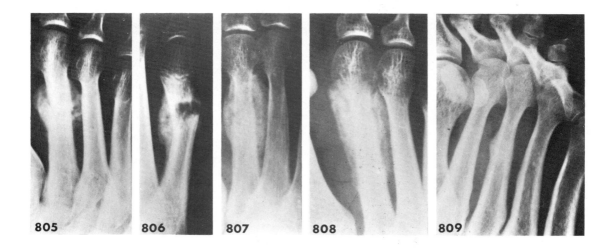

805. March fracture of the second metatarsal shaft : fragmentary type with swelling callus.

806. Pathologic fracture at the level of enchodroma of the fifth metatarsal head.

807, 808. Fatigue fracture of the second metatarsal shaft. **807.** Fusiform and heterogeneous callus. **808.** Pronounced hypertrophic callus.

809. Fatigue fracture of the third metatarsal diaphysis, linear type : fine interruption of the cortex.

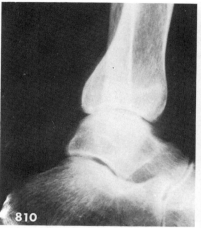
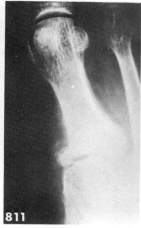
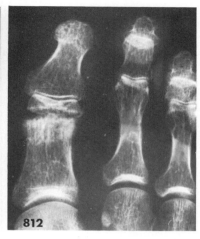

810. March fracture of the tibial epiphysis : osteosclerotic line of the tibial distal spongiosa, showing the fracture. Posterior periosteal elevation due to a subperiosteal hematoma.

811. Fatigue fracture of the first metatarsal proximal end : lamellar periosteal apposition regular, at the outer aspect of the diaphysis, and spicular at the inner one.

812. Fatigue fracture of the distal phalanx of the great toe. Transversal radiolucent band and laminated periosteal elevation.

813, 814. Infantile cortical hyperostosis of Caffey-Silverman, unknown etiology, characterized by oscillating fever spikes with swelling of the soft tissues, developing in stages from birth to adult age (very rare in the adult).

Radiologically, there is periosteal hyperostosis at the level of the diaphyses. At every new burst, either the same diaphysis may be involved once more, with remodeling of the previous periostosis or other bones, previously unaffected, may be involved. The cortical thickening may also completely disappear.

813. Four-year-old girl ; cortical hyperostosis of the second, third and fourth metatarsal shafts.

814. Radiograph 1 year later : normal picture.

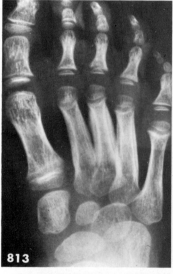
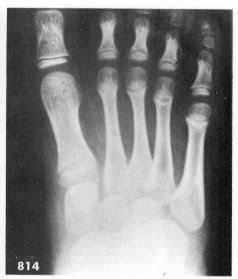

815. Diaphyseal periostosis and sclerotic island of the adjacent metatarsal, unknown etiology.

816. Muscular insertion crests on the metatarsal shafts

817. Hypertrophic muscular insertion ridge or periostosis ? Unknown etiology.

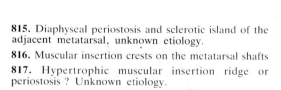
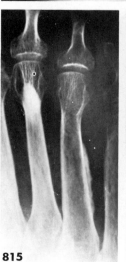
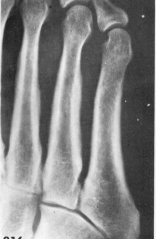
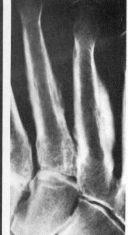

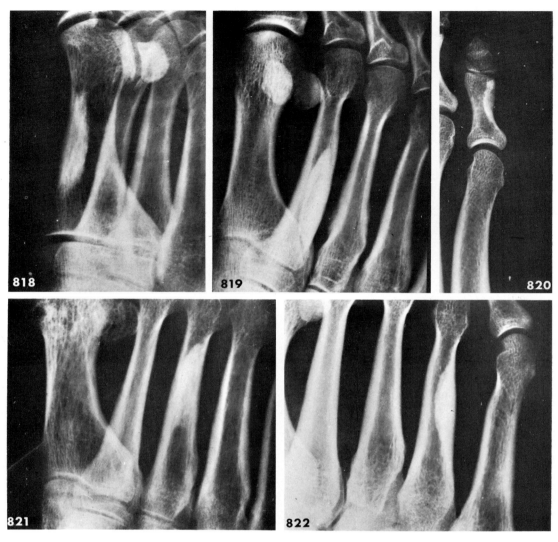

818, 822. Endosteal hyperostosis, unknown etiology, involving rather frequently the metatarsals and the phalanges. This condition resembles the melorheostosis of Leri.

818. First metatarsal shaft.

819. Second metatarsal diaphysis.

820. Phalangeal localization.

821. Third metatarsal diaphysis.

822. Fourth metatarsal shaft.

PERIOSTOSES - HYPEROSTOSES

Acquired generalized periostoses

    Cooley anemia
    Cornelia de Lange syndrome
    Cusching disease
    Fluorosis
    Gaucher disease
    Histiocytosis X
    Hypertrophic osteoarthropathy (see page 132)
    Hypervitaminosis A
    Hypoparathyroidism of the newborn
    Infantile cortical hyperostosis (Caffey)
    Leukemia
    Pachydermoperiostosis
    Scurvy
    Sickle-cell anemia
    Syphilis, congenital
    Thyroid osteosis (thyroid acropachy)
    Tuberous sclerosis
    Varices

Acquired localized periostoses

    Acromegaly
    Bone crests of muscular insertions
    Bone tumors, benign and malignant
    Endosteal hyperostosis, unknown etiology
    Hemophilia
    Infective periosteal elevations (osteoarthritis, perforating ulcer)

    Inflammatory rheumatisms
    Leprosy
    Osteoid osteoma
    Osteomyelitis
    Pagetoid changes after trauma
    Paget disease
    Physiologic, of the newborn
    Polyarteritis nodosa
    Post-traumatic periosteal elevations : callus of fracture, burn, eschars.
    Rickets, healing
    Rubella

Osteochondrodysplasia

    Irregular thickening of the bone cortical structure :
        Craniodiaphyseal dysplasia
        Craniometaphyseal dysplasia (Jackson)
        Diaphyseal dysplasia (Camurati-Engelmann)
        Frontometaphyseal dysplasia
        Oculo-dental-osseous dysplasia
        Osteodysplasia (Melnick-Needles)
        Osteoectasia with hyperphosphatasia
        Metaphyseal dysplasia (Pyle)

    Regular thickening of bone cortical structure :
        Endosteal hyperostosis (Worth-Van Buchem)
        Sclerosteosis (Hansen)
        Tubular stenosis (Kenny-Caffey)

7

REGIONAL OR GENERALIZED OSTEOPENIA

RADIOGRAPHIC APPEARANCES OF GENERALIZED OSTEOPOROSES

They may have five osteoporotic radiological appearances :
— uniform lucency caused by diffusely rarefied osseous structure ;
— reticular areas of radiolucency caused by fibrillar network of rarefaction ;
— patchy lucent foci caused by spotty demineralization of variable size and appearance : large geographic well delineated or punched-out bone defects, moth-eaten or permeated bony architecture ;
— complete effacement of bony architecture : vitreous-like appearence ;
— mixed types.

The bone rarefaction is more apparent when unilateral by comparison with the other foot.

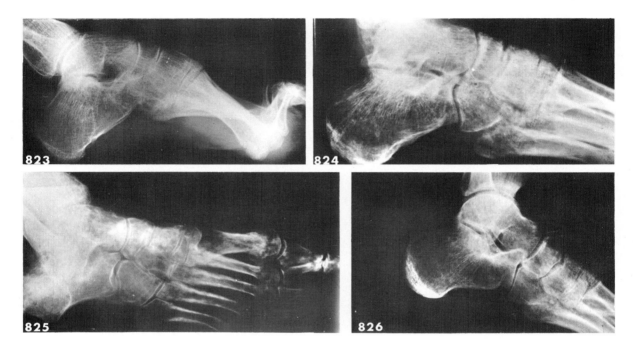

823. Simple bone rarefaction : the bone as a whole is less opaque, the trabecular pattern appears more clearly, as if schematic.

824 → 826. Spotty rarefaction. Multiple round or oval bony radiolucent areas of varying size **(824)** : dapple-like demineralization **(825)**, miliary-like rarefaction **(826)**.

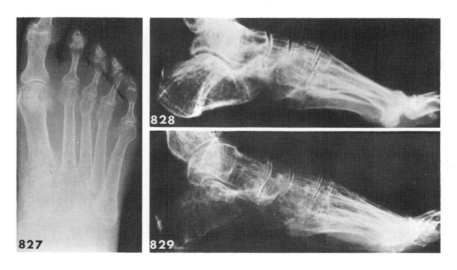

827. Vitreous-like rarefaction : complete effacement of osseous architecture. The cortical border-lines are blurred, pourly delineated (wash-drawing-like radiographic appearence). Sometimes, on the contrary, they are well-defined, dense, contrasted, surrounding the bone like an ink outline drawing.

828. Uniformity decreased bone density with coarsening of osseous architecture.

829. Mixed radiographic findings.

RADIOGRAPHIC APPEARANCES OF REGIONAL OSTEOPOROSES

Metaphyseal or diaphysometaphyseal rarefaction. Two radiographic shapes :
— circumscribed areas of radiolucency with blurred contours never with a sclerotic border,
— transverse lucent bands.

Epiphyseal rarefaction : subchondral demineralization.

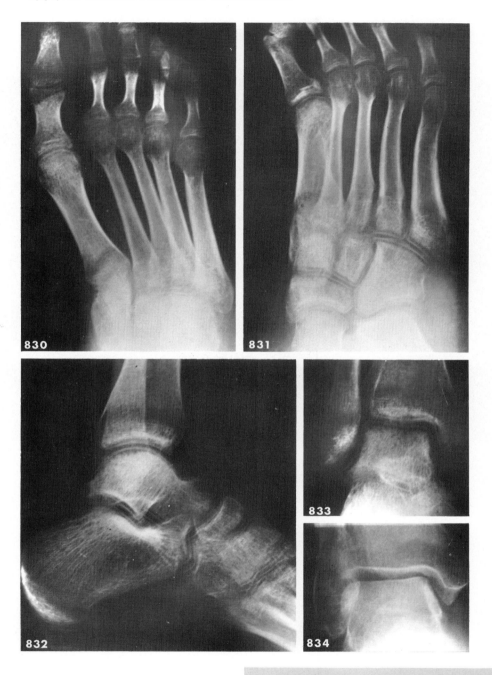

830. Transverse radiolucencies in growing metaphyses.

831. Rarefied subchondral osseous structures underlining the articular margins.

832. Same radiographic appearence and osteoporotic metaphyseal transverse band of the tibia.

833. Subchondral demineralization and transverse metaphyseal radiolucent band of the tibia.

834. Larger subchondral rarefaction.

RADIOLUCENT METAPHYSEAL BANDS

Cushing syndrome
Hypervitaminosis D
Leukemia
Metastatic neoplasm (esp. neuroblastoma)
Normal variant (esp. in neonate)
Osteogenesis imperfecta
Osteopetrosis
Postnatal infection (eg. brucellosis)
Scurvy
Systemic illness or stress in infancy or in utero
Transplacental infection (eg. toxoplasmosis, rubella, cytomegalic inclusion disease, herpes, syphilis)

PRIMITIVE GENERALIZED OSTEOPOROSIS

Common osteoporosis (after the 55th year) : menopause, senile (**835**).

Congenital osteoporosis :
    — Hajdu and Cheney syndrome.
    — Juvenile idiopathic.
    — Osteogenesis imperfecta congenita-Porak-Durante disease (**836, 837, 838**).
    — Osteogenesis imperfecta tarda-Lobstein disease (**839**).
    — Severe osteochondrodysplasia.

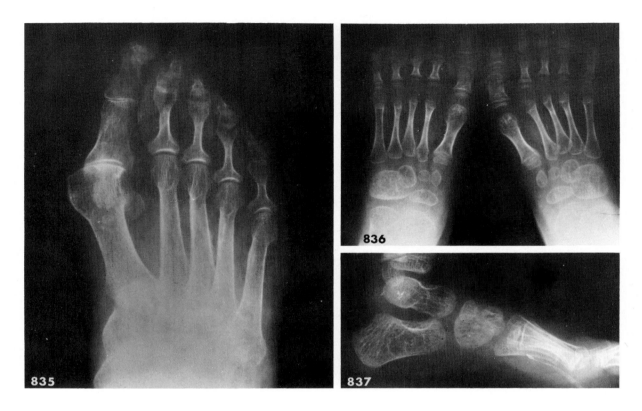

835. Common primary osteoporosis : foot of a centenarian.

836→837. Osteogenesis imperfecta congenita letalis (Porak-Durante-Vrolik disease). Inherited osteochondrodysplasia manifesting itself in forms of various severity, from simple osteopenia to osseous deformities with multiple fractures.

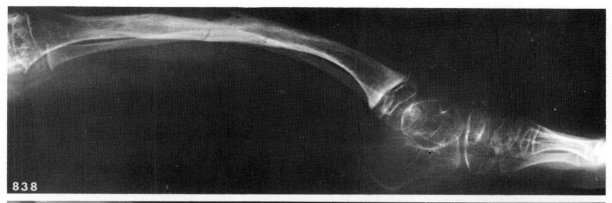

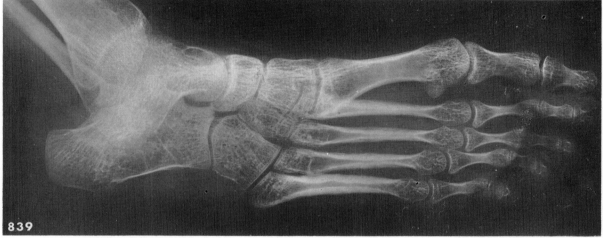

838, 839. Osteogenesis imperfecta tarda or osteopsathyrosis (Lobstein disease). Inherited osteochondrodysplasia characterized by the clinical triad of Van der Hoeve : blue sclerae, deafness and osseous abnormalities (demineralization, bone fragility, and fracture). The fibrillar bone rarefaction of the tarsus contrasts with an endosteal hyperostosis of the metatarsal shafts (**781**).

GENERALIZED SECONDARY OSTEOPOROSIS

Chromosome aberrations : Turner syndrome (**656**).

Congenital syphilis (**854, 855, 856**).

Dermatomyositis, Chronic atrophic polychondritis (**834**).

Endocrinopathies : Cushing disease, excessive steroid therapy, Addison disease, hyperthyroidism.

Hemopathies : Multiple pyeloma, acute leukemia, hemophilia (**862**), anemia (**840**), thalassemia (**845**), sickle-cell anemia (**846, 847**).

Idiopathic disorders of the bone growth : dwarfisms, Marfan disease (**844, 863**). Ehlers-Danlos disease, progeria, Werner syndrome.

Metabolic disorders : diabetes, mucolipidosis, hemochromatosis, mucopolysaccharidosis, homocystinuria.

Miscellaneous neuromuscular diseases.

Rheumatoid arthritis (**857, 859, 861**).

Weightlessness.

GENERALIZED SECONDARY OSTEOPOROSIS

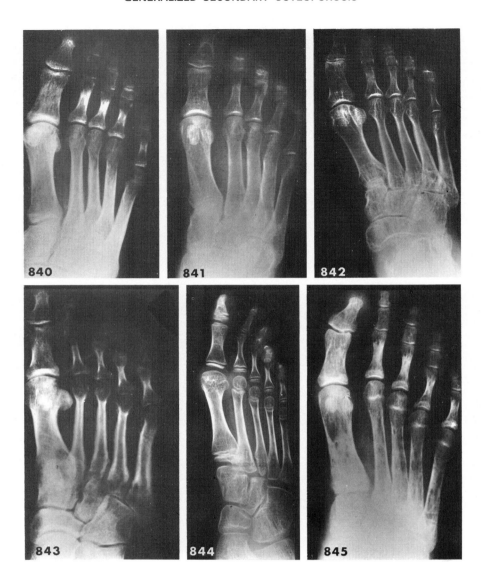

840. Anemia : simple decalcification.

841. Primary hyperparathyroidism in a 26-year-old patient. Simple rarefaction and thinning down of the cortex.

842. Hyperthyroidism : fibrillar osteopenia.

843. Chronic atrophic polychondritis : unknown disease of the cartilage characterized by inflammation, followed by atrophy of the cartilaginous structures producing a bizarre form of arthritis (**1173**) with deformities of the nose, tracheobronchial tree and ears. Note the epiphyseal band-like rarefaction.

844. Marfan disease - arachnodactyly : long slender metatarsals, simple osteopenia.

845. Thalassemia (Cooley anemia) : hereditary disease characterized by a fetal hemoglobin found in the blood with hypochromatic microcytic anemia, splenomegaly, hepatomegaly, arthralgia, and osseous disorders. Fibrillar and patchy rarefaction.

SPLAYING OR FLARING OF THE METAPHYSES

Chronic hemolytic anemia (eg, sicklemia, thalassemia)
Enchondromatosis (Ollier disease)
Fracture
Histiocytosis X
Hypophosphatasia
Kniest disease
Lead poisoning
Lipid storage disorders (esp. Gaucher disease, Neimann-Pick disease)
Metaphyseal chondrodysplasia (types Jansen, McKusick, Schmid)
Metaphyseal dysplasia (Pyle disease)
Metatrophic dwarfism
Mucoviscidosis
Multiple cartilaginous exostoses
Normal variant
Osteodysplasia (Melnick-Needles)
Osteopetrosis
Rickets, including renal osteodystrophy and biliary rickets
Spondyloepiphyseal dysplasia (congenita or pseudo-achondroplastic types)
Thanatophoric dwarfism

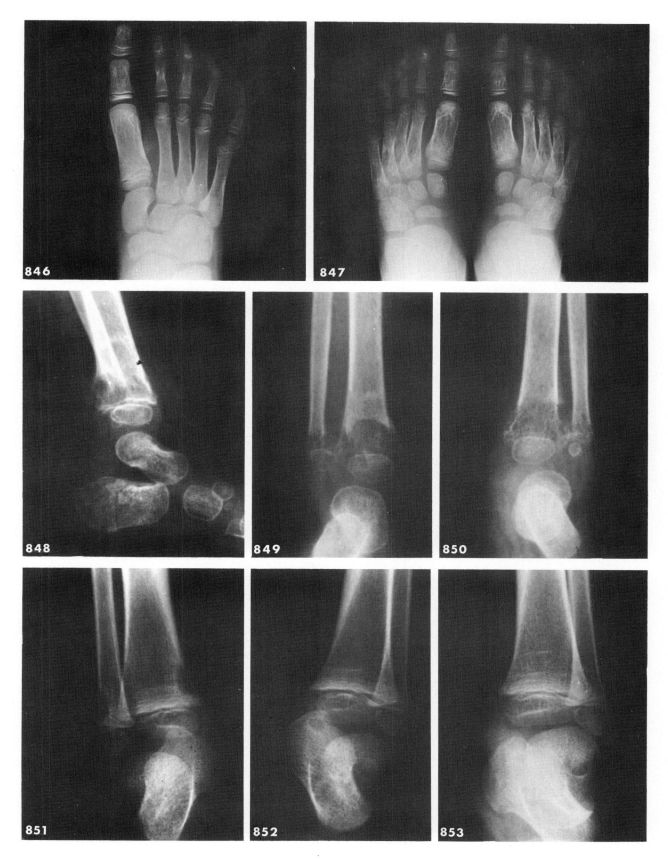

846. Drepanocytosis (sickle cell anemia) : small fine circumscribed cystic radiolucencies.

847. Drepanocytosis : diffuse fibrillar rarefaction.

848→850. Acute leukemia : metaphyseal band-like radiolucency with periosteal apposition.

851→853. Acute leukemia. **851, 852.** Cyst-like rarefied osseous structure of both malleoli and of the calcaneus. **853.** After specific treatment, these lytic lesions disappear.

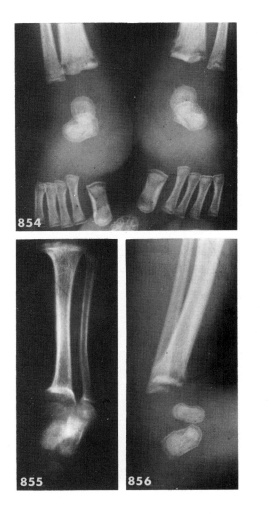

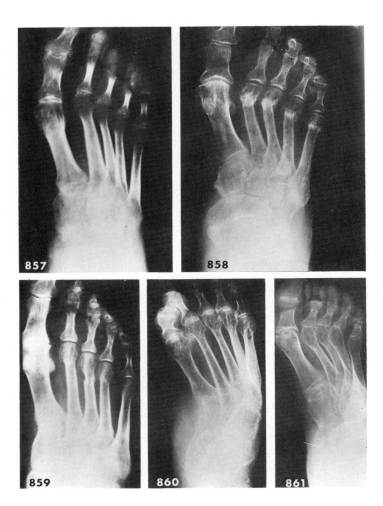

854→856. Congenital syphilis : a condition caused by placental inoculation directly in the secondary phase of the disease, it produces total body disorders (skeletal and visceral changes).

Increased density of the epiphyseal growth cartilage with metaphyseal band-like radiolucent underlying zone. The bone rarefaction also involves the proximal metatarsal epiphyses, the talus and the calcaneus which frequently present with a sclerotic ring-like shape (« rosette » appearance).

Likewise radiographic findings may exist of periosteal reaction or osteochondritis. The degenerative hypertrophic metaphyseal spur formations and the transverse diaphyseal band-like bone condensations are radiological pictures of recovery or sequelae. Cyst-like osteoporosis of the medial border of the proximal metaphyses of the tibia is the pathognomonic (« Wimberger sign »).

857. Rheumatoid arthritis epiphyseal transverse band-like osteoporosis of the metatarsals. Decrease in height of the joint spaces.

858. Osteoporosis : 80-year-old female. Demineralization. Fracture of the four metatarsal necks.

859. Rheumatoid arthritis : simple osseous rarefaction without joint involvment. Spontaneous fracture of the third metatarsal diaphysis after cortisone therapy.

860 Poliomyelitis : diffuse osteoporosis by muscular hypofunction (talipes equinovarus).

861. Juvenile rheumatoid arthritis in a 15-year-old girl : diffuse vitreous decalcification, narrowing of the metatarsophalangeal joint spaces. Cyst-like radiolucency and erosions of the first metatarsal head.

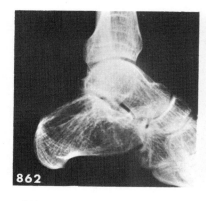 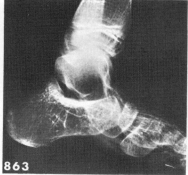 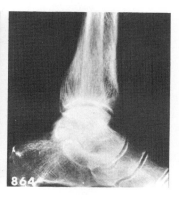

862. Hemophilia : diffuse fibular bone rarefaction. Metaphyseal growth lines of Harris.

863. Marfan disease : widespread demineralization. Vertical talus with flat foot.

864. Paget disease : simple decalcification of the tibia.

LOCALIZED SECONDARY OSTEOPOROSIS

Acute and chronic osteomyelitis.
Algodystrophia.
Benign tumors. Malignant tumors, primary or secondary.
Burn. Frostbite.
By hypofunction (poliomyelitis, **860**, paralyses) or by inactivity (post traumatic immobilization).
Fibrous dysplasia.
Fractures : malposition, pseudoarthrosis, sepsis, **866.**
Local hemorrhage (trauma, hemophilia).
Metastases.
Neurotrophic disorders (Leprosy).
Rheumatisms, diabetes, Paget disease **864.**
Vascular compression (arterial, venous, lymphatic) extra- or intra-osseous (**1512-1515**).

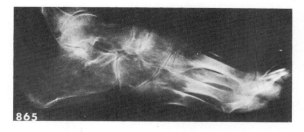

Algodystrophy : painful syndrome, commonly unilateral, characterized by vasomotor and trophic disorders with osteoporosis. Radiologically, the early sign is a diffuse rarefaction in the distal part of the foot. Gradually, the osteoporosis extends to the entire foot, giving the bone a moth-eaten or multivacuolated appearance.

In a very advanced stage, vitreous rarefaction may supervene. In the healing phase, normal osseous structure reappears. In this condition, there is never osteolysis, and the joints are never involved. The sharpness of the pain in this sympathetic reflex syndrome has no reference to the severity of the initiating causal agent which remains unknown in 25 % to 50 % of cases (idiopathic painful decalcified foot of J.P.Ravault). The radiologic examination must always be bilateral for comparison. One must search for any spreading to other skeletal parts (knees, hips) with or without guidance by a scintigram.

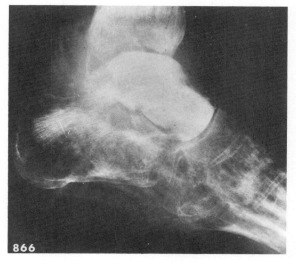

865. Algodystrophy : mixed type. Note the contrast between the diffuse proximal demineralization and the normal radiolucency of the metatarsal shafts.

866. Post-traumatic osteoporosis : fibrillar bone rarefaction of the calcaneus (combed-like appearance). Patchy osseous demineralization of the tarsus (dapple-like aspect). Metaphyseal band-like radiolucent zone of the tibia. These findings contrast with the dense osteosclerotic and necrotic talus (open fracture-dislocation of the ankle).

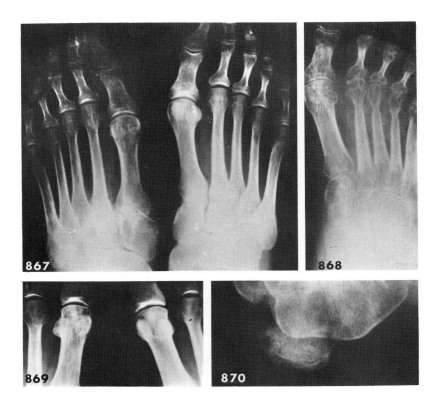

867. Algodystrophy. Left inversion sprain of the ankle. Diffuse rarefaction.

868. Algodystrophy. Fracture of the ankle. Moth-eaten osseous structure.

869. Algodystrophy. Unknown etiology. Localized osteoporosis of the first metatarsal.

870. Algodystrophy. Vacuolar rarefaction of the first metatarsal head and medial sesamoïd after surgical ablation of the lateral sesamoid in the MacBride procedure for treatment of hallux valgus.

OSTEOMALACIA WITH VITAMIN D DEFICIENCY

Food and sunshine deficiency.
Late congenital rickets
Vitamin D malabsorption

Biliary insufficiency
Chronic pancreatic insufficiency
Enteritis : sprue, Crohn disease, Whipple disease, intoxication by lactose or gluten, gammaglobulin deficiency.
Postoperative gastric or small bowel resection

OSTEOMALACIA WITHOUT VITAMIN D DEFICIENCY

Glomerular and tubular nephropathies
Hypercalciuria, idiopathic or secondary
Idiopathic vitamin D resistant rickets : early pseudodeficiency rickets (Prader, Royer), hypophosphatemic familial rickets, late pseudodeficiency rickets
Scurvy

SYMPATHETIC REFLEX ALGODYSTROPHY OF THE LOWER LIMB

Primary
Secondary

Diabetes
Iatrogenic : anticonvulsivant drugs, excessive steroid therapy, tuberculotherapy
Long confinent to bed
Lumbago-Radiculalgia
Pregnancy
Traumatism
Vascular disorders : arteritis, hemiplegia, phlebitis.

8

CYST-LIKE BONE LESIONS

ANKLE JOINT

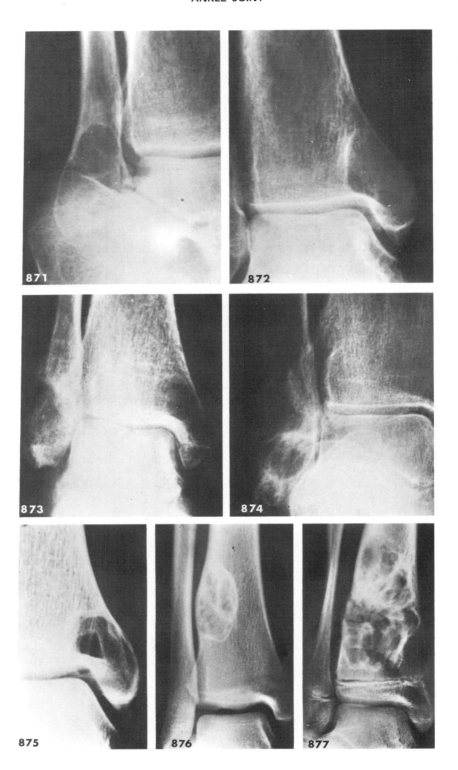

871. Rheumatoid arthritis : large homogeneous cyst-like bone defect with sharp, finely sclerotic borders at the level of the lateral malleolus. The ankle joint is not involved. Such a tumor-like lesion is an uncommon radiographic appearance of this disease.

872. Rheumatoid arthritis : same radiographic picture at the level of the medial malleolus. Joint space not narrowed, but there are small subchondral cyst formations on the talar medial side.

873. Tuberculous arthritis : large homogeneous cyst-like radiolucencies, with hazy borders of both malleoli.

874. Gout : large homogeneous cyst-like lytic lesion, with sharp sclerotic borders and blister bone appearance of the lateral malleolus.

875. Necrobiotic lesion of bone (ischemic bone defect) : unknown etiology, large cyst-like radiolucency with fine well-delineated sclerotic borders of the medial malleolus.

876→877. Nonossifying fibroma (fibrous cortical defect) : benign fibrocystic bone lesion of childhood, usually situated in the metaphysodiaphyseal zone, asymptomatic, casually detected and which usually heals spontaneously. A polyostotic variety is possible.

876. Nonossifying fibroma affecting the lateral cortex of the tibia : oval radiolucent bone defect, ballooning the cortex, multilocular with fine septae internally, sharply demarcated with scalloped sclerotic borders.

877. Giant nonossifying fibroma revealed by a pathologic fracture.

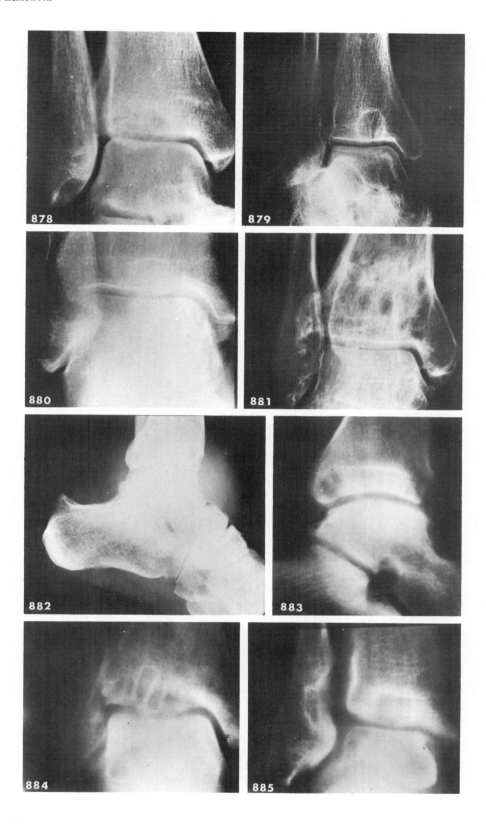

878. Von Willebrand-Jurgens disease : hereditary constitutional thrombopathy with hemarthrosis of the knee and ankle, as in hemophilia. Small homogeneous pseudocystic tibial areas of subchondral bone resorption, with well-circumscribed sclerotic borders.

879. Dystrophic subchondral lytic lesion of bone : casually detected solitary, round or oval, well delimited and finely delineated cyst-like lytic lesion of the juxta-articular subchondral osseous tissue. Questionable etiology : necrobiotic bone defect, or synovial tissue misplaced in osseous structures by inclusion, or invagination.

880. Ochronosis : hereditary disorder in the metabolism of homogentisic acid (alkapton) accumulating in the mesenchymal tissues with dark-colored urine and sweat, pigmented skin and other tissues, such as cartilage, causing arthrosis and calcification of intervertebral discs.

Small, oval, homogeneous, subchondral bone cyst-like lesions with well-delimited sclerotic borders. Interarticular space not involved.

881. Paget strutural change after a fracture of the ankle.

882 → 885. Pigmented villonodular synovitis : diffuse benign outgrowths of the articular synovial membrane, composed of synovial pigmented villi producing a chronic monoarthritis. Uncommon localization in the ankle.

882. Hypertrophic synovium and hemarthrosis causing a soft tissue density in front of the joint and producing behind it pressure erosion of the superior aspect of the calcaneus.

883 → 885. Same patient. Tomograms. Homogeneous subchondral cyst-like bone defect, sharply circumscribed with sclerotic margins, sometimes eroding the cartilage, opening into the joint space.

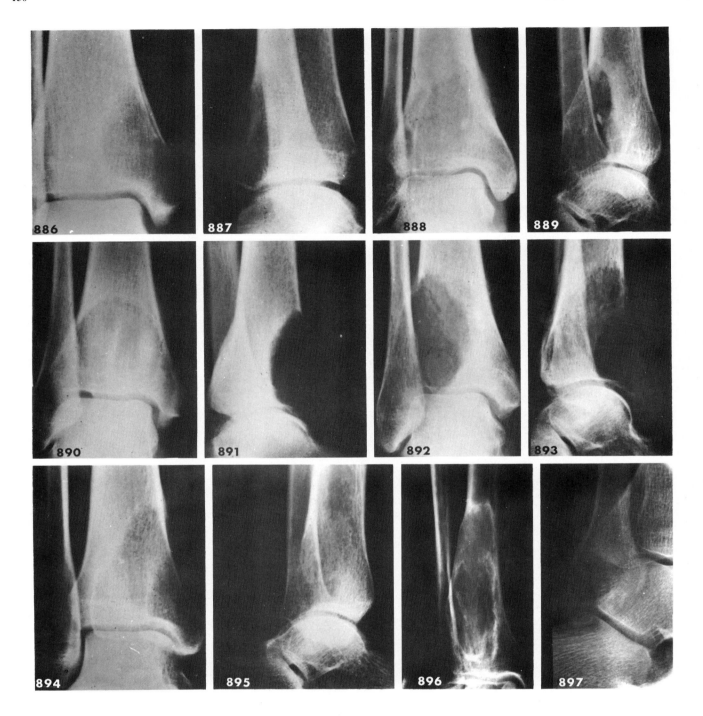

886 → 895. Giant-cell tumors (myeloplaques). Bone tumor occurring between the 20th and the 40th years, uncommon in the foot, and situated in the epiphysometaphyseal zones. The radiographic findings do not accurately reflect the malignant or benign character of a particular giant-cell tumor.

886, 887. Giant-cell tumor of the lower tibial epiphysis : oval, homogeneous cyst-like radiolucent zone with regular and well-delimited margins. Uncommon long parallel layers of periosteal reaction.

888, 889. Giant-cell tumor of the lower tibial epiphysis, same radiographic appearance but larger size and some fine trabecular partitions.

890, 891. Giant-cell tumor of the tibial distal end, same radiographic picture with complete effacement of the anterior margin.

892, 893. Giant-cell tumor of the lower tibial epiphysis : same radiographic appearance but more marked bone destruction.

894, 895. Giant-cell tumor of the tibial distal end : same radiographic picture with complete effacement of the posterior malleolus and periosteal roughened reaction with spicules.

896. Fibrous dysplasia of the tibia : large, homogeneous, metaphysodiaphyseal cyst-like ballooning bone lesion, well circumscribed with sharped sclerotic borders.

897. Tuberculous osteitis of the lateral malleolus. Epiphyseal cyst-like bone lesion, with blurred margins. Laminated periosteal elevation.

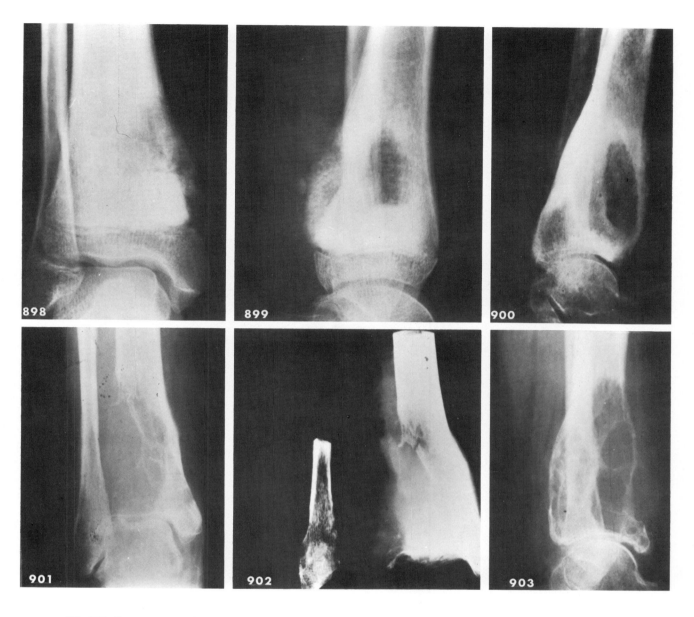

898, 899. Osteosarcoma of the distal end of the tibia located in the diaphysometaphyseal zone and not involving the growth cartilage. Large cyst-like lytic bone lesion with blurred borders, surrounded by heterogeneous osteosclerosis. This malignant tumor spreads through the cortex and invades the soft tissues, with periosteal appositions.

900. Tuberculous osteitis of the distal end of the tibia : large, well-demarcated cyst-like bone defect and marked osteosclerosis deforming the bone.

901→903. Giant-cell tumor. Same patient. Large, well-delimited cyst-like lytic lesion with inner septae. Destruction of the cortex with extension into the soft tissues. **902.** Anatomical specimen.

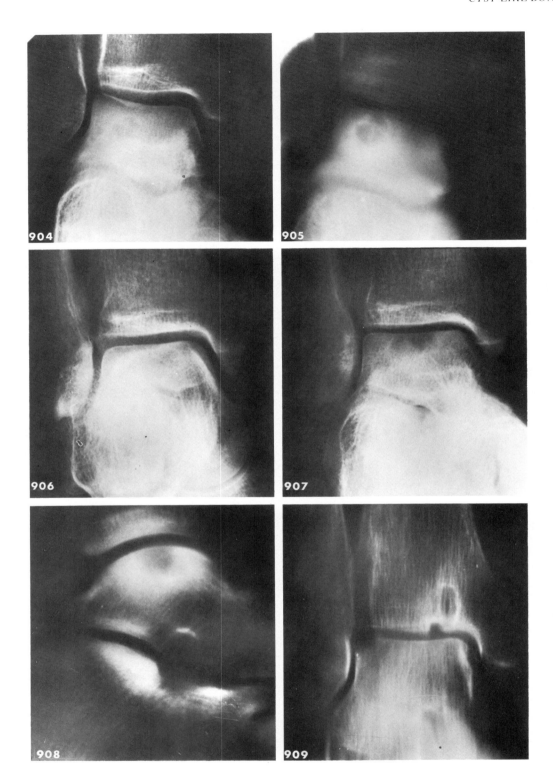

904, 905. Brodie abscess (see page 156) affecting the body of the talus : cyst-like, round bone defect, heterogeneous (including small sequestra) with well-delimited and marked sclerotic margins. **905.** Tomograph.

906, 907, 908. Talar cyst-like bone lesion due to a synovial tumor. **906.** Dorsal flexion. **907.** Plantar flexion : the damage is more visible. **908.** Lateral tomogram.

909. Subchondral cyst-like lesion of arthrosis (frontal tomogram of the ankle).

TARSUS

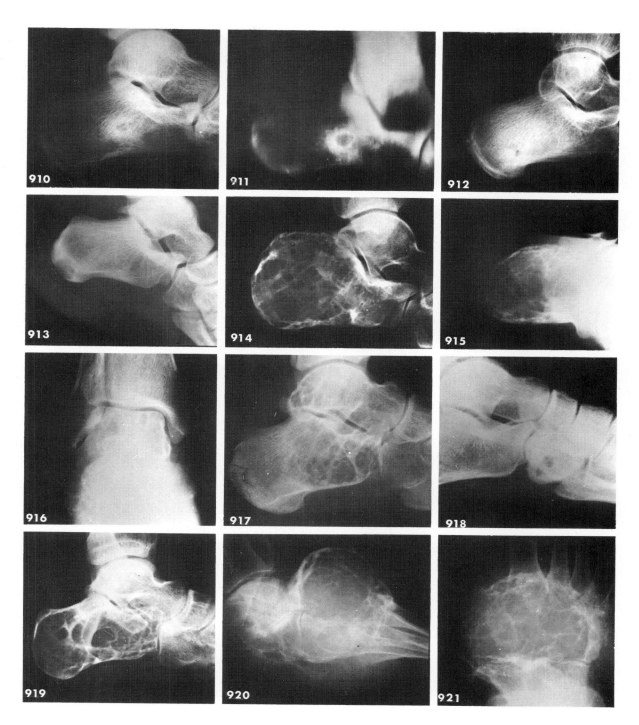

910, 911. Osteoid osteoma of the calcaneus. Radiograph and tomogram. Oval, homogeneous cyst-like radiolucency measuring 10 mm with well-delineated borders, and surrounded by an osteosclerotic zone.

912. Inoculated osteitis : osteosclerotic area around a small radiolucency representing the course of a pin passed through the calcaneus for skeletal traction.

913. Benign chondroblastoma of the tuber calcanei. Rare cartilaginous tumor, arising usually in the epiphyses of bones in young people, with clinically night bone pains. In this 15-year-old boy, peculiar but classical localization at the level of a tuberosity. Round homogeneous cyst-like lucent bone defect, without surrounding bone condensation, well circumscribed but with an opening into the soft tissues of the heel.

914, 915. Aneurysmal bone cyst. It is a benign osteolytic lesion of adolescence, mostly in females, occurring particularly in long bones and vertebrae. Uncommon involvement of the foot. **914.** Aneurysmal cyst ballooning

the calcaneus, well circumscribed, with inner fine septae (« soap-bubble » appearance), consisting of blood-filled spaces, not visualized on the arteriogram, after injection of a radiopaque contrast medium. **915.** Same patient. Axial radiograph of the calcaneus.

916, 917. Hemangioblastoma. Rare benign tumor, derived from blood vessels, and involving usually many adjoining bones. Multiple cyst-like bone lesions of talus and calcaneus, varying in size and shape, without neighboring periosteal reaction, osteolysis or osteosclerosis.

918. Osteomyelitis of the cuboid : homogeneous cyst-like lytic lesions with blurred margins, surrounded by an irregular osteosclerotic zone.

919. Giant-cell tumor of the calcaneus. Large, cyst-like, multilocular sharply defined bone defect.

920, 921. Giant-cell tumor of the navicular. Grossly expanded,ballooning cyst-like lytic lesion with adjoining bone destruction.

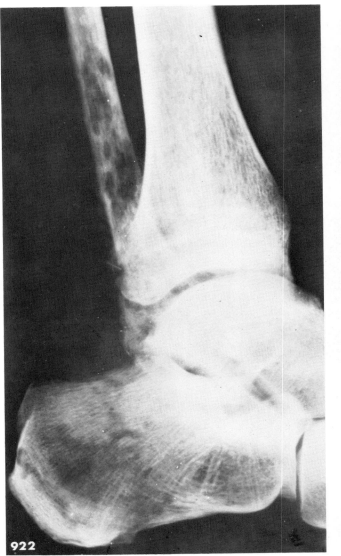

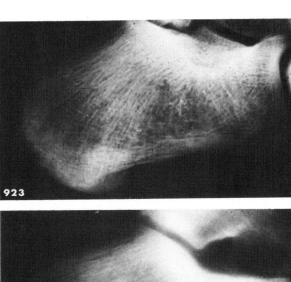

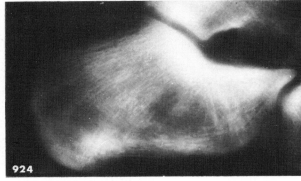

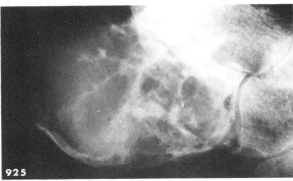

922. Cytosteatonecrosis : necrosis of adipose tissues, sometimes complicating a pancreatitis and inducing an aseptic necrosis of the bones (osteolysis and sequestra). Hindfoot and ankle : multiple round or oval cyst-like lytic lesions, varying in size, poorly defined with hazy borders or very easily discernible without sclerotic margins (punched-out bone defects). This multicystic osteolysis results in a moth-eaten or permeated appearance of the bones with erosions or breaks of the cortex. Absent periosteal reaction and no involvement of the joints simultaneously with clinical signs of arthritis.

923, 924. Osteosarcoma : primary malignant bone tumor with the greatest incidence in the age group between 8 and 35 years, involving mostly the male (70 % of the cases) and affecting chiefly the ends of long bones (90 % of the cases). Foot occurrence is rare. Radiologically, one describes three types of osteosarcoma : osteolytic, osteosclerosing and mixed. Osteosarcoma of the calcaneus. Radiograph and tomogram : slightly ill-defined spotted radiolucencies.

925. Aneurysmal bone cyst : ballooning cyst-like bone lesions with fine inner septae (« soap-bubble » appearance) and regular slightly sclerotic borders.

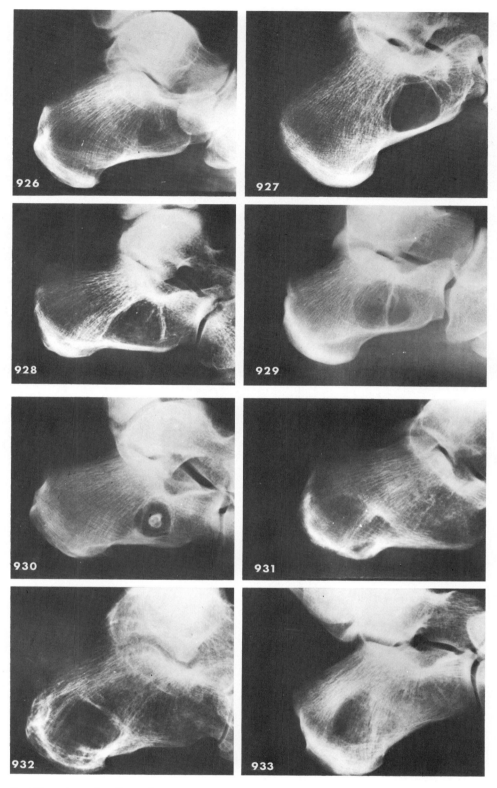

926 → 933. Cyst-like calcaneal radiographs.
The normal structure of the spongiosa of the calcaneal body presents four discernible areas of peculiar trabecular architecture : posterior complex continuing the fibers of the Achille's tendon ; anterior and posterior sustentacular complexes formed by radiating fan-like osseous trabeculae circumscribing, together with the fourth complex (plantar), a triangular zone of rarefied bone structure, of which the marked radiolucency simulates a true pathologic cyst.

926 → 930. Simulated calcaneal cyst : typical sites and various shapes.

926. Normal variant : area of indistinct structural detail within the spongiosa, located at the great calcanean apophysiseal level ; **927.** Simulated calcaneal cyst. Optical illusion of an entirely void space ; **928.** Simulated calcaneal cyst : only a few trabeculae are visible ; **929.** Simulated calcaneal cyst : with inner fine septae ; **930.** Simulated calcaneal cyst with an inner lipomatous and calcified inclusion (histological verification).

931. Rheumatoid arthritis : large cyst-like lytic lesion of the tuber calcanei.

932. Pagetoid structural change after fracture of the ankle : wide-meshed, coarsely reticulated trabecular architecture and large area of osteolysis of the calcaneal tuberosity.

933. Calcaneal osteitis : cyst-like bone defect with blurred borders and small central round radiolucency representing the course through the bone of a pin for skeletal traction.

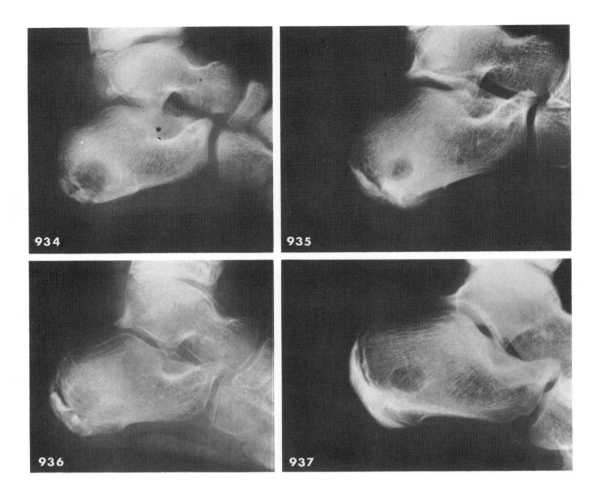

934 → 937. Osseous central abscess (Brodies abscess) : it is a rare and peculiar form of staphylococcal osteitis. This entity is characterized usually by a sharp round focal area of radiolucency, well-defined, located right in the middle of the bone, varying in size, surrounded by a thick reactive zone of sclerosis.

Various radiological shapes are possible : cyst-like radiolucent bone lesion with poorly-delineated, blurred borders, or with inside sequestra or a multilocular lytic cavity or a subperiosteal form with periosteal layering reaction, etc. All radiological appearances may simulate several diseases : dystrophic, infective, tumorous, etc.

Clinical course of a calcanean Brodie abscess in a child.

934. Initial radiograph : cyst-like lytic lesion, well circumscribed surrounded by an area of bone condensation.

935. Radiological picture 2-months after an antibiotic treatment.

936. Two years later, another medical group examines the same child who again has clinical manifestations viz bone night pain, relieved by aspirin. This suggested the diagnosis of osteoid osteoma which was not corroborated by surgery : curettage of the cavity, removing altered tissues of an intraosseous abscess.

937. One year later : persistence of the cyst-like bone defect and disappearance of the osteosclerosis.

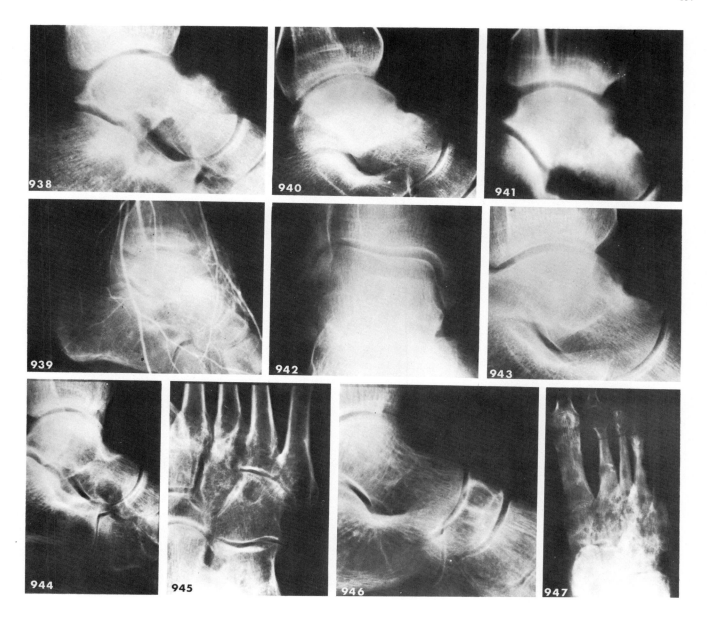

938, 939. Osteoid osteoma in the talar neck. Local tumefaction and osteosclerotic zone surrounding a patchy round osteolytic area, measuring 5 mm in diameter and getting opaque at the time of arteriography (nidus).

940, 941. Osteoid osteoma of the talar neck. Radiograph and tomogram : small area of osteolysis with sclerotic margins, surrounded by a zone of osteosclerosis enclosing a central compact bone (rosette).

942, 943. Benign osteoblastoma. Very uncommon benign tumor, occurring most frequently in the spine of young people. It resembles, clinically and histologically, an osteoid osteoma, but, radiologically, it is an entirely different type of lesion more especially the larger area of osteolysis (exceeding 1 cm) and the less widespread and less dense osteosclerosis.

942. Benign osteoblastoma of the talar neck around area of osteolysis, sharply circumscribed by fine sclerotic borders with a central patchy osseous condensation (rosette appearance).

943. Same patient : lateral view.

944. Rheumatoid arthritis : round, homogeneous cyst-like lytic lesion, well delineated, located in the lower part of the talar head with narrowed opposite joint space.

945. Multiple myeloma : homogeneous cyst-like punched-out bone defect of the cuboid.

946. Paget disease of the navicular ; cyst-like sharply delineated areas of osteolysis in the midst of a coarsely reticulated bony trabeculation.

947. Mycetoma : multiple round and oval areas of osteolysis, varying in size with hazy or well-defined borders. Destruction of the tarsal joints. Widened metatarsals with effacement of their cortex and diaphyseal erosions.

METATARSUS

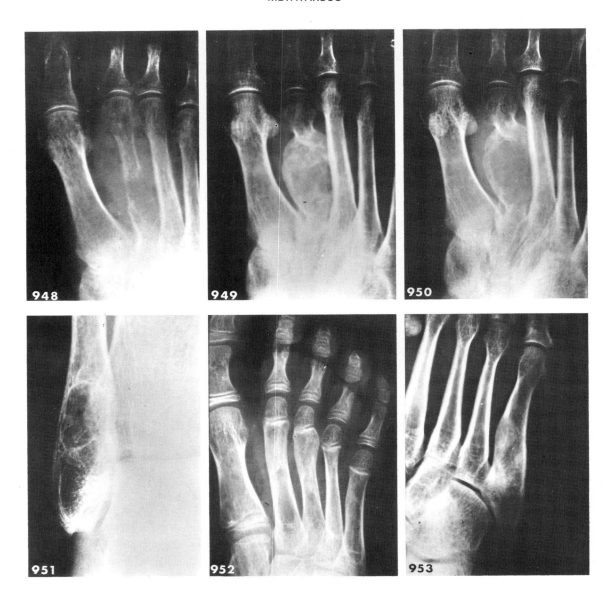

948 → 951. Primary hyperparathyroidism (parathyroid osteosis, also named Von Recklinghausen disease of bone
or generalized osteitis fibrosa cystica). Clinical features
are : fatigue, digestive disorders (eg ulcer), renal disorders
(eg lithiasis), osseous disorders (eg pains, marked diffuse
osteoporosis, pathologic fracture, tumors, etc.) and biolo-
gical disorders (elevated serum calcium, decreased serum
phosphorus). The marked endosteal demineralization
widens the medullary spaces, effaces the osseous architecture and punches the cortex like a postage-stamp. The cyst
formations and brown tumors produce a large circumscribed rarefaction, homogeneous or partitioned (honeycomb-like appearance) with circinate borders.

In the same patient, clinical course of a tumor-like form
of parathyroid osteosis at the level of the second metatarsal.

948. Diffuse demineralization, ill-defined areas of osteolysis, effacement of the external cortex of the metatarsal
base. Swelling of the soft tissues.

949. Ten months later : heterogeneous osteosclerosis cyst-
like bone lesion expanding the shaft, well delimited, not
breaking the cortex.

950. One month later : increased osteolysis with enlargement of the cyst-like bone defect. Based upon this
radiological change, a surgical amputation of the second
metatarsal was performed.

951. Shortly later, at the level of the lateral malleolus
appeared an oval cyst-like bone lesion, well delineated,
with fine sclerotic borders. Blood chemistry exam revealed
hypercalcemia and at subsequent surgery a tumor of the
right parathyroid weighing 5 g was removed.

952. Albright syndrome : precocious puberty and skin
pigmentation associated with fibrous dysplasia (953). In an
8-year-old girl, demineralization, thickened and bowed
metatarsal shafts.

953. Fibrous dysplasia of bone (Jaffé-Lichtenstein disease) : disturbance of medullary bone maintenance with
an abnormal proliferation of fibrous tissue. Mostly sympto-
matic, this condition shows various radiographic findings :
plaque-like areas of osteolysis ; solitary « pseudocystic » or
multilocular « cavities » in the bone. Osteosclerosis of the
vertebrae and the base of the skull. Irregular inner layers of
the cortical bone with widened or obliterated medullary
spaces. Protrusions from the normal contours of the bone,
bowed shafts and spontaneous fractures. Epiphyses always
remain intact (896). The carpus and the tarsus are said to be
never involved but expansion to one digit of the hand or
foot is possible (monomelic topography). Localization on
the fifth metatarsal, thinned bone cortex, osseous rarefaction, bent and thickened shaft.

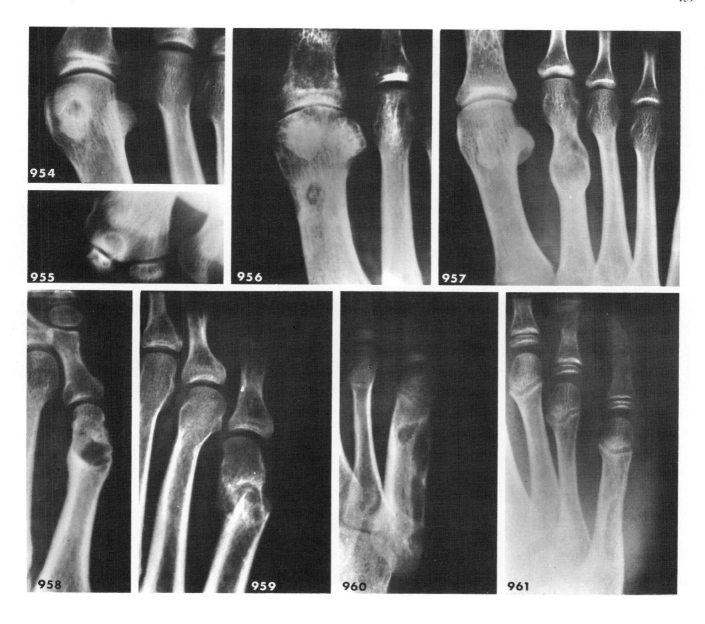

954. Cyst-like degenerative lesion : in the antero-posterior view, this lesion is projected on the medial sesamoid.

955. Same patient : in the axial projection of the sesamoids there is a homogeneous well-circumscribed cyst-like subchondral bone defect with fine sclerotic borders in the first metatarsal head. One sees also small cyst-like bone lesions of the medial sesamoid with subchondral osteosclerosis.

956. Staphylococcal osteomyelitis of the first metatarsal : cyst-like lytic lesion with a sequestrum.

957, 958. Solitary enchondroma : very common benign cartilaginous tumor, especially located in the short tubular bones of the hands and feet, revealing itself at any time of life, often by a fracture (966, 967). The typical radiographic picture is a round or oval cyst-like lucency, usually located centrally, sometimes peripherally. This type of lesion is often expansible but doesn't invade the cortex. It is homogeneous or includes numerous punctate areas of calcification.

957. Enchondroma of the second metatarsal : cystic bone expansion, heterogeneous (cloud-like and with septae), with normal appearance of the rest of the shaft.

958. Enchondroma of the fifth metatarsal : homogeneous, well-defined cyst-like bone lesion distorting the shaft.

959. Leprose osteitis of the fifth metatarsal : diffuse demineralization and pathologic fracture through a cyst-like lytic lesion.

960. Tuberculous osteitis of the fifth metatarsal : thickened diaphysis with homogeneous multilocular cyst-like lytic lesions, sharply circumscribed (spina ventosa).

961. Malignant synovioma of the fifth metatarsal shaft : oval, sharply delimitated area of osteolysis with swelling of the soft tissues (1426).

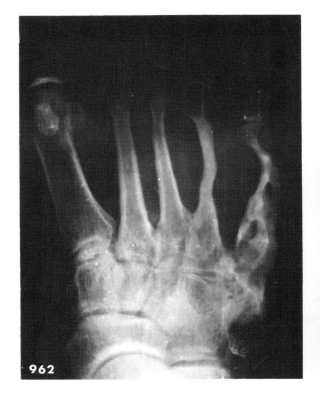

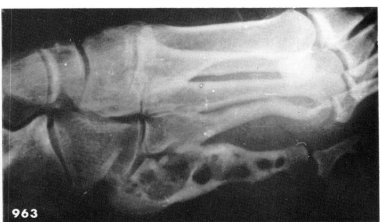

962, 963. Mycetoma. Typical Madura foot in a 47-year-old man. Radiographic appearance at the second year of the disease. Fourth metatarsal : swelling and increased density of the soft tissues ; thinned, osteosclerotic, bowed shaft with large pressure erosion. Fifth metatarsal : punched-out diaphyseal bone defects, which constitute the orifices of tunnels bored through the osseous tissue by the fungal mycelium. At the level of this metatarsal base, large cyst-like lytic lesion with smaller cystic defects showing the hollows of this large lesion : laminated periosteal reaction on the styloid tuberosity (*Madurella mycetomi*).

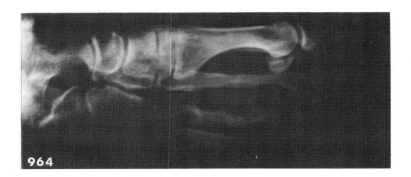

964. Mycetoma : radiographic appearance at the fourth year of the disease ; adjacent pressure erosions producing two large notches (1 cm in diameter) in the fourth metatarsal shaft (*Madurella mycetomi*).

PHALANGES

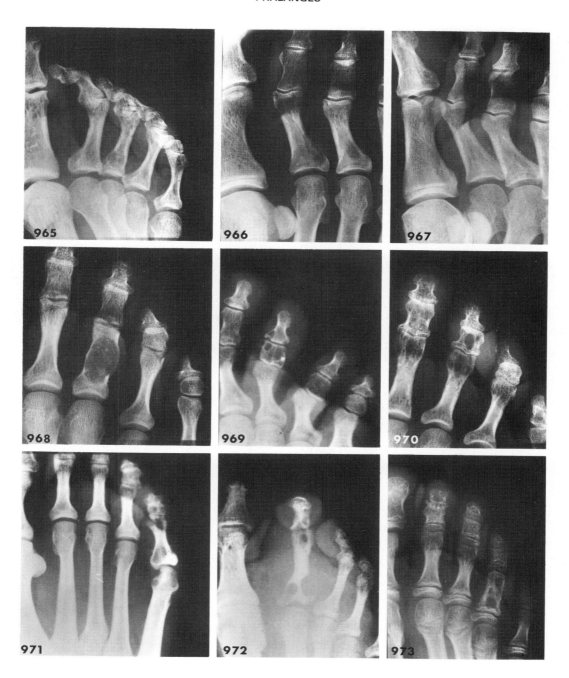

965. Solitary enchondroma : at the proximal phalanx of the third toe, round, well-circumscribed cyst-like bone defects, including punctate areas of calcification.

966. Solitary juxtacortical enchondroma : round, subperiosteal cyst-like lytic area with pathological fracture.

967. Same patient : 5 months later, because of a fracture, spontaneous healing.

968. Solitary enchondroma of the proximal phalanx of the third toe : cyst-like bone lesion ballooning the cortex, including a sowing of calcium deposits.

969. Villonodular synovitis : polyhedral sharply well-circumscribed cyst-like bone lesions of the middle phalanx of the third toe. Breaks in the articular cartilage of the distal phalangeal base.

970. Sarcoidosis (Perthes-Jungling disease or Besnier-Bœck-Schaumann disease) : systemic granulomatosis disease of the young adult (benign lymphogranulomatosis) characterized by nodular granulomas involving the lungs, skin, lymph nodes and bones (20 % to 30 % of the cases), especially at the level of the phalangeal bones. Jungling has depicted five structural changes, successive or simultaneous :

— type 1 : bleb-like radiolucent zone ballooning the bone ;

— type 2 : oval well-delimited punched-out bone radiolucencies (proximal and middle phalanges of the third toe) ;
— type 3 : meshed reticulated osteoporosis ;
— type 4 : diffuse small multicystic osteolysis (middle phalanx of the second toe) ;
— type 5 : osteosclerosing form with osteophytes.

971. Ollier disease : osteochondrodysplasia characterized by multiple enchondromas involving especially the ends of the limbs, which may distort the bones or produce abnormalities of skeletal development. The classical radiographic picture is identical with that of the solitary enchondroma homogeneous, well circumscribed and sharply marginated cyst-like bone defects of the proximal and middle phalanx of the fifth metatarsal and breaks in its head. One may also find large metaphyseal radiolucent areas with sclerotic streaks as in the osteopathia striata of Voorhoeve. Exostoses are often associated with enchondromae.

972. Mycetoma of the second toe : swelling of the soft tissues. Cyst-like punched-out bone lesions and pressure erosions notching the proximal phalangeal base.

973. Sarcoidosis in a 12-year-old girl (rare occurrence at this age) : cyst-like bone lesions (type 2 of Jungling) of the proximal phalanx of the fourth toe.

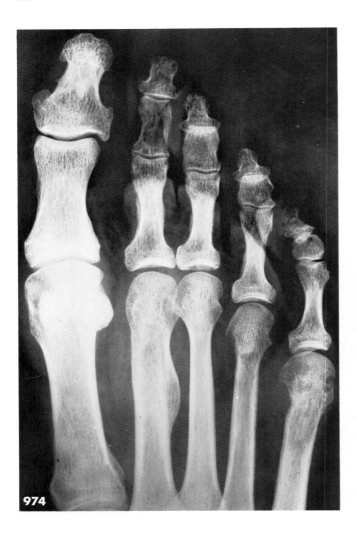

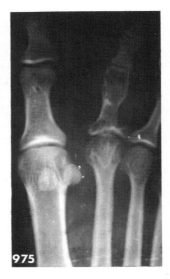

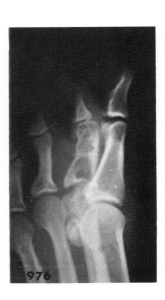

974. Cytosteatonecrosis (see **922**) : small cyst-like radiolucencies disseminated in the metatarsal heads. Callus of a fracture of the second metatarsal shaft.

975, 976. Mycetoma : radiographic appearance at the second year of the disease. Isolated involvement first phalanx of the second toe : small disseminated cyst-like lytic lesions, 3 to 4 mm in diameter (*Streptomyces pelletieri*) ; larger cyst-like ballooning bone defect with punched-out pressure erosion of the phalangeal base.

CYST-LIKE LESION IN A PHALANX ((SOLITARY OR MULTIPLE)

Arthritis (esp. gout, rheumatoid arthritis, osteoarthritis)
Angioma
Bone cyst
Chondromyxoid fibroma
Chondroblastoma, chondrosarcoma
Cystic osteomyelitis
Enchondroma
Epidermoid inclusion cyst (distal phalanx)
Giant cell tumor
Giant cell tumor of tendon sheath
Glomus tumor (distal phalanx)
Hemophilic pseudotumor
Leprosy (leproma)
Metastasis (esp. lung, breast)
Myeloma
Sarcoidosis
Tuberculosis (« spina ventosa »)
Tuberous sclerosis
Villonodular synovitis
Wilson disease.

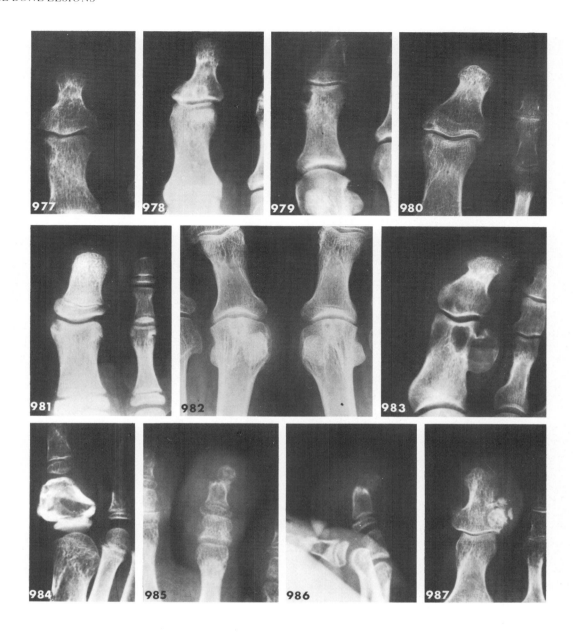

977. Cyst-like radiolucent juxtacortical medial zone of the proximal phalanx of the great toe with articular notch and narrowed joint space. On the lateral side, simple bone rarefaction : possible arthrosis.

978. Two fine marginated radiolucent areas of the distal phalangeal base of the great toe : possible arthrosis.

979. Gout : well-delineated cyst-like bone lesion, ballooning the medial cortex of the head of the first phalanx.

980. Rheumatoid arthritis : demineralization, cyst-like bone lesions with blurred borders on both sides of the inner part of the interphalangeal joint space of the great toe. No narrowing of the articular space.

981. 14-year-old child : cortical erosion of the medical side of the proximal phalangeal head (note the clefts and see **508, 509**). Surgery : intraosseous angioma.

982. Subchondral pseudocystic areas with fine sclerotic borders of the metatarsal head of both great toes : early pathologic findings of hallux rigidus.

983. Ollier disease.

984. Hydatid cyst* : exceptional osseous localization of an echinococcus cyst in the proximal phalanx of the great toe in a 6-year-old girl. Surgery corroborated the presence of hydatid vesicles.

985, 986. Glomus tumor (see **992**) in a 10-year-old boy. Swelling of the soft tissues of the third toe with erosion and fracture of the distal phalanx.

987. Epidermal cyst : a benign tumor formed of a mass of epidermal cells which, as a result of trauma, has been pushed beneath the epidermis in the osseous tissue, especially at the level of the distal phalanx. This inclusion cyst produces a small swelling of the toe and a mild pain. This cyst contains concentric layers of keratin which may calcify. Round, sharply marginated implantation cyst containing concentric layers of calcified keratin expanding in the soft tissues.

* By courtesy of the Prs. M. Jeddi and H.A. Gharbi.

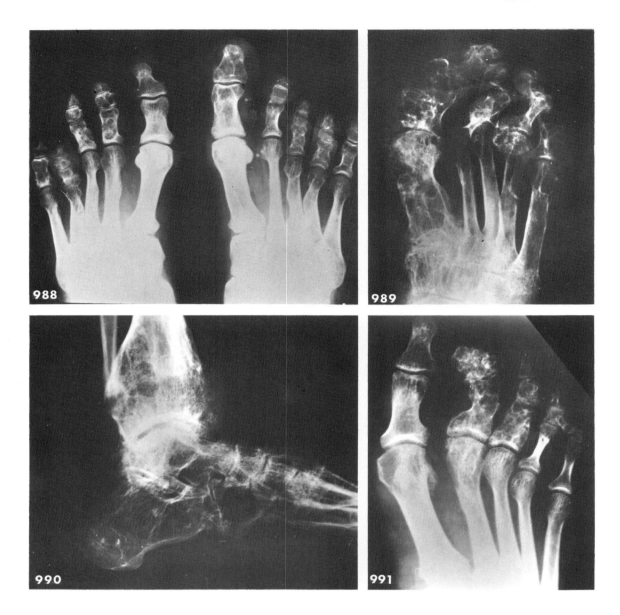

988. Maffuci syndrome : enchondromatosis **(971)** with multiple cavernous hemangiomas. Numerous phalangeal enchondromas. Shortening of the metatarsals, swelling of the soft tissues with radiopaque phleboliths in angiomas.

989. Ollier disease : diffuse rarefaction of the whole forefoot ; multiple cyst-like bone lesions of varying size deforming the shafts.

990. Ollier disease : large, heterogeneous cyst-like radiolucent areas of the tibial metaphysis and fibrillar reticulated demineralization. Large cyst-like bone defect entirely occupying the cuboid.

991. Ollier disease : multiple cyst-like radiolucencies deforming the phalanges of the second and third toe.

992. Glomus tumor : subcutaneous neoplasm originating in a tiny neuromyoarteriolo-venular body (Masson glomus). This exquisitely tender spot causes sharp pains, intensified by pressure and thermal variations. This occurs in the skin of the distal phalanx of a digit, and may lead to cortical erosions **(985, 986)**. Exceptionally, such as in this case, it may produce a notch or a punched-out bone defect.

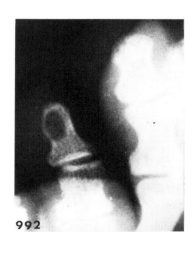

9

EXPANDING BONE LESIONS

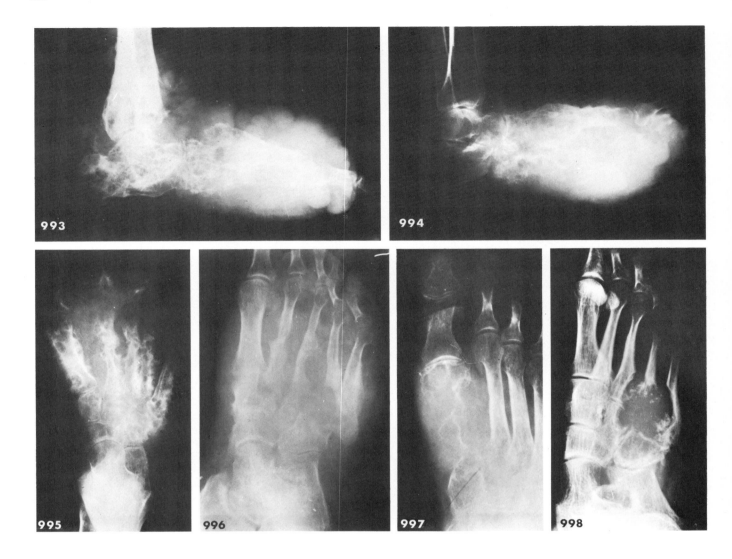

993, 994. Mycetoma. Huge Madura foot : considerable swelling of the soft tissues with draining sinuses. Cyst-like areas of osteolysis, large pressure erosions (*Madurella mycetomi*), complete phalangeal resorption.

995. Mycetoma. Madura foot. Multiple cyst-like bone lesions. Large pressure erosions notching the metatarsal shafts, periosteal reaction of the first and fifth metatarsal, joint and phalangeal resorption.

996. Mycetoma. Madura foot. Swelling of the soft tissues. Large eroding notches of the metatarsal shafts.

997. Osteosarcoma. Osteolytic form with complete destruction of the first metatarsal shaft, invasion of the soft tissues and demineralization of adjoining bones.

998. Chondromyxoid fibroma. Uncommon benign cartilaginous slow-growing tumor of young adults. The typical radiographic change is a round metaphyseal cyst-like radiolucent area, well circumscribed with sclerotic margins, producing, in the small bones, a radiographic appearance quite similar to the picture of an enchondroma. In this patient, there is a large expanding cyst-like bone lesion of the fourth metatarsal base, with invasion and destruction of the cortex of the adjacent bones.

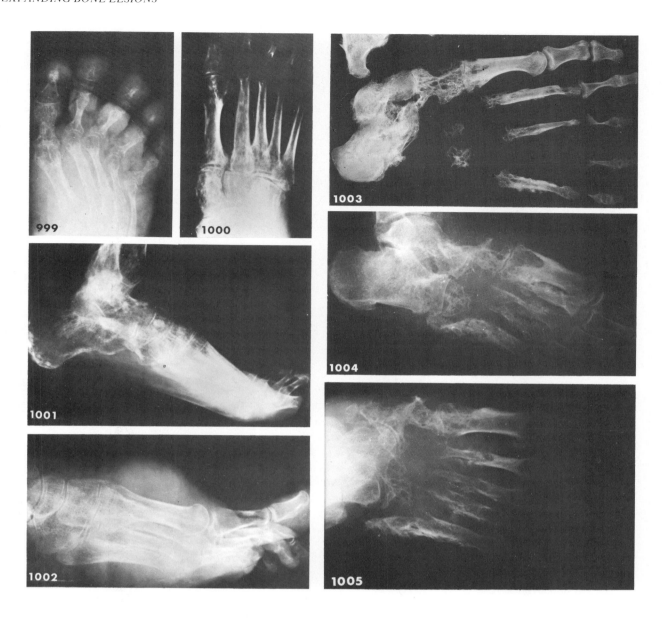

999. Venous angioma. Swelling of the soft tissues with small vascular calcification. Considerable generalized deformity of the metatarsal shafts by concentric bone resorption.

1000. Breast carcinoma. Diffuse small cyst-like areas of osteolysis.

1001. Prostate carcinoma. Diffuse fibrillar and cystic osteolysis.

1002. Ewing sarcoma of the second metatarsal : primary malignant bone tumor in which the cell of origin is controversial, but probably derived from the reticulum of the bone marrow. This neoplasm occurs usually before the age of 30 years ; it may involve any bone and often presents clinical signs.
Swelling of the soft tissues. Diffuse rarefaction of the whole foot. Laminated periosteal elevation of the shaft.

1003. Mycetoma (amputated specimen). *Cephalosporium.* Radiographic picture at the tenth year of the disease.

1004, 1005. Mycetoma. Madura foot. Radiographic picture at the fifth year of the disease. Diffuse rarefaction of the whole foot. Bone destruction in the intermediate and lateral cuneiforms and the second, third and fourth metatarsal bases. Other bones are pitted with multiple circumscribed radiolucencies (honeycomb-like rarefaction). *Streptomyces pelletieri.*

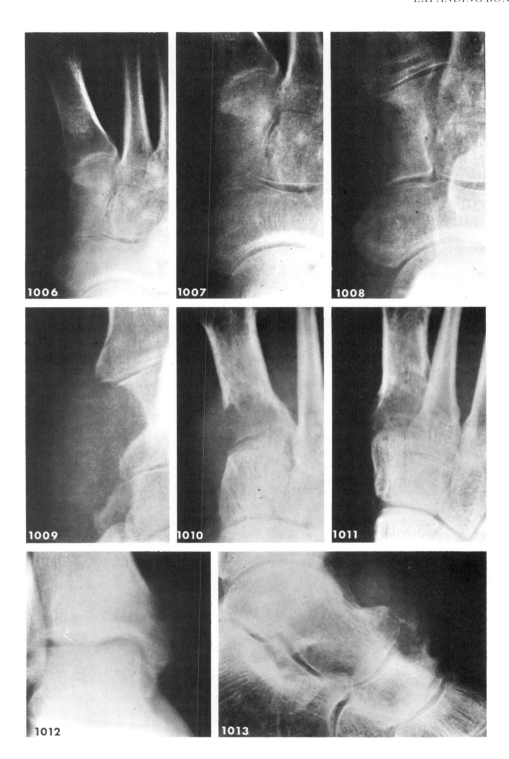

1006 → 1009. Chondrosarcoma malignant neoplasm. The primary type derived from cartilage cells, occurring most frequently in middle-aged males, slow growing, is situated in the central or peripheral part of the bone. The secondary type results from a malignant transformation of a preexisting osteochondroma (1 % of case). Same patient. These four radiographs were taken on the same day.

1006. Slight rarefaction of the bony architecture of the medial cuneiform.

1007, 1008, 1009. Close-up view in various radiographic projections : large notch of the inferior aspect of the medial cuneiform with swelling of the soft tissues and granular calcifications.

1010, 1011. Malignant synovioma : A malignant tumor of synovial origin involving the joints or the tendon sheaths, extending into adjacent bones. Approximately one-third show radiographic evidence of calcification. Notch of the cortex of the first metatarsal base and invasion of the soft tissues.

1012. Mycetoma : cortical extrinsic erosions of the medial malleolus and periosteal reaction.

1013. Gouty tophus originating in the talar neck and navicular bone, expanding into the soft tissues and destroying the tendons of the extensor muscles.

10

BONE RESORPTIONS

Some diseases produce peculiar osteolyses simulating the melting of a piece of ice, and ending in complete disappearance, at various times, of the involved bone. Usually, they occur at the distal part of the bone.

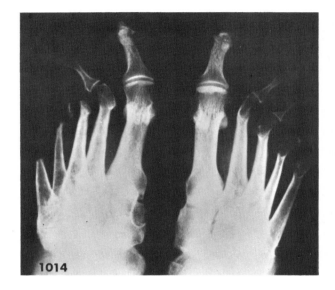

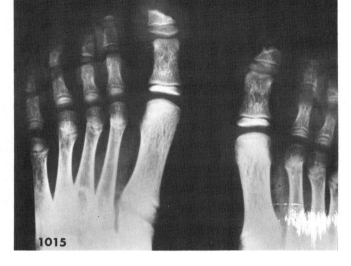

1014. Idiopathic acro-osteolysis (phalangeal type). Hereditary disease due to a recessive or dominant gene, progressing since childhood in a 53-year-old female : phalangeal resorption ; typical changes in metatarsal shafts ; pencil-like or candlestick deformity.

1015. Idiopathic distal acro-osteolysis in a 9-year-old boy, son of the woman cited in **1014** ; beginning of osteolysis in the distal phalanx of both great toes.

ACRO-OSTEOLYSIS CONFINED TO ONE DIGIT

Angiomatous malformation
Carcinomas
Epidermoid cyst
Fibroma
Giant cell tumor of tendon sheath
Glomus tumor
Infection (eg, whitlow, osteomyelitis)
Metastasis ; lymphoma
Neurofibroma

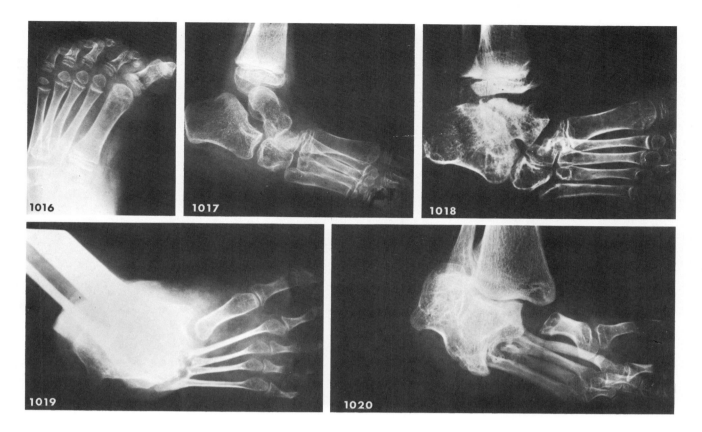

1016 → 1020. Idiopathic osteolysis of Julien Marie and Derot (tarsocarpal form). Hereditary disease characterized by a proximal osteolysis of the extremities with nephropathy. Early radiographic and clinical signs occur in the carpus and the tarsus. For a long time, the digits are spared.

1016, 1017. Five-year-old girl : rarefaction of the bone structure. Resorption of two cuneiforms.

1018. One year later : same radiographic appearance.

1019, 1020. Seven and nine years later : complete destruction of the anterior tarsus with an empty space between the metatarsals and the posterior bone block fusion (arthrodesis to enable weight-bearing erect position). Same clinical course for the other foot and both wrists.

EROSION OF MULTIPLE TERMINAL PHALANGEAL TUFTS (ACRO-OSTEOLYSIS)

Arteriosclerosis obliterans
Brachydactyly B
Buerger disease
Burn, thermal or electrical
Congenital (familial) acro-osteolysis (eg, Hajdu-Cheney S.)
Congenital indifference to pain
Diabetic gangrene
Disseminated lipogranulomatosis
Drug therapy (eg, dilantin, phenobarbital, ergot)
Ectodermal dysplasia
Epidermolysis bullosa
Frostbite
Gout
Hereditary sensory radiculopathy (Thevenard)
Hyperparathyroidism, primary or secondary
Idiopathic osteolysis (Jackson-Gorham)
Leprosy
Lesch-Nyhan S. (mental defective finger biting)
Neurotrophic disease
Osteomalacia (eg. malabsorption syndromes)
Osteopetrosis

Pachydermoperiostosis
Peripheral nerve injury
Pityriasis rubra
Polyvinyl chloride osteolysis
Porphyria
Progeria ; Werner S.
Pseudoxanthoma elasticum
Psoriasis
Pyknodysostosis
Raynaud disease
Reticulohistiocytoma (lipoid dermatoarthritis)
Rheumatoid arthritis
Rothmund S.
Sarcoidosis
Scleroderma, dermatomyositis
Sjögren syndrome
Streeter congenital amniotic bands
Tabes dorsalis
Thromboangiitis obliterans
Trauma
Trophic ulcer

PHALANGES

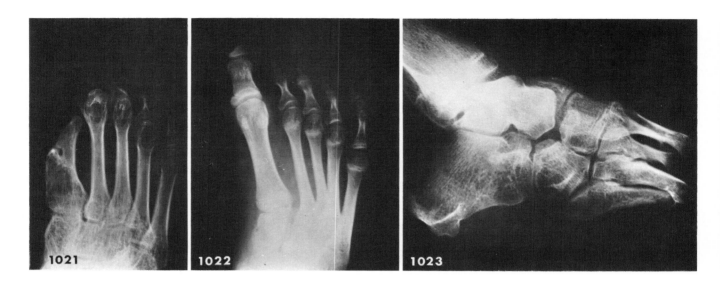

1021. Idiopathic osteolysis of the five toes after a benign injury of the foot.

1022. Idiopathic osteolysis of the distal phalanx of the right great toe. (Bilateral involvement).

1023. Amniotic disease : congenital intrauterine amputation of the toes attributed to the pressure of adventitious constricting bands, more recently regarded as the result of an intrinsic deficency of embryonic tissue.

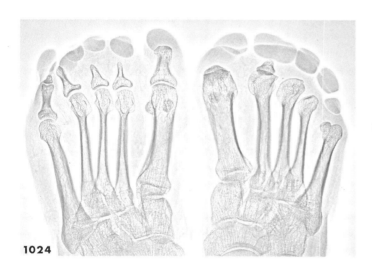

1024. Congenital aphalangia (see page 85).

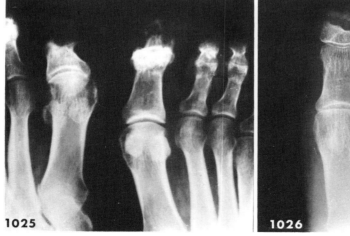

1025. Arteritis : phalangeal osteolysis leading to amputation.

1026. Arteritis : the two typical radiographic findings of acro-osteolysis are : 1) longitudinal osteolysis pointing and spindling the distal end of the bone (pencil-like or candlestick shape of shafts) ; 2) transversal osteolysis cleavage.

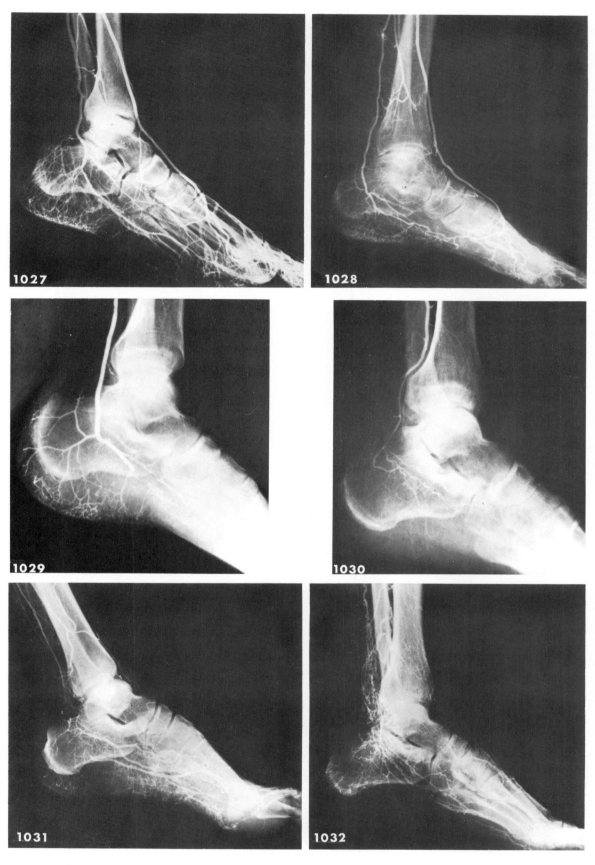

1027 → 1032. Arteritis - Angiograms.

1027. Deep plantar-arch thrombosis. Atheromatous parietal defect of the medial plantar artery. Terminal arteriolitis.

1028. Peroneal artery thrombosis.

1029. Thrombosis of the anterior tibial artery, peroneal artery and medial plantar artery.

1030. Thrombosis of the anterior tibial artery, peroneal artery and posterior tibial artery.

1031. More advanced arteritis.

1032. Thrombosis of all the arterial trunks of the foot.

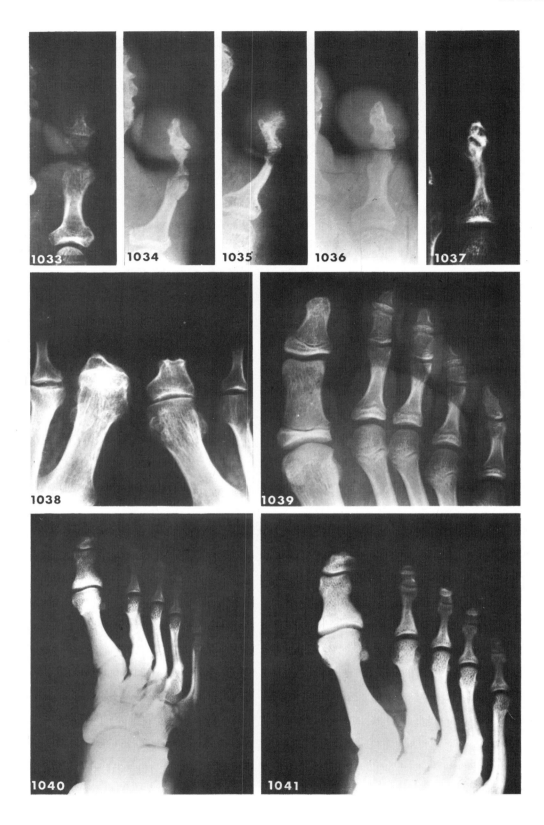

1033 → 1036. Ainhum : disease of unknown cause affecting male Negroes, especially characterized by a constricting scleroderma of the toe (usually the little toe) and gradually resulting in spontaneous amputation of this toe. Strangulating cutaneous ring and osteolysis of the fifth toe : various radiographic changes.

1037. Leprosy. Concentric diaphyseal osteolysis of the proximal phalanx of the fifth toe.

1038, 1039. Frostbites : they produce osteolyses of various severity involving all of the toes or a part of them.

1038. Absorption of the distal end of both great toes.

1039. Partial absorption of the tufts of the terminal phalanges in the second and third toes.

1040. Pyknodysostosis : marked generalized osteosclerosis (see 720).

1041. Same case : close-up view. The osteolysis of the distal phalanx of the great toes is a typical clinical sign of this disease.

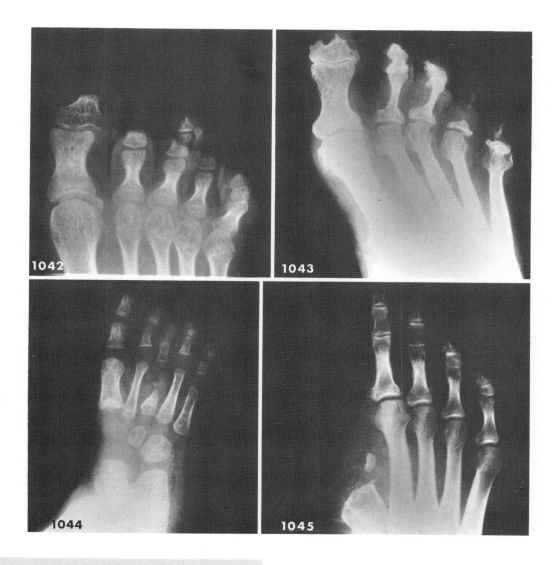

**NEUROTROPHIC BONE CHANGES
(POINTED OR SPINDLED BONES)
IN THE FEET**

Acro-osteolysis (see page 171)
Amputation (congenital, traumatic, or surgical)
Arteriosclerosis obliterans
Burn, thermal or electric ; frostbite
Congenital indifference to pain
Diabetes
Ergot intoxication
Leprosy
Peripheral nerve injury
Porphyria
Psoriatic arthritis
Raynaud disease ; Buerger disease
Rheumatoid arthritis
Scleroderma, dermatomyositis
Spinal cord trauma or disease (eg, pernicious anemia, syringomyelia, spina-bifida, meningo-myelocele neoplams)
Tabes dorsalis
Trophic ulcer of soft tissue with underlying destruction

1042. Spina-bifida in a 13-year-old child. Osteolysis of the distal phalanx of the great toe (see the calcanei of this same patient **1083, 1084**).

1043. Diabetes mellitus. Acro-osteolysis : incomplete amputation of the proximal phalanx of the great toe. Subtotal absorption of the phalanges of the fourth and fifth toes.

1044. Sickle-cell anemia : areolar structure of the bones. Lysis of the distal part of the third metatarsal.

1045. Buerger disease : thromboangiitis obliterans, in young and middle-aged (heavy smokers) Israeli men, characterized by arterial and venous thrombotic occlusions, commonly resulting in gangrene with iterative amputations, Subtotal resorption of the first ray.

METATARSUS

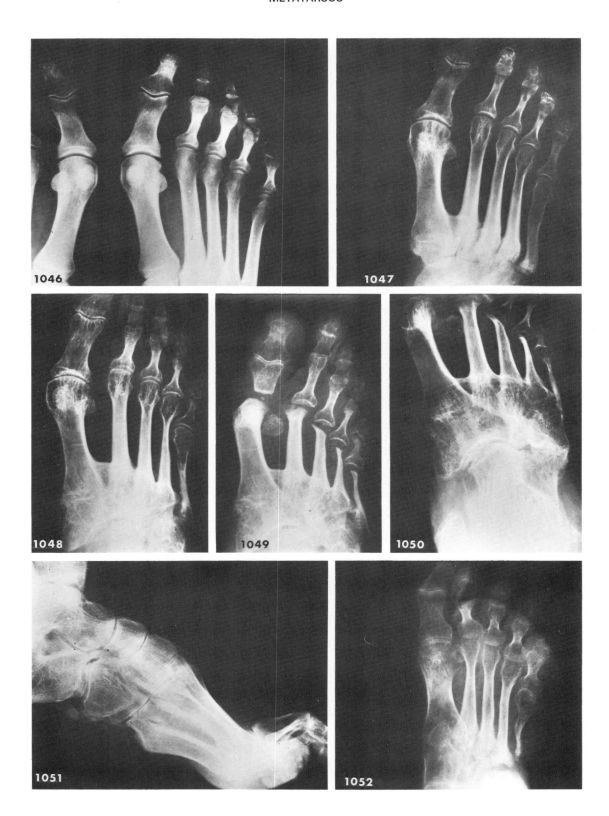

1046 → 1050. Course of a case of metatarsal osteolysis.

1046. Initial radiograph.

1047. One year after a metatarsectomy for pes cavus : cyst-like osteolysis of the metatarsal heads and bowing of the fifth metatarsal shaft.

1048. Four years later : osteolysis of the fourth and fifth metatarsal shafts.

1049. Two years later : the shafts have become thread-like, after surgical removal of the metatarsal heads.

1050. Ten years later, stationary condition. Ankylosis of the tarsus anterior.

1051. Destruction of the base of the fifth metatarsal in a 44-year-old male showing a spina-bifida.

1052. Same patient. Advanced stage : cuboideo-metatarsal arthritis with complete destruction of the fifth metatarsal and generalized demineralization of the foot.

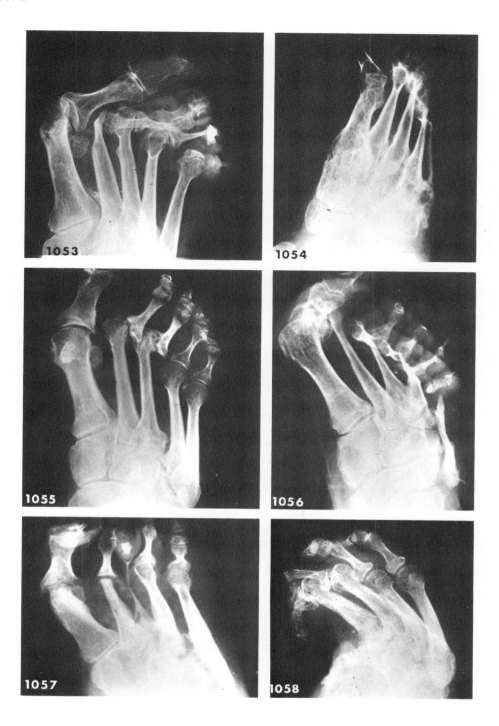

1053. Rheumatoid arthritis : absorption of the second metatarsal head, generalized diffuse bone rarefaction, dislocation of the phalanges, which look as if they were bent outward by the wind (« fibular-gust »).

1054. Paralysis of the common peroneal nerve after traumatic dislocation of the knee 2 years ago : demineralization, longitudinal osteolysis of the diaphyses. Absorption of the fifth toe, with extreme thinning of the fifth metatarsal shaft. Ankylosis of the anterior tarsus.

1055, 1056. Thevenard syndrome (familial ulceration of the extremities) : hereditary sensory neuropathy, characterized by a pseudosyringomyelic syndrome of the lower limbs, trophic cutaneous disorders, (perforating ulcer) and bone lesions (acro-osteolysis).

1055. Early osteolysis of the metatarsal heads with dislocation of the phalanges.

1056. Longitudinal osteolysis of the second, third, fourth metatarsal shafts with dislocation of the toes. The fifth metatarsal is reduced to a detached, dislocated, small osseous tongue.

1057. Complex neuropathy, unknown cause. Diaphyseal osteolysis of the third metatarsal with complete destruction of the phalanges, crushing of the anterior tarsus : diaphyseal periosteal reaction of the fifth metatarsal. Arthroplasty of the first and second metatarsophalangeal joints.

1058. Osteolysis after radiotherapy on the plantar surface : complete absorption of the first ray. Bending of the metatarsal bony spur formation on the anterior tarsus. Hypertrophic changes of the ankle and subtalar joints.

Arteriographic study of the foot in hereditary sensory radicular neuropathy and in diabetic arthropathy shows, similar radiographic pictures :

— early appearance of arterial network and quick venous return,

— hypervascularization around the progressive bone lesions.

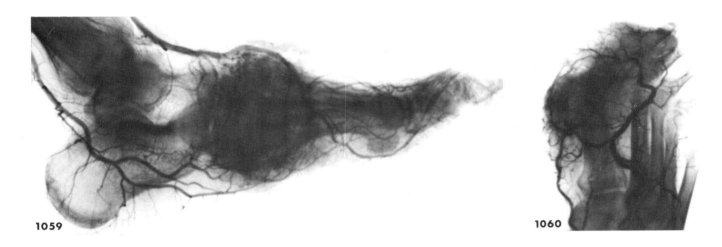

1059   1060

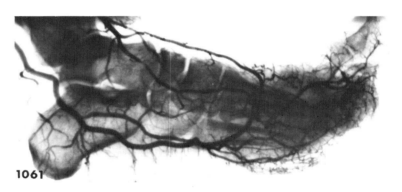

1061

1059 → 1061. Hereditary sensory radicular neuropathy of the Burreau-Barrière type (see 1067). Arteriography (arterial time) : localized hypervascularization at the level of the progressive bone lesions, metatarsophalangeals (1061), tarsals (1059) and of the great toe (1060).

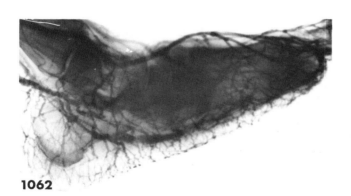

1062

1062. Diabetes mellitus. Chronological disturbance : at the sixth second a large widened plantar vein appears with numerous « flames of fire » shapes at the level of the heel.

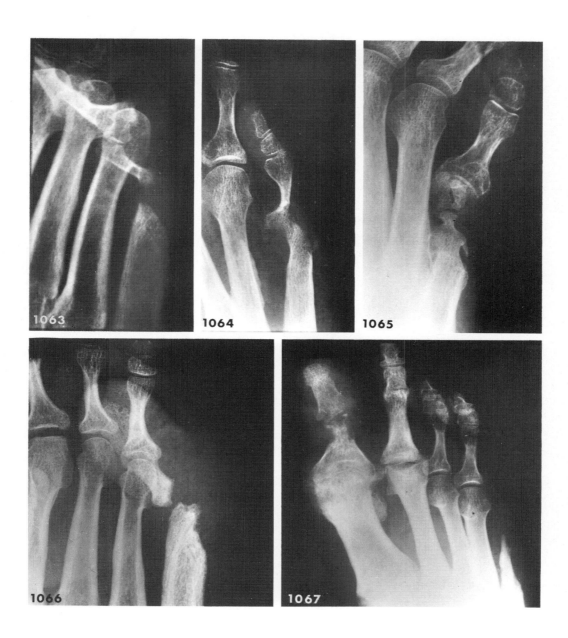

1063 → 1067. Lysis of the fifth metatarsal head.

1063. Psoriasis.

1064. Perforating ulcer.

1065. Gout.

1066. Spina bifida.

1067. Bureau-Barrière disease. A nonfamilial condition affecting especially males, characterized by a sensory neuropathy of the lower limbs with trophic cutaneous disorders (perforating ulcer) and bone destructions, but with hypertrophic bone formations during the intermittent quiesant periods. Concentric osteolysis of the proximal phalanx of the great toe. Pointed, spindled fifth metatarsal shaft. Necrosis of the second metatarsal head.

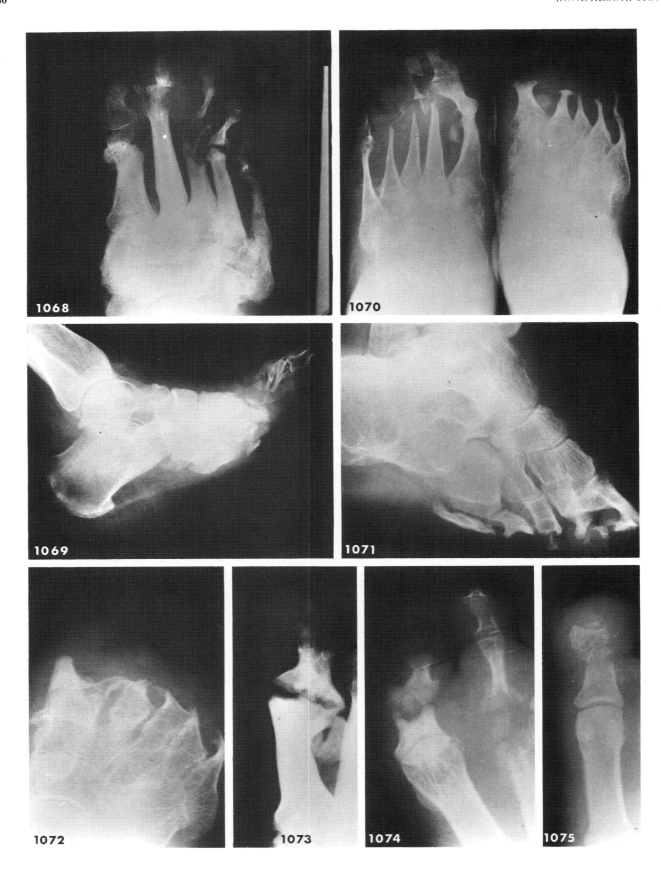

1068, 1069. Diabetes mellitus, same patient. Resorption of the metatarsal shafts. This radiographic appearance contrasts with the osteosclerosis of the uninvolved second metatarsal.

1070. Leprosy. Marked longitudinal osteolysis of the metatarsals, spontaneous amputation of all the phalanges of the right foot.

1071. Leprosy.

1072. Leprosy.

1073. Leprosy. Phalangeal absorption concomitant with metatarsophalangeal leprous arthritis.

1074. Leprosy. Leprous arthritis destroying the interphalangeal joint of the great toe and the metatarsophalangeal joint of the second toe.

1075. Leprosy. Spontaneous distal phalangeal amputation and transverse band-like radiolucent bone destruction of the proximal phalanx of the great toe.

TARSUS

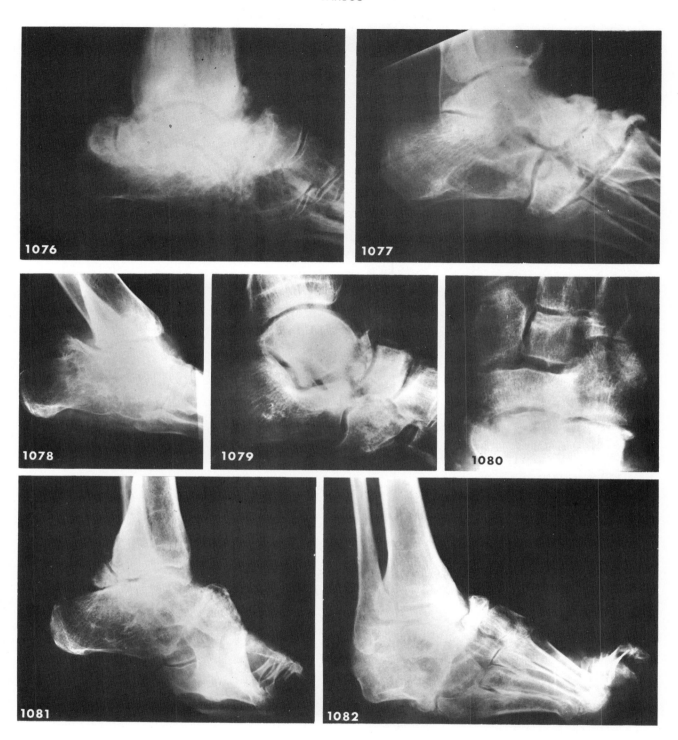

1076. Diabetic osteo-arthropathy (tabes diabetica type) : marked hypertrophic osseous formations (osteophytes - osteochondromatosis, tibial periosteal reaction), associated with talar crushing and flatness of the plantar arch of the foot producing a radiographie appearance similar to Charcot joint.

1077, 1078. Tabes dorsalis. Midtarsal form of Alajouanine, involving especially the talonavicular joint. **1077.** Crushed navicular and destruction of the talar head : the subtalar and cuboideocalcanean joints may be initially

spared. When involved, the tarsus becomes completely destroyed (**1078**).

1079, 1080. Familial ulceration of the extremities (Thevenard syndrome). Osteolysis of the talar head.

1081. Tabes dorsalis : cubic foot of Charcot and Ferré. Generalized osteoarticular lesions with crushing of the bones and dislocations of the joints, producing a telescopic shortening of the foot.

1082. Same patient. Opposite foot : the forefoot is spared.

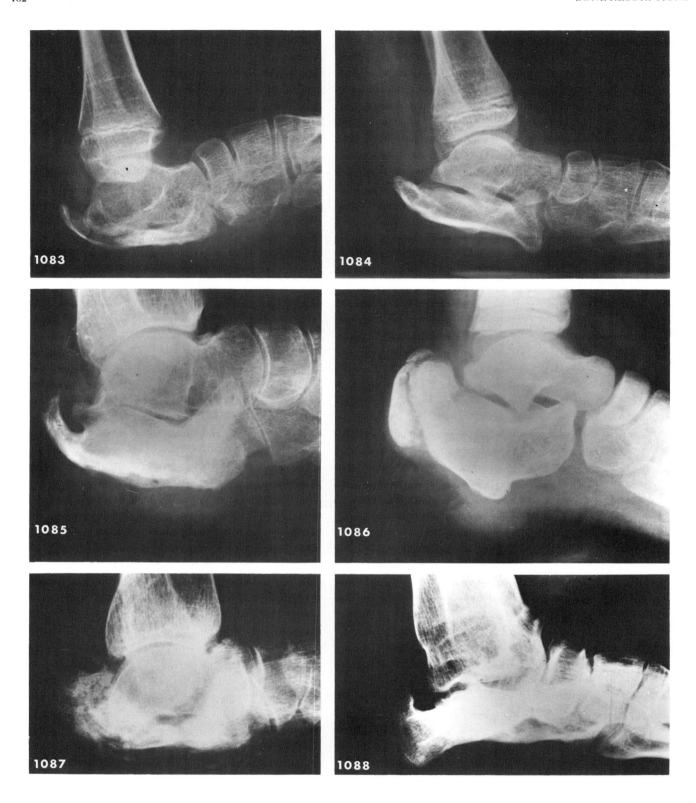

1083, 1084. Spina-bifida. Same patient as **1042**. Marked osteolysis of bone calcanei.

1085. Syringomyelia. A condition characterized by the presence in the spinal cord of a longitudinal cavity, interrupting the spinal thalamic tract and therefore producing thermoanesthesia and analgesia of the limbs, but sparing the tactile sense. The lunar segment of the spinal cord is not usually involved. Osteolysis of the calcaneus.

1086. Thevenard disease. Osteolysis of the calcaneus.

1087. Sequela of a calcanean fracture.

1088. Osteomyelitis occurred in a 6-year-old child and was treated by talectomy.

11

PICTURES OF OSTEONECROSIS

FOCAL ASEPTIC NECROSIS OF BONE

Idiopathic (**1089**).

Secondary : trauma, caisson disease, pancreatitis, steroid therapy, collagen
disease (eg. lupus), sickle cell anemia, Gaucher disease, leukosis,
radiation therapy, frostbite, burns, articular chondrocalcinosis, etc.

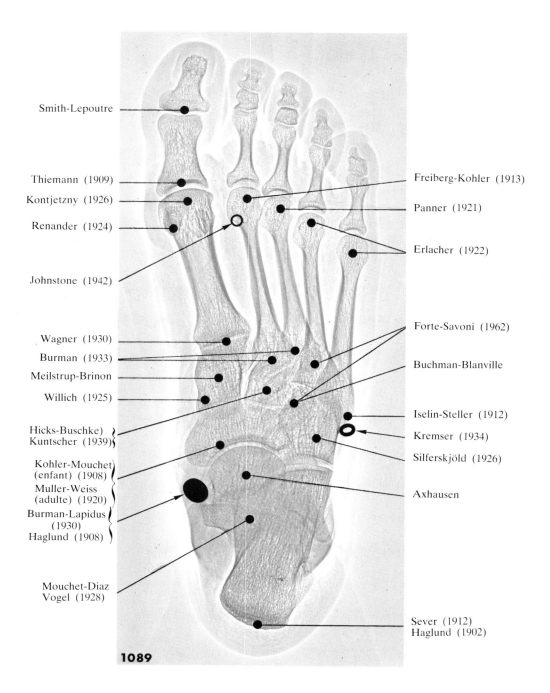

1089. Diagram of the sites of predilection and
eponyms for aseptic necrosis.

TALUS

Osteochondritis dissecans of the talus. Incomplete necrosis of the medial, lateral and superior joint surfaces of the trochlea - usually caused by trauma and often unrecognized in its early stage. It is interesting to radiograph the ankle bent in valgus or varus and in dorsi or plantar flexion, to clear the margins of the talar trochlea.

Usually, the osteochondritis dissecans of the talar trochlea does not lead to hypertrophic arthritis.

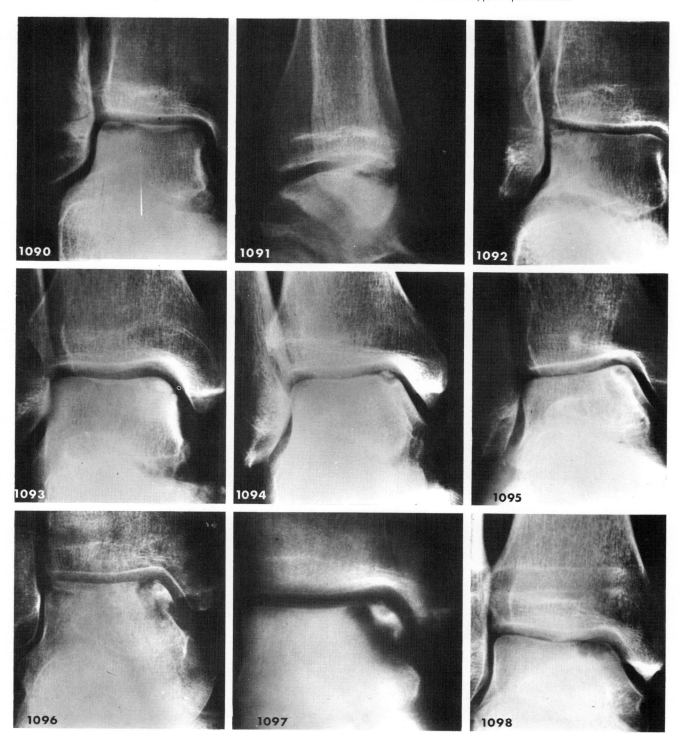

1090 → 1092. Osteochondritis dissecans of the lateral articular margin of the talar trochlea.

1090, 1091. Island of subchondral bone surrounded by an area of rarefaction. Otherwise normal articular space of the malleolar mortise.

1092. Same localization : separated fragment of bone.

1093 → 1098. Osteochondritis dissecans of the medial articular margin of the talar trochlea.

1093. Subchondral bony defect.

1094. Completely separated bone fragment.

1095. Cyst-like subchondral area of osteolysis.

1096, 1097. Radiograph and tomogram : necrosis and sequestrum with diffuse rarefaction of the ankle.

1098. Subchondral area of osteolysis supervening after a traumatic diastasis of the ankle treated by osteosynthesis with a screw, the course of which is still visible through the tibial epiphysis.

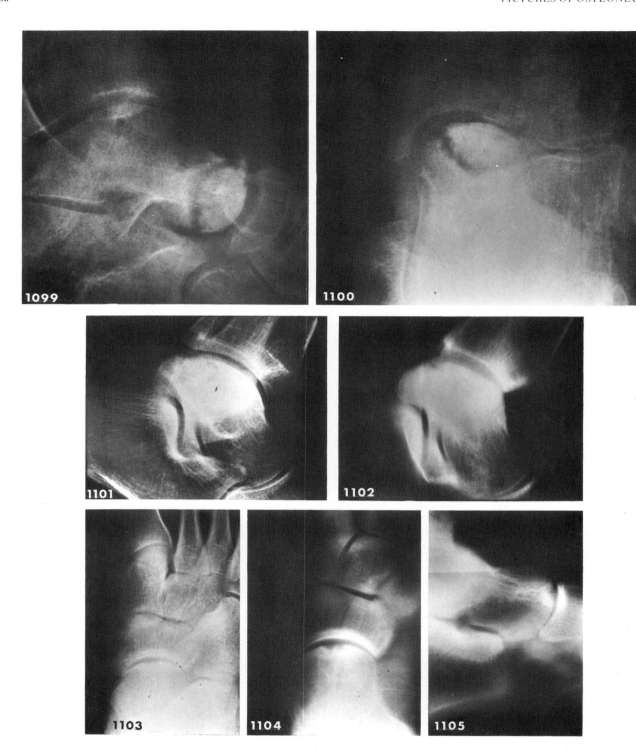

1099, 1100. Tuberculous osteitis : osteosclerotic, necrotic talar head, separated from the body of the talus by a semicircular radiolucent strand of osteolysis.

1101, 1102. Necrosis of the posterior part of the talar trochlea. Radiograph and tomogram.

1103 → 1105. Osteochondritis dissecans of the talar head. The tomograms show small cyst-like bone lesions lying under the subchondral defect.

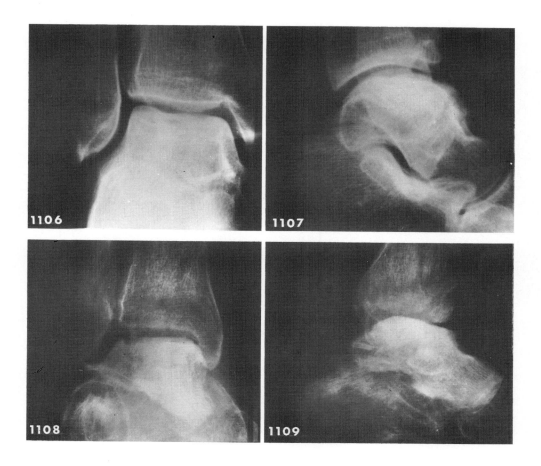

1106, 1107. Large necrosis of the talar trochlea with dense, osteosclerotic bone structure. Trauma 3 years ago.

1108, 1109. Complete necrosis of the talus. Post-traumatic origin with sepsis. The osteosclerotic talus contrasts with the diffuse demineralization of the calcaneus and the ankle.

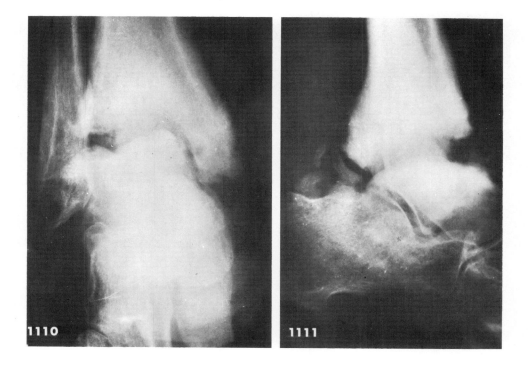

1110, 1111. Diabetic arthropathy of the ankle in a 20-year-old untreated male. Massive destruction of the ankle and remodeling by the diabetic osteonecrosis. Tibial and peroneal periosteal reaction.

NAVICULAR

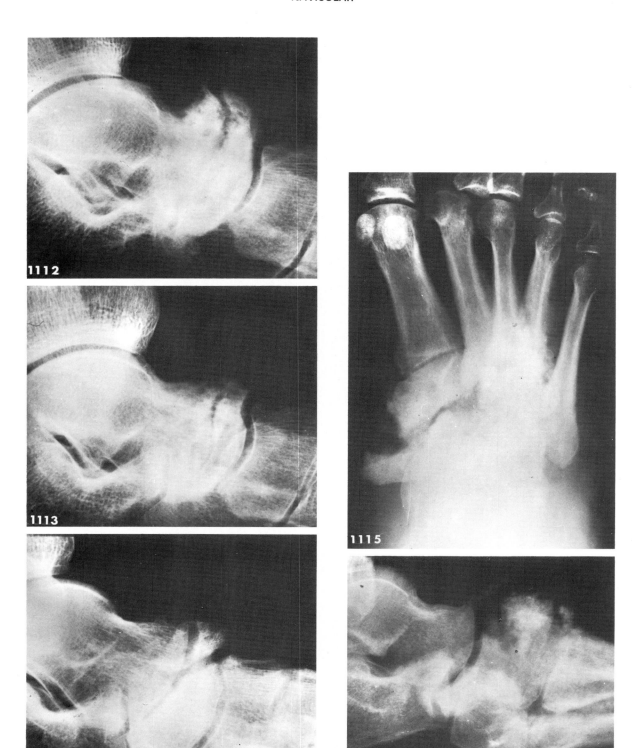

1112, 1113. Muller-Weiss disease (scaphoidolisthesis of Brailsford). Aseptic necrosis of the navicular of the adult, the origin of which is still debated : fatigue fracture (Mansart and Ruffie), sequela of an aseptic necrosis of childhood (Viladot), bipartite navicular (Köhler and Zimmer). Two cases of Muller-Weiss disease with degenerative changes of the talonavicular joint.

1114. Necrosis of the navicular bone and of the talar head associated with a chondrocalcinosis, proved by the pathological anatomy.

1115, 1116. Diabetic osteoarthropathy : the dense and necrotic navicular is enucleated : periosteal reaction at the metatarsal bases.

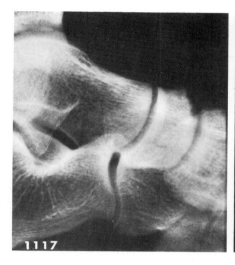

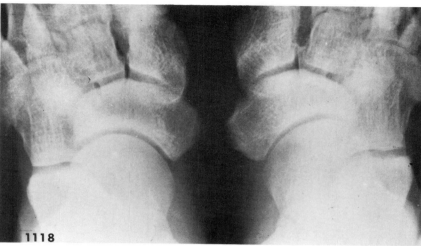

1117, 1118. Muller-Weiss disease : bilateral form in a record-holding runner (steeple), incomplete medial enucleation of the navicular body between the talar head and the cunei- forms. The lateral part of the navicular is dense, sclerotic and thinned.

CALCANEUS

1119. Cytosteatonecrosis (see **922**) : disseminated cyst-like areas of osteolysis, varying in size, without surrounding osteosclerosis, showing a permeated radiographic appearance of the bone. Sequestrum of the tuber calcanei.

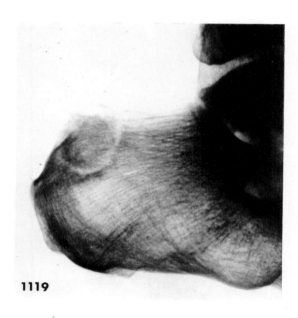

SESAMOIDS

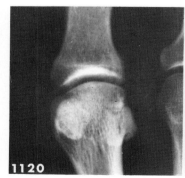

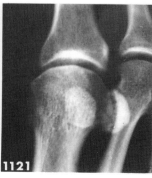

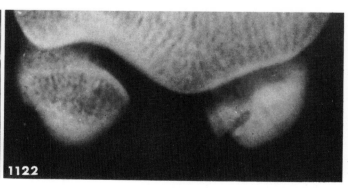

1120 → 1122. Renander disease : aseptic necrosis of sesamoids of the right great toe : longitudinal cleft of the lateral sesamoid contrary to the cleft, generally trans- verse of the bipartite sesamoid. In the bipartition, the medial sesamoid is most frequently involved

Frequency of the bipartition : lateral sesamoid 1 %, medial sesamoid 30 % of the cases (after Kewanter).

METATARSALS

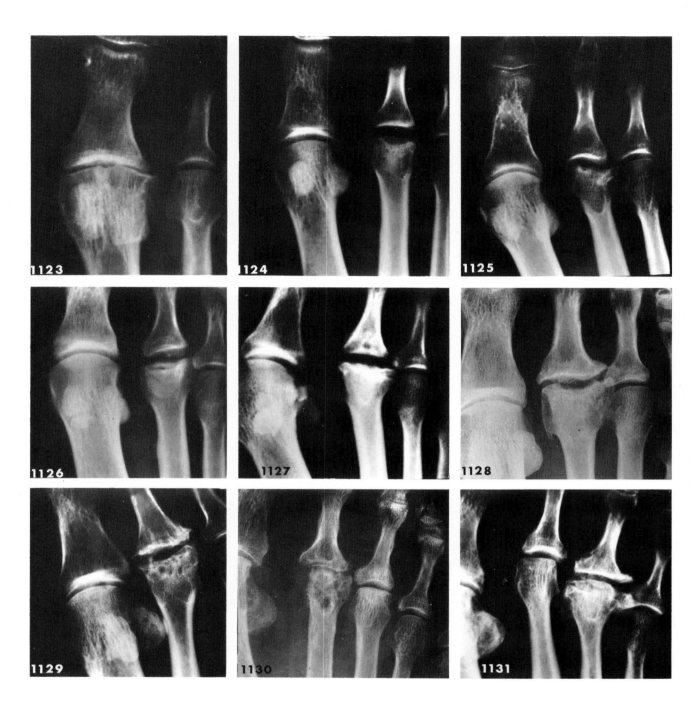

1123. Hallux rigidus (see **1344**) : narrowed metatarso-phalangeal joint space, with subchondral cyst formation, surrounded by a thick osteosclerotic margin, notching the first metatarsal head. Some authors suggest that the subchondral cyst is a true osteochondritis dissecans of the first metatarsal head, later obscured by secondary degenerative changes.

1124 → 1128. Freiberg-Köhlers disease : aseptic necrosis of the second metatarsal shaft. Various radiographic findings from an early stage to an advanced one.

1124. Widening of the joint space. Slight flattening of the second metatarsal head. Fine line of osteosclerosis.

1125. Irregular, flattened second metatarsal head.

1126. Concave head with sequestrum, slight degenerative changes affecting the opposite phalangeal base.

1127. More deformed metatarsal head. Slight degenerative changes of the adjacent phalangeal base.

1128. Sequela of Freiberg disease : arthrosis of the crushed metatarsal head with marked osteophyte formations on both sides of the joint.

1129, 1130. Rheumatoid arthritis in an old Freiberg disease : cyst-like areas of osteolysis and bone rarefaction.

1131. Degenerative changes of the third metatarsophalangeal joint in an old juvenile aseptic necrosis (Panner disease).

12

BONE AND JOINT DESTRUCTION

In this chapter, are described miscellaneous inflammatory, individual or multiple, joint diseases.

The associated radiographic findings may include :

— narrowing of the joint space
— involvement of both sides of the joint : demineralization, subchondral cyst-formations and cartilage erosion, extending bone destructions of the epiphyses
— dislocations.

The sites of occurrence and the number of involved joints are often indicative of the cause of the disease. Other noninflammatory arthropathies have been included under this caption, because of their similar radiographic appearances.

ANKLE JOINT

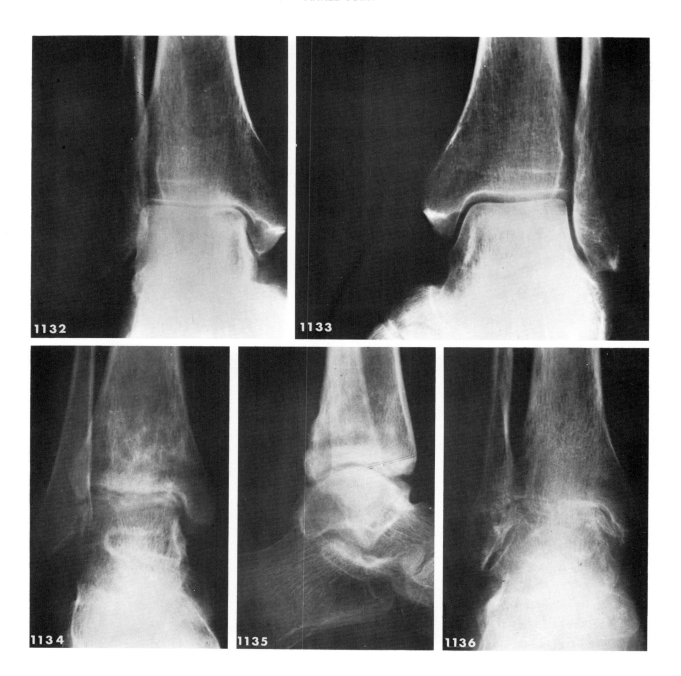

1132 → 1136. Pyogenic arthritis.

1132, 1133. Pyogenic arthritis, early radiographic findings. **1132.** Uniform narrowing of the whole joint space. Compare with the normal opposite ankle (**1133**).

1134, 1135. Pyogenic arthritis (staphylococcus). Entirely narrowed joint space with hazy margins : cyst-like areas of osteolysis and radiolucent transverse metaphyseal band.

1136. Pyogenic arthritis. Uniform narrowing of the whole joint space.

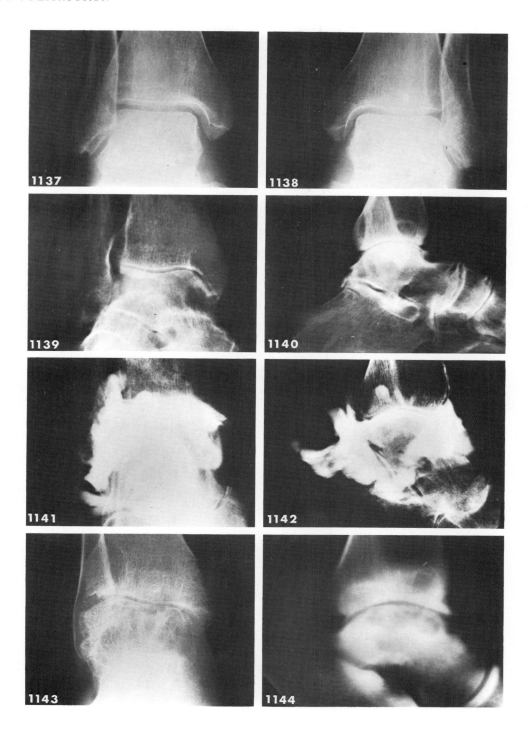

1137 → 1144. Rheumatoid arthritis. A systemic disease, especially common in women, with a progressive course, characterized by a chronic synovitis with proliferation of granulation tissue (pannus) which symmetrically destroys cartilage, bone, and ligaments.

1137, 1138. Rheumatoid arthritis. Early radiographic findings : narrowing of the left ankle joint space (1138). Compare with the normal right ankle (1037).

1139, 1140. Rheumatoid arthritis : advanced stage, more marked, narrowing of the ankle joint space, diffuse osteoporosis, subchondral cyst formations. The talo-navicular, subtalar and cuneo-navicular joints are also involved.

1141, 1142. Rheumatoid arthritis. Arthrography performed at the time of a synoviorthesis, shows the synovial proliferation, destroying the joint : the contrast agent opacifies the cavities carved out by the pannus (see normal arthrogram page 241).

1143, 1144. Hemophilic arthritis. Radiograph and tomogram. The bones and joints are more frequently involved in hemophilia A than in hemophilia B (Christmas disease). The early stages of this disease are recurrent hemarthrosis. The degenerative arthropathy occurs later and bony ankylosis may ensue. Narrowing of the ankle joint space and cartilage erosions, cyst-like areas of osteolysis due to intraosseous hemorrhages.

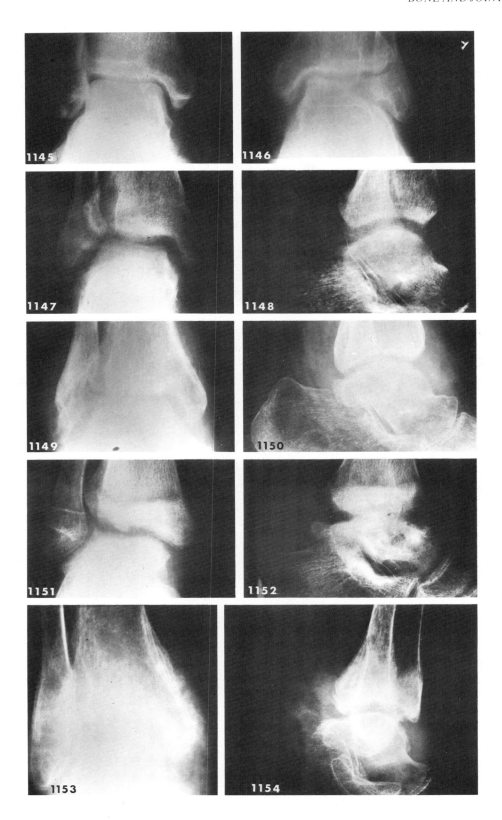

1145, 1146. Tuberculous arthritis. **1145.** Uninvolved right foot. **1146.** Normal intra-articular space but its margins are hazy. Cyst-like radiolucent areas in the lateral malleolus.

1147, 1148. Tuberculous arthritis : capsular swelling at the level of the posterior aspect of the ankle joint. Bony rarefaction. Widening of the joint cavity with blurred margins.

1149, 1150. Tuberculous arthritis : swelling of the posterior and anterior capsular articular recesses.

1151, 1152. Tuberculous arthritis : bony rarefaction, destruction of the joint space, necrosis of the talar trochlea.

1153, 1154. Actinomycotic arthritis : marked swelling of the soft tissues. Erosions of the articular margins of the ankle joint. Laminated periosteal elevation and thick bush-like spicular bony outgrowths are characteristic of this disease.

SUBTALAR JOINT

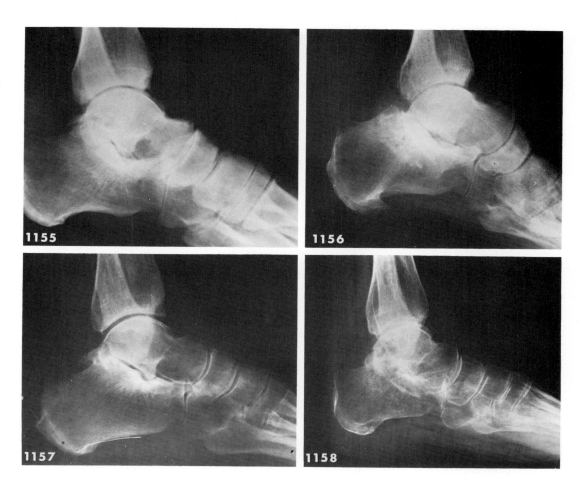

1155. Rheumatoid arthritis : narrowing of the posterior talocalcanean joint.

1156. Psoriasis. In 9 % of cases, psoriasis becomes complicated with an inflammatory arthritis, either of the axial type (same as in the ankylosing spondylitis), or of the peripheral type, distal, asymmetric and less frequent. This condition is characterized by a fibrous proliferative synovitis, without pannus, occurring especially in males. The bone and joint involvement may precede the psoriatic dermatitis and it progresses with specific bouts, bearing no relation to the clinical course or gravity of the skin changes. Involvement of the ankle joint and mostly of the subtalar joint. Calcanean psoriatic bone lesions (see **1266, 1267**).

1157. Tuberculous arthritis : demineralization of the whole foot. Slight narrowing of the posterior talo-calcanean joint. Small cyst-like areas of bone rarefaction.

1158. Tuberculous arthritis. More advanced stage : narrowing of the whole joint space. Cystic osteolysis of the talus.

TARSUS ANTERIOR

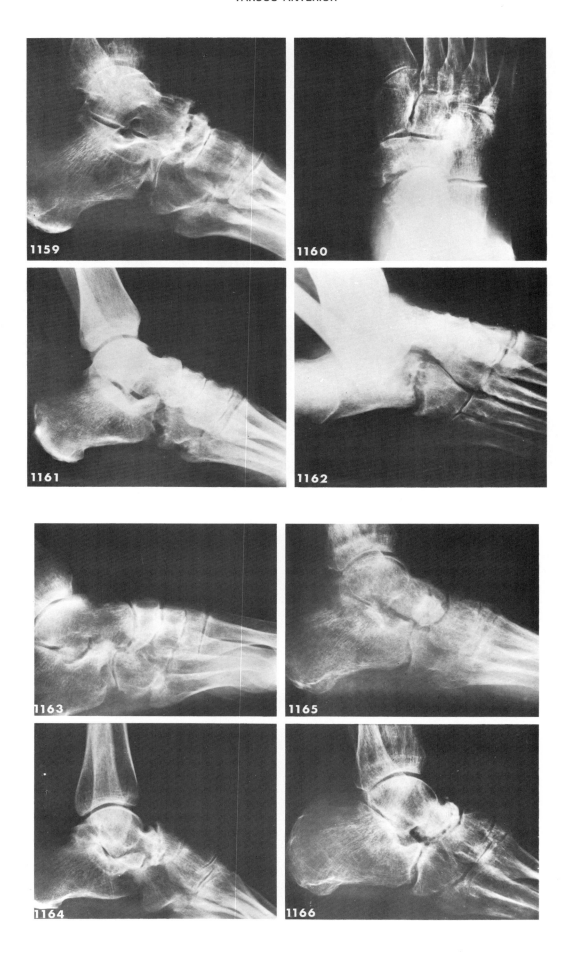

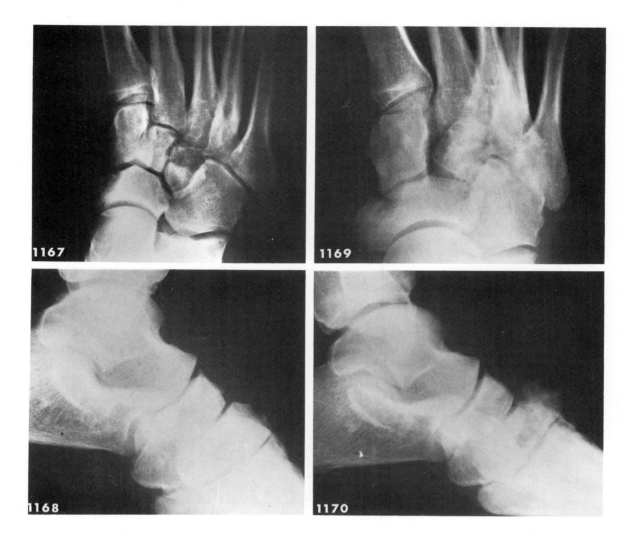

1159 → 1162. Rheumatoid arthritis.

1159. Rheumatoid arthritis : demineralization of the entire foot. Cartilage erosions of the articular margins of the talonavicular joint and disappearance of the joint cavity. Cyst-like radiolucent areas of the talar neck. Necrotic changes of the navicular bone. Narrowing of other joint spaces.

1160. Rheumatoid arthritis : frontal view. Narrowing of the lateral part of the talonavicular joint and cartilaginous erosions of its margins. Cyst-like radiolucent bone lesions of the navicular.

1161, 1162. Rheumatoid arthritis. Lateral and oblique views. Chopart joint : complete narrowing of the talonavicular joint ; erosions of both articular margins of the calcaneocuboid joint with widening of the interarticular space.

1163. Psoriasis : diffuse bone rarefaction of the whole foot. The intraarticular spaces of the talonavicular and cuneonavicular joints are irregular.

1164. Rheumatoid arthritis in a 30-year-old woman. Cyst-like radiolucent areas of the talus, narrowing of the subtalar joint : talar head deformed, talonavicular joint narrowed with erosions of both its articular margins.

1165, 1166. Tuberculosis.

1165. Generalized bony rarefaction, cystic osteolysis and transverse radiolucent metaphyseal bands in the tibia. Scrappy navicular. Narrowing of the superior part of the calcaneocuboid joint.

1166. Radiograph 2 years later. Bony remineralization. Osteosclerosis of both sides of the calcaneocuboid joint which itself is spared. Collapse of the talar head and complete necrosis of the navicular.

1167 → 1170. Diabetic arthropathy.

1167, 1168. Gout and diabetes mellitus in a 50-year-old man, inadequately treated. Lisfranc joint is narrowed and irregular. Cyst-like bone lesions of the navicular ; articular puncture by needle removes an aseptic exudate.

1169, 1170. Same patient. Advanced stage 1 month later. Destruction of the tarsus with enucleation of the second cuneiform ; another puncture is aseptic.

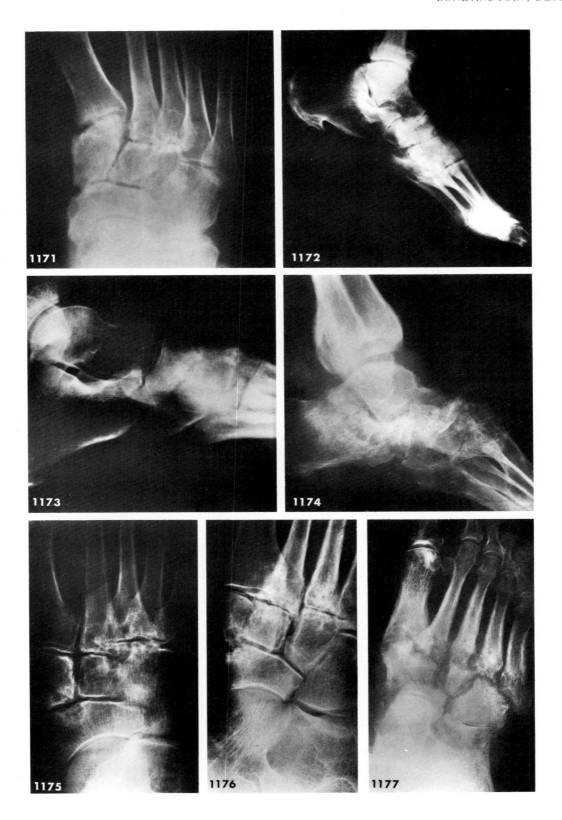

1171. Rheumatoid arthritis : narrowed interarticular spaces with irregular and hazy margins.

1172. Rheumatoid arthritis : all joint spaces of the anterior tarsus are involved.

1173. Chronic atrophic polychondritis : bone rarefaction, involvement of the cuneonavicular and Lisfranc joints with subchondral osteosclerosis.

1174. Tuberculosis : diffuse demineralization, swelling of the soft tissues, tarsal destruction and tibial periosteal reaction.

1175, 1176. Tuberculous arthritis : cyst-like bone lesions, cartilage destruction, narrowing of the interarticular spaces of the cuneonavicular and cuneometatarsal joints, but with well-delineated borders. No periosteal reaction. These early radiographic appearances are misleading.

1177. Diabetes mellitus : extensive bone and joint destruction of the anterior tarsus.

METATARSOPHALANGEAL JOINT OF THE GREAT TOE

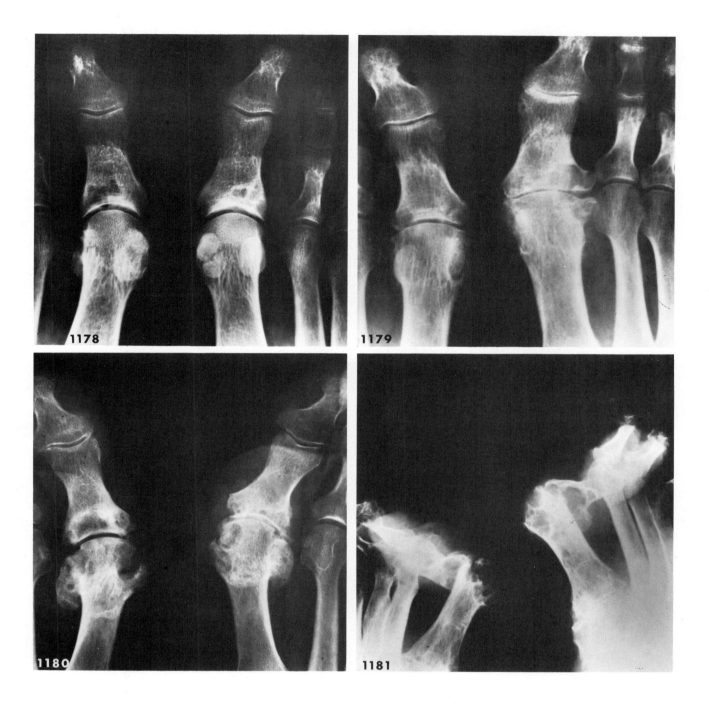

1178 → 1181. Gout : the primary gouty form occurs especially in men, the secondary form in various metabolic disorders. This condition is characterized by deposition of crystalline sodium urate in poorly vascularized tissues, like the tendons or the articular cartilage which are first eroded, then destroyed. The metatarsophalangeal joint of the great toe is especially involved.

1178. Gout : cyst-like bone lesions of the base of the proximal phalanx of the great toe. No articular narrowing. No osteoporosis.

1179. Gout : subchondral cyst-like bone lesions of both sides of the first metatarsophalangeal joint. Note the radiographic appearance of the right foot simulating a chondroma. Narrowing of the joint spaces. No demineralization.

1180. Gout : cyst-like intraosseous lesions and bony erosions. Destruction of the joint. Preservation of mineralization. Tophus in the soft tissues.

1181. Gout : large punched-out joint. Marginal defects. Destruction of the epiphyses and dislocation.

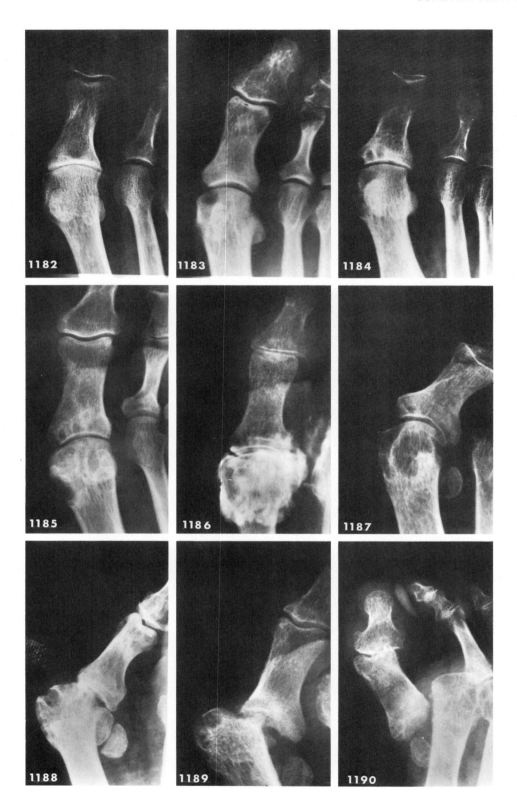

1182 → 1190. Rheumatoid arthritis.

1182. Complete narrowing of the joint space.

1183. Cystic resorption in the subchondral bone. The interarticular space is spared.

1184. Cystic bone rarefaction and cortical erosions, narrowing of the joint space.

1185. Subchondral bone cysts. Cortical erosions, narrowing of the joint cavity.

1186. Arthrography at the time of a synoviorthesis : irregularities of the articular capsule due to the proliferative synovitis.

1187. Pseudocystic subchondral bone lesions of the first metatarsal head with outward angulation of the phalanx. Uninvolved joint space.

1188. Multiple metatarsal cyst-like bone lesions and erosions. Hallux valgus.

1189. Epiphyseal cystic osteolysis and destruction with outward dislocation in valgus.

1190. Epiphyseal destruction and complete inward dislocation in varus.

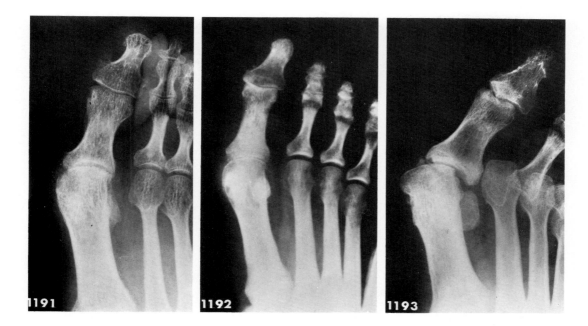

1191. Ankylosing spondylitis (Strümpell-Marie disease). Inflammatory axial rheumatism affecting young adults and progressing to bony ankylosis. This condition is primary. A similar condition is associated with psoriasis, Reiter syndrome, or intestinal disorders. In these disorders, the extremities are more frequently involved. In the initial phase of the disease, the foot is involved in 20 % of the cases, especially the metatarso-phalangeal joints and the calcaneus (**1264, 1265**).

Ankylosing spondylitis in a 32-year-old man : diffuse rarefaction, narrowing of the joint space of the great toe. Small bone erosions of the head of the first metatarsal and the proximal phalanx.

1192. Chronic atrophic polychondritis. Radiolucent bands of osteolysis, complete narrowing of the metatarsophalangeal and interphalangeal joints of the great toe.

1193. Psoriasis : narrowing of the metatarsophalangeal and interphalangeal joints of the great toe, small bone erosions, valgus angulation, dislocation of the second toe.

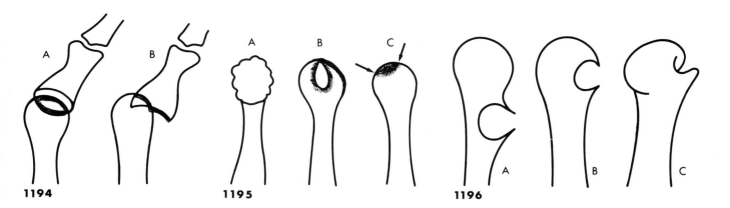

1194. A - Static clawing of a toe. B - Subluxation (rheumatoid polyarthritis) : seagull sign.

1195. A - Aseptic necrosis. B - Degenerative cyst-like bone lesion. C - Osteochondritis (the arrow shows the stress lines).

1196. A. - Gout : extraarticular cyst-like bone defect. B. - Inflammatory or infective granuloma : intraarticular cyst-like bone lesion. C - Picture of an apparent cystic lesion : tubercle for insertion of the lateral ligament on the metatarsal head (oblique view).

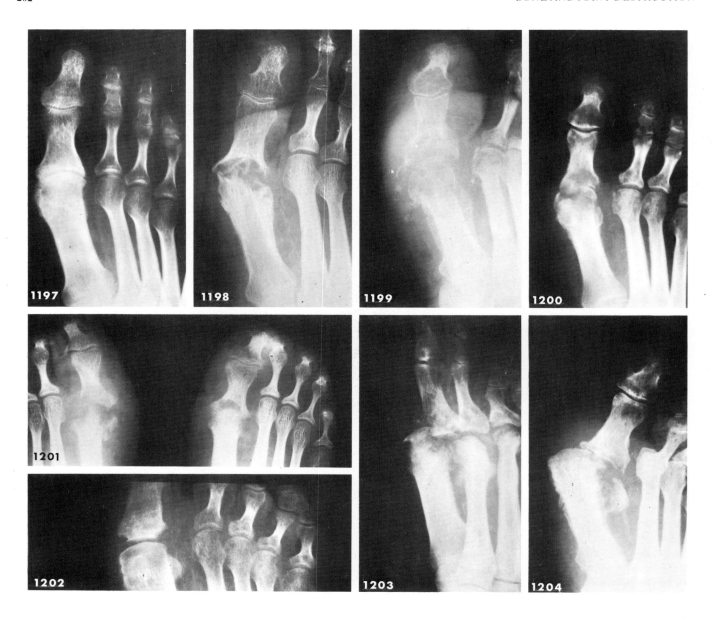

1197. Polyarteritis nodosa (Kussmaul-Maier disease) : a condition characterized by inflammation and necrosis of medium-sized and small arteries. Small cyst-like bone lesions of the first metatarsal head with complete narrowing of the joint space.

1198. Diabetes : septic arthritis following a wound. Destruction of the first metatarsal head and the opposite phalangeal base. Periosteal hyperostosis of the diaphyses. Arterial calcification.

1199. Thevenard disease : arthritis associated with a perforating ulcer. Marked swelling of the soft tissues of the great toe. Cyst-like areas of osteolysis and disappearance of the metatarsophalangeal joints. Diaphyseal periosteal reaction of the first metatarsal. Early involvement of the second ray.

1200. Pyogenic arthritis of the metatarsophalangeal joint of the great toe. Bony rarefaction, cystic osteolysis, disappearance of the joint space.

1201. Brucellosis : undulant fever (melitococcosis) is a universal endemic bacterial disease displaying two kinds of clinical manifestations : either acute septicemia or a subacute form with visceral, articular and osseous localizations. Arthritis of both metatarsophalangeal joints. Swelling of the soft tissues, bony destruction, disappearance of the joint spaces.

1202. Tuberculous arthritis of the first metatarsophalangeal joint. Swelling of soft tissues. Diffuse rarefaction of the forefoot. Cystic osteolysis of the first metatarsal head with bone erosions of the opposite phalangeal base. No narrowing of the joint space of which the margins are spared and well-delineated : misleading radiographic findings.

1203. Mycosis. Small cyst-like bone lesions of the distal phalanx of the great toe with destruction and dislocation of the metatarsophalangeal joint. Diaphyseal erosions and periosteal reaction. Involvement of the adjacent joints and osteosclerosis of the second metatarsal shaft.

1204. Mycosis : another case.

FIFTH METATARSOPHALANGEAL JOINT

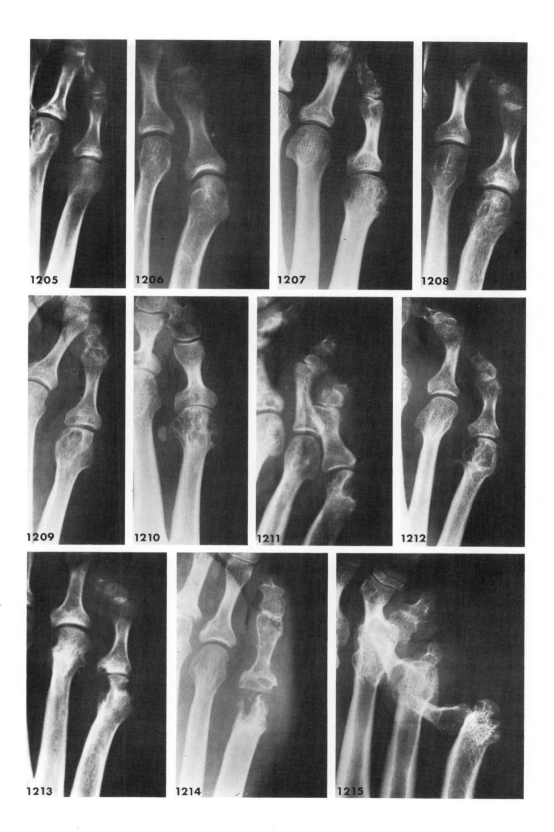

1205 → 1215. Rheumatoid arthritis. The involvement of the fifth metatarsal head is frequent, is often an early radiographic finding and is sometimes the only visible bone lesion (Coste-Braun).

1205. Stage 1 : simple osteoporosis in the lateral and plantar sides of the condyle of the fifth metatarsal.

1206, 1207. Stage 2 : cyst-like bone lesions of varying size.

1208 → 1210. Stage 3 : cyst-like bone defects and erosions giving a nibbled appearance to the metatarsal head.

1211 → 1213. Stage 4 : large bone erosions, leading to incomplete destruction of the metatarsal head.

1214, 1215. Stage 5 : complete destruction of the metatarsal head and dislocation.

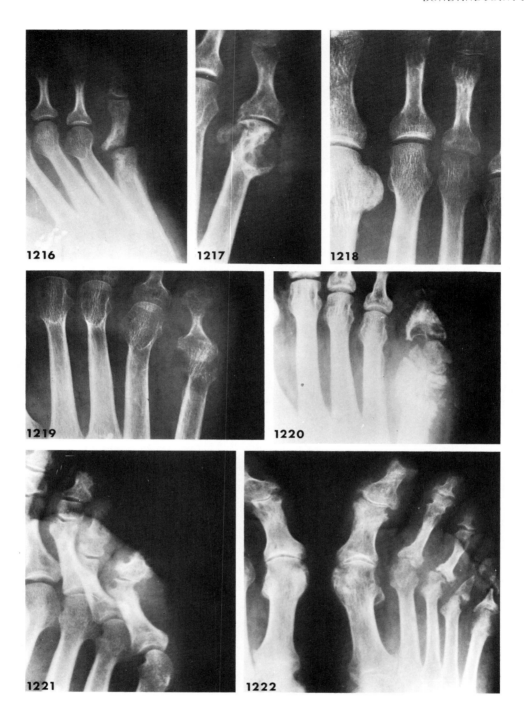

1216. Diabetes : perforating ulcer with pyogenic arthritis destroying the metatarsophalangeal joint of the fifth toe with diaphyseal laminated periosteal elevation.

1217. Gout : small cyst-like bone resorption and deep erosive notch of the fifth metatarsal head with large tophus in the soft tissues.

1218. Septic arthritis of the third metatarsophalangeal joint : diffuse rarefaction of both sides of the narrowed joint space.

1219. Septic arthritis by anaerobic organism : destruction of the fifth metatarsal head with gaseous radiolucent areas in the soft tissues (see same case 1453).

1220. Tertiary syphilitic osteitis : admixture of osteosclerotic and osteolytic lesions of the fifth toe. Cystic punched-out bone defects of the phalangeal base, destruction of the metatarsal head with periosteal reaction and hypertrophic bone formation.

1221. Psoriasis : interphalangeal distal arthritis of the fifth toe. Punched-out bone notches of the proximal phalangeal head. Pagoda-like cortical hyperostosis of the distal phalanx.

1222. Psoriasis : demineralization of the whole foot. Destruction of the interphalangeal joints of the fourth and fifth toes with tapered proximal phalanx and flared distal phalanx : « pencil-pointing and cupping » shape. Ankylosis of the interphalangeal joint of the second and third toes. The admixture of interphalangeal destructive arthritides and ankyloses at the same forefoot is pathognomonic of psoriasis (A. Fournié).

INTERPHALANGEAL JOINTS

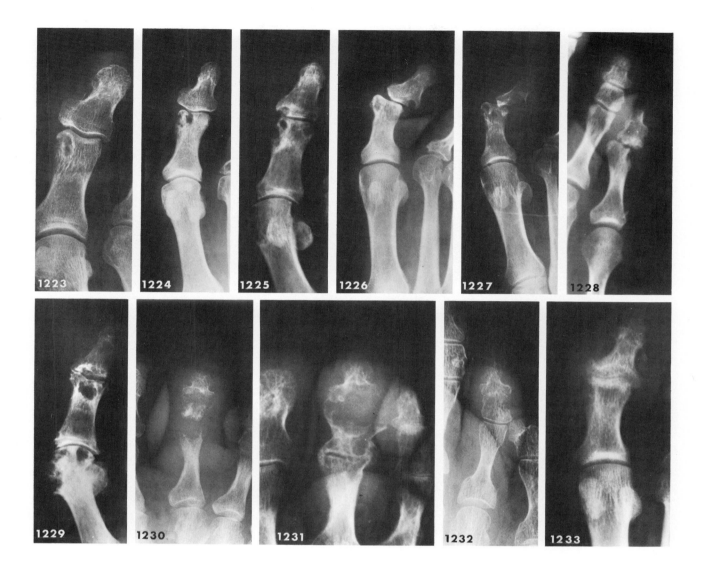

1223 → 1225. Rheumatoid arthritis : involvement of the interphalangeal joint of the great toe. Various radiographic findings.

1223. Solitary cyst-like area of radiolucency surrounded by a fine osteosclerotic border.

1224. Punched-out cortical defect of the head of the proximal phalanx and cartilage erosion.

1225. Multiple cystic bone lesions and erosions of both sides of the joint. Similar radiographic appeareances at the level of the metatarsophalangeal joint.

1226, 1227. Psoriasis : involvement of the interphalangeal joint of the great toe.

1226. Cyst-like bone defects of the head of the proximal phalanx. Erosions of the base of the distal phalanx with dislocation.

1227. Same patient, 2 years later.

1228. Rheumatoid arthritis of the proximal interphalangeal joint of the fifth toe. Juxta-articular erosions, narrowing of the joint space and subluxation.

1229 → 1231. Gout.

1229. Cystic bone lesions and punched-out erosions of the metatarsophalangeal and interphalangeal joints of the great toe. Narrowing of the joint spaces. No bone rarefaction.

1230. Second toe : swelling of the soft tissues with joint destruction.

1231. Second toe : large cystic punched-out erosion, with bone expansion giving a blister-like shape to the middle and distal phalanges. This radiographic appearance is characteristic of gouty lesions.

1232. Felon of the fourth toe with secondary septic arthritis. Swelling of soft tissues, bone rarefaction and cystic osteolysis of the middle and distal phalanges, disappearance of the joint cavity.

1233. Staphylococcal arthritis of the interphalangeal joint of the great toe. Bone rarefaction, narrowing of the joint space of which the margins are hazy.

GENERAL PATTERN OF RHEUMATOID LESIONS OF THE FOOT

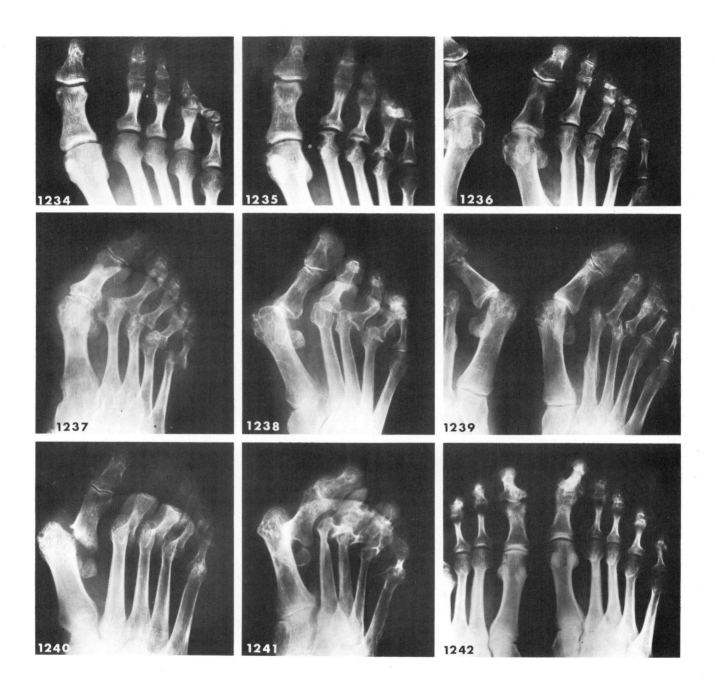

1234, 1235. Example of radiological changes in a polyarthritis involving the metatarsal heads. Fourteen months between these two radiographs.

1236. Rheumatoid arthritis : multiple cystic bone lesions of the metatarsal heads. Joints uninvolved. No dislocation.

1237. Rheumatoid arthritis : at the level of metatarsal heads, one sees cystic bone lesions, erosions, notching bone defects, bone resorption. At the level of joints, various pathologic appearances : simple narrowing or complete destruction of the joint space.

The toes are dislocated and outwardly angulated as if they were bent by the wind (« fibular blast »).

1238. Rheumatoid arthritis in a triangular static forefoot : small cystic-bone lesions and erosions of the metatarsal heads. Dislocation of the third and fourth toes.

1239. Rheumatoid arthritis : typical metatarsophalangeal joint lesions. Callus of a diaphyseal fracture of both second toes (due to osteoporosis by corticotherapy).

1240, 1241. Rheumatoid arthritis : marked destruction and dislocations.

1242. Psoriatic arthritis of the interphalangeal joint of both great toes : combined ankylosis and bone resorption.

BONY ANKYLOSES

Acquired disappearance of the intraarticular space between two adjacent bones. This fusion
results from numerous causes : above all the arthritides.

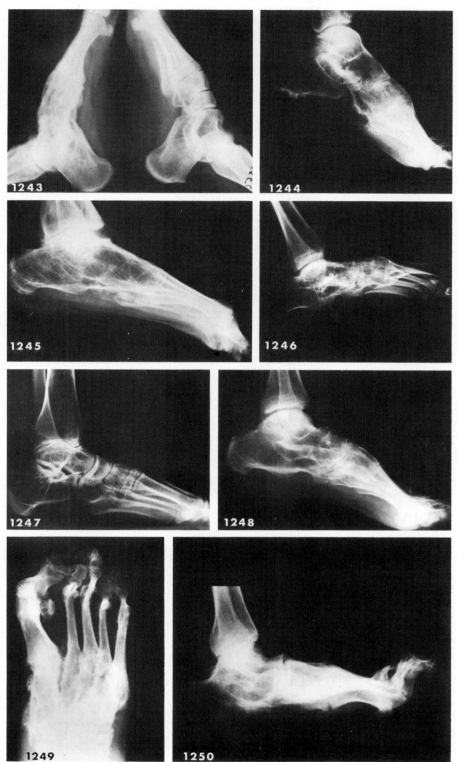

1243 → 1245. Rheumatoid arthritis : bony ankyloses.

1243. Fusion of the anterior and posterior tarsus of the left foot. Right foot normal.

1244. Fusion of the anterior tarsus with fibrillar reticulated trabecular architecture. Plantar calcaneal spur formation.

1245. Fusion of the anterior and posterior tarsus. Fibrillar and cyst-like bony architecture.

1246. Cerebral palsy : tarsal fusion.

1247. Sequela of tuberculosis : incomplete ankylosis of the ankle.

1248. Rheumatoid arthritis : fusion of the subtalar, Chopart and Lisfranc joint spaces. Talonavicular arthritis in process of fusion.

1249, 1250. Fiessinger-Leroy-Reiter disease.

This condition may be caused by a germ of *Bedsonia* species and is characterized by diarrhea, urethritis, iridocyclitis and arthritis, which appear in that order. The bone and joint localizations of this disease are axial or peripheral, progressing slowly to ankylosis of the involved joints.

Bone fusions with osteosclerosis and hyperostosis. The radiographic findings were formerly considered sequelae of gonococcal polyarthritis. Note also the calcaneal cystic osteolysis.

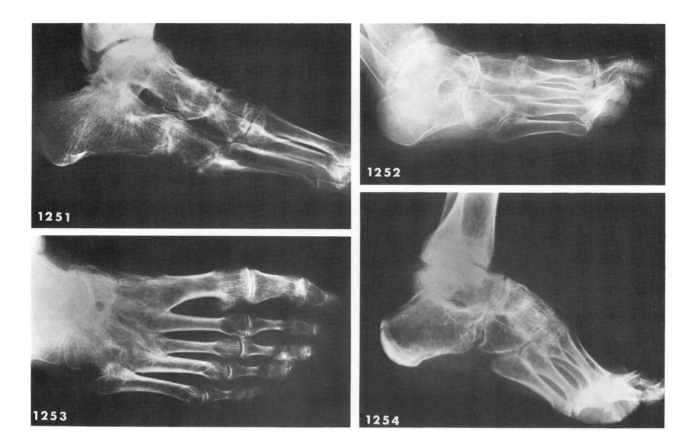

1251. Ankylosis of the talo-navicular, calcaneo-cuboid and postero-talo-calcanean joints, 2 years after an open fracture of the ankle.

1252. Sequela in a 15-year-old child with juvenile rheumatoid arthritis : ankylosis of the tarsometatarsal joints.

1253. Sequela in a 24-year-old patient with juvenile rheumatoid arthritis : pes cavus due to ankylosis of the anterior tarsus. Arthritis of the ankle, the subtalar and Chopart joints.

1254. Poliomyelitis : tarsometatarsal ankylosis.

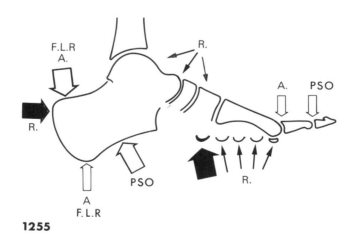

1255. Diagram which illustrates the more important and characteristic foci of inflammatory arthritis involving the foot.
F.L.R. : Fiessinger - Leroy - Reiter.
R. : Rheumatoid arthritis.
PSO : Psoriasis.
A. : Ankylosis, arthritis.

13

HYPERTROPHIC BONY CHANGES AND EROSIONS OF THE TUBER CALCANEI

The unique anatomy of the calcaneus with its tuber calcanei where the Achilles tendon inserts, and with its numerous subtendinous synovial bursae, explains the frequency of involvement of this bone with both inflammatory and degenerative disorders of the foot.

INFLAMMATORY CALCANEITIS

1256 → 1261. Rheumatoid arthritis.

The rheumatoid pannus involves the plantar bursa of Lenoir or the Achilles bursa in about 20 % of cases, but only the invasion of adjacent bones produces radiographic changes (14 % of cases). The talalgia is the first sign of the disease in 1 to 2 % of cases. The Achilles bursitis is the most characteristic.

Its radiological features are, first, a localized bone rarefaction, later a cyst-like osteolysis of the posterior edge of the tuber calcanei, sparing its superior margin and giving it a capped appearance. The absence of periosteal reaction and of hypertrophic bone formation differentiate this rheumatoid calcaneitis from the other calcaneal bone lesions. The plantar bursitis is less frequent.

1256. Posterior calcaneitis : single bone erosion, well-delineated by a fine line of osteosclerosis.

1257. Postero-superior calcaneitis : posterior bone erosion adjacent to normal overhanging bone, and superior second bone erosion.

1258. Posterior calcaneitis : cystic osteolysis.

1259. Plantar calcaneitis ; cyst-like bone defects between which uninvolved bone persists, simulating spur formation.

1260, 1261. Posterior calcaneitis. **1260.** Bone notch crowned by the « calcaneal ». **1261.** At the time of a synoviorthesis, opacification of the Achilles bursa was responsible for the bone erosion.

1262, 1263. Reiter disease.

This condition affects the foot in 78 % of cases, the most frequent localization being the calcaneus (62 % of cases) and the metatarsus (16 % of cases).

The combination of the two clinical symptoms talalgia-metatarsalgia is almost pathognomonic. At the level of the calcaneus, the radiographic findings are an admixture of osteolysis and plantar and posteriorly oriented bony spurring similar to the calcaneal alteration of ankylosing spondylitis.

1262. Reiter disease : calcaneitis with mixed radiographic changes. Posterosuperior bone erosion. Inferior bone erosion with plantar periosteal reaction.

1263. Reiter disease : same changes. Posterosuperior bone erosion. Inferior periosteal reaction with a coated osteosclerotic plantar aspect of the calcaneus.

1264, 1265. Ankylosing spondylitis. The talalgia, isolated or associated with a rachialgia, is a very frequent early sign of this condition. The calcanean radiographic findings are the following :

— various, nonspecific, structural osseous alterations : bony rarefaction or osteosclerosis, flat bony erosion or cystic osteolysis ;

— growing bone formation, more suggestive :

• calcaneal spurs : posterior and mostly plantar, irregular, illdefined. Their unexpected appearance in a young subject and their heterogenous appearance allow differentiation from the common calcaneal spurs of the older patients ;

• periostitis : downy laminated periosteal elevation (shaggy bearded calcaneus of Forestier) or irregular corticoperiosteal thickening of the calcanean posterior border (armour-plate shape) and of the calcaneal plantar aspect (coating-shape).

1264. Posterior calcaneitis : osteosclerosis and cystic osteolysis.

1265. Posterior calcaneitis : cystic osteolysis, posterior calcanean armour, plantar calcaneal spur.

1266, 1267. Psoriasis : the psoriatic osseous lesions are frequent in the foot, especially at the level of the forefoot and the calcaneus. The calcaneal radiographic changes are varied and nonspecific, the growing bone formations prevailing over the bone destruction, eg the irregular, « bristly » calcaneus of A. Fournie. One may see posterior and plantar calcanean spurs with an inflammatory radiographic appearance, erosions, irregular armour-like thickening, etc.

1266. Bone erosions of the posterior aspect of the calcaneus. Plantar calcaneal spur.

1267. Posterior and plantar calcaneal spurs, coating-like thickening of the posterior edge of the calcaneus and armour-like rough thickening of its plantar aspect.

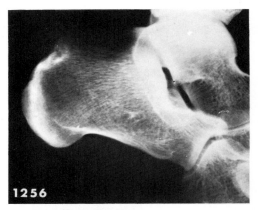

1256

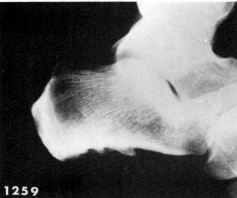

1259

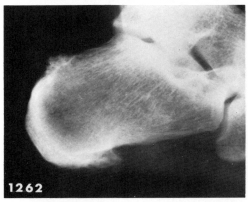

1262

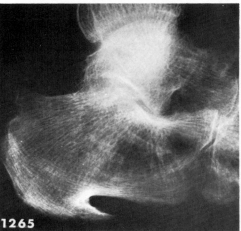

1265

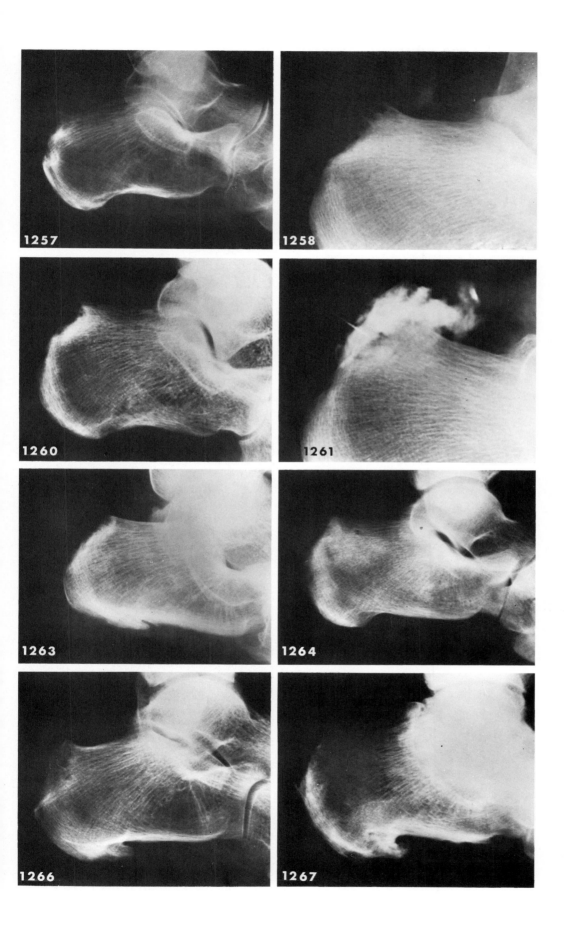

RADIOGRAPHIC APPEARANCE
OF METABOLIC CHANGES
IN THE CALCANEUS

1268, 1269. Chondrocalcinosis (pseudogout) : associated with the calcification of cartilage. Tendinous and aponeurotic calcifications are often described and bring up the nosologic problem of differentiation from other calcifying diseases : periarthritis, tumoral calcinosis, hydroxyapatite deposition.

1268. Chondrocalcinosis with hemochromatosis : linear deposit of calcium salts along the anterior border of the Achille tendon.

1269. Chondrocalcinosis : advanced stage.

1270. Calcifying polyperiarthritis : a condition characterized by acute arthralgia simulating gout, with hydroxyapatite crystals in the synovial fluid (hydroxyapatite rheumatism of B. Amor). The X-ray examination shows periarticular and tendinous calcifications. Calcification of the tendinous insertions on the posterior tuberosity of the calcaneus with shield-like corticoperiosteal reaction.

1271 → 1275. Gout : this condition involves the calcaneus less frequently than the forefoot, producing characteristic sharp osteophytes and sometimes an armoured posterior aspect of the calcaneus.

1276. Localized nodular deposits of calcium salts in the sole of the foot during chronic renal insufficiency.

1277. Gout : tophus eroding the superior edge of the calcaneus.

INFECTIVE CALCANEITIS

1278. Infective streptococcal calcaneitis.

1279. Subcalcaneal perforating ulcer : « bristle-like » periosteal reaction.

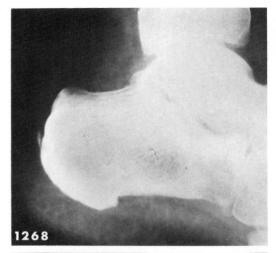
1268

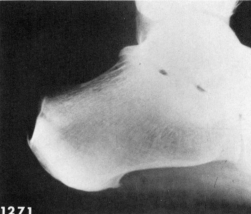
1271

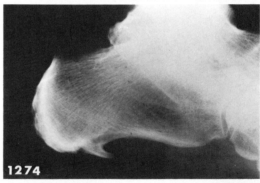
1274

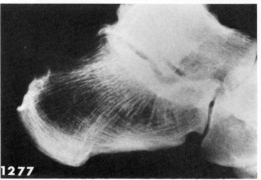
1277

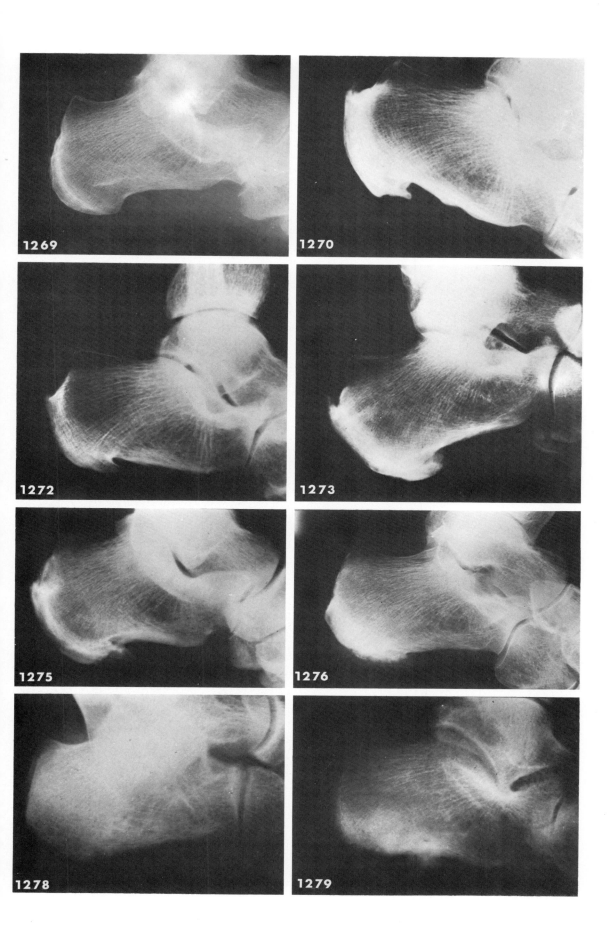

OSTEOPHYTES AT THE MYOTENDINOUS INSERTIONS LEVEL

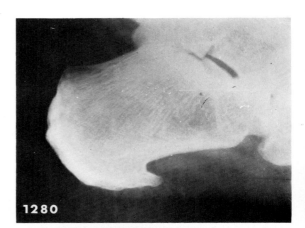

1280 → 1283. The common calcaneal exostosis of the adult gives a picture of a growing *bone* spur with a cortex and a marrow. This characteristic distinguishes it from the paraosseous ossifications or calcifications : tendinous, aponeurotic or ligamentous (see page 250). This exostosis is implanted on the calcaneal inferior aspect at the insertion of the plantar aponeurosis (plantar calcaneal spur), or on its posterior aspect at the Achilles tendon insertion (posterior calcanean spur).

1284. Acromegaly : plantar spur and armoured posterior aspect of the calcaneus. Thickening of the plantar pad (see 1455).

1285. Large posterior calcaneal spur.

1286. Gross plantar calcaneal spur.

1287, 1288. Incomplete fracture of the tuber calcanei : 1287. The lateral view may lead to misinterpretation : calcaneal spur ; 1288. The axial view shows the fracture.

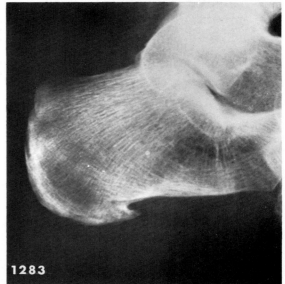

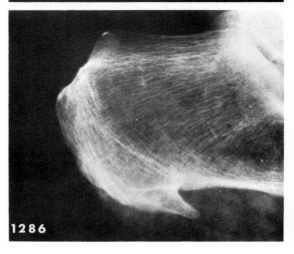

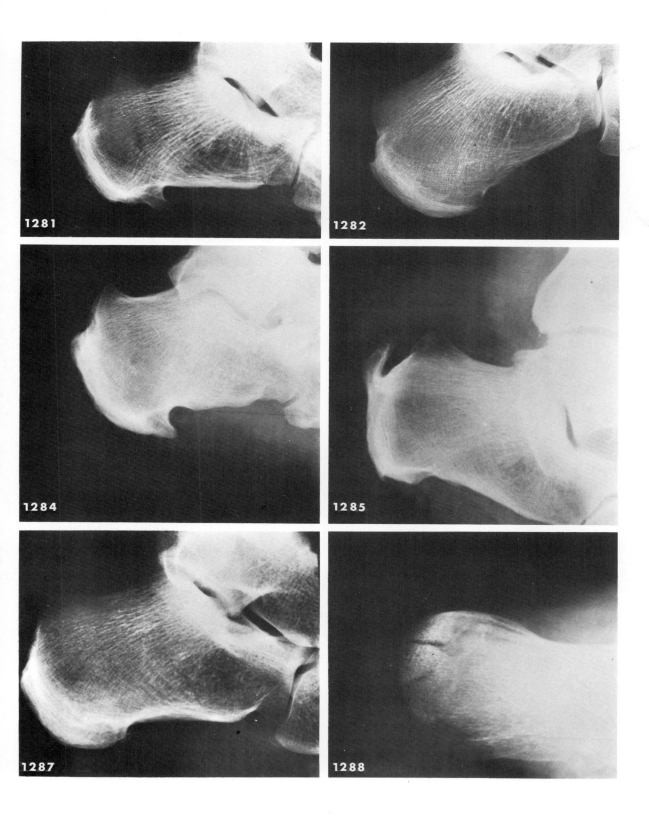

VARIOUS SHAPES

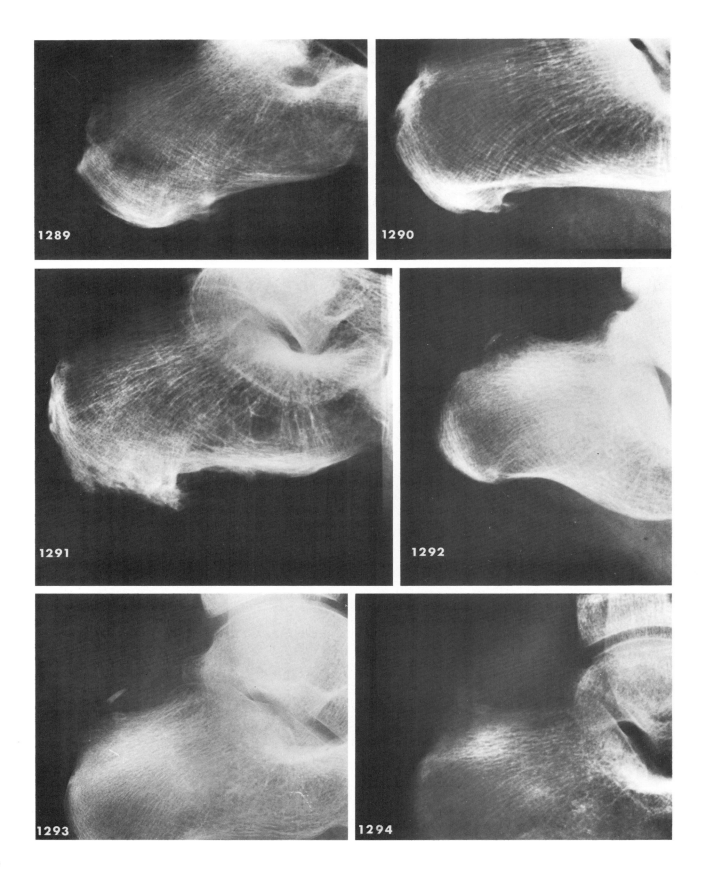

1289, 1290. Fracture of a subcalcanean spur.

1291. Irregular subcalcanean armoured and coated hyperostosis. Unknown etiology.

1292 → 1294. Staphylococcal posterosuperior calcanean osteomyelitis : detached sequestrum, evolution in 2-months.

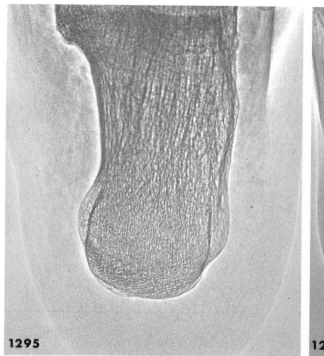
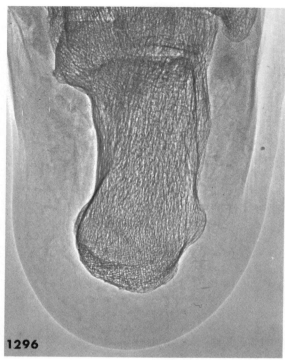

1295, 1296. Strict axial view of the calcaneus.

1295. Normal calcaneus.

1296. Postero-lateral exostosis.

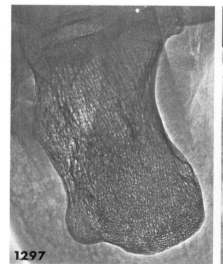
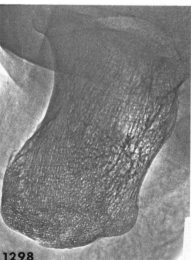
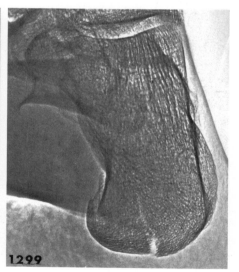

1297 → 1299. Axial view of the calcaneus (same patient).

1297, 1298. Inferior postero-lateral tuberosity of the calcaneus visible when the heels are placed in varus (false exostosis).

1299. A more marked varus shows the fracture of the right tuber calcanei.

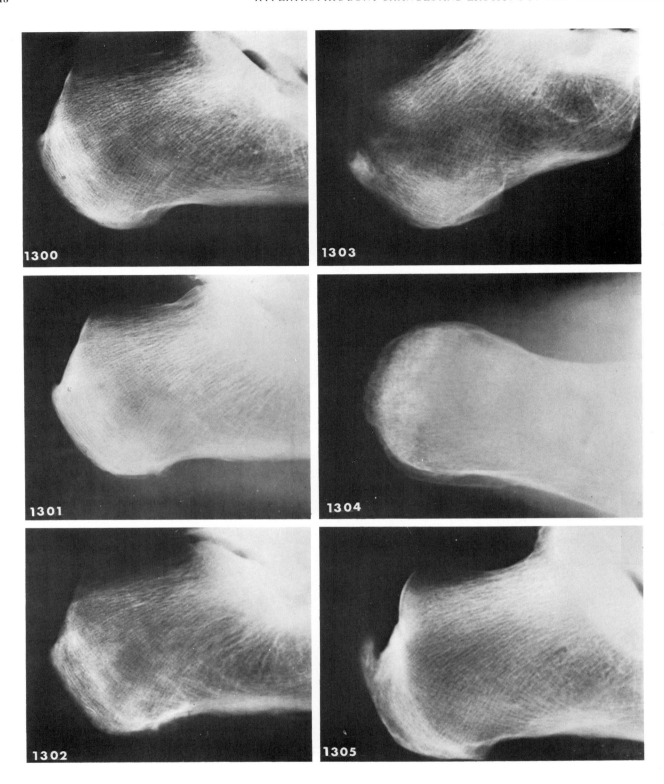

Examples showing the need for various radiographic projections

1300 → 1302. Same case.

1300. *Latero-medial* projection : normal picture.

1301. *Medio-lateral* projection : early detectable change.

1302. Latero-medial projection, 1 year later : plantar periostitis.

1303 → 1305. Same case, patient suffering from a talalgia.

1303. Lateral radiograph with the patient in *erect position :* postero-superior erosion of the calcaneus.

1304. Axial view : posterior osteosclerosis.

1305. Lateral radiograph with the *patient recumbent :* large posterior calcaneal exostosis with « bristly » corticoperiosteal reaction.

14

HYPERTROPHIC DEGENERATIVE CHANGES

This chapter unites the osseous or osseocartilaginous formations either situated far from the joints, eg the exostoses, or periarticular and intraarticular, eg the osteophytes of the arthritides.

These last bony outgrowths proceed from endochondral ossification of preformed cartilaginous tissue, with or without subperiosteal periarticular osteogenesis. These degenerative hypertrophic bone changes associated with cartilage erosion, subchondral bone osteosclerosis and cyst-like areas in epiphyseal spongiosa substantia characterize degenerative osteoarthritis. The radiologic findings in degenerative osteoarthritis are narrowing of the joint space, subchondral osteosclerosis, cyst-like areas, and osteophytes.

ANKLE JOINT

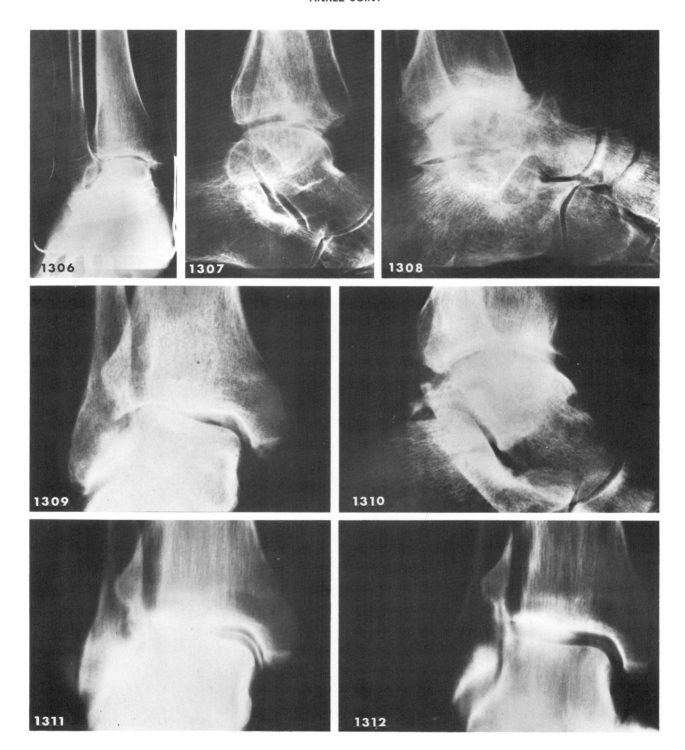

The arthrosis of the ankle is rare, always secondary, often post-traumatic.

1306. Arthrosis of the ankle joint in a 26-year-old patient, complicating healed juvenile rheumatoid arthritis.

1307. Early arthrosis of the ankle joint following posterior marginal fracture of the tibia with displaced fragments. Narrowing of the anterior part of the joint space with osteophytes.

1308. Marked arthrosis of the ankle joint after crush injury of the talus due to a fall from a height of 6 meters.

1309 → 1312. Same case. Arthrosis complicating repeated sprains in a 55-year-old sportsman.

1309. Frontal view : narrowing of the lateral part of the joint space.

1310. Lateral view : marginal osteophytes.

1311, 1312. Arthrogram : **1311.** Localized thinning of the articular cartilage (lateral part) ; **1312.** Stress film demonstrating the loss of cartilaginous substance.

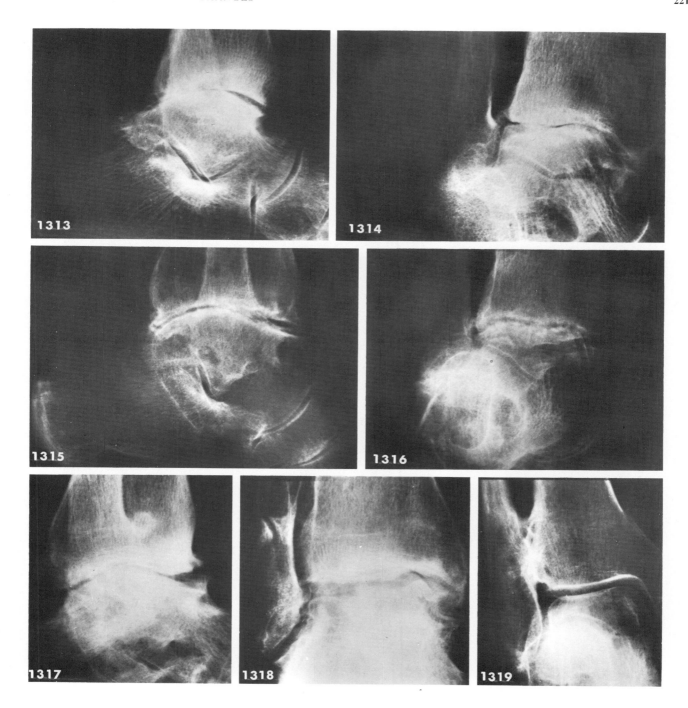

1313, 1314. Arthrosis of the ankle joint, frontal and lateral view. Narrowing of the joint space, more marked posteriorly. Subchondral osteosclerosis and cyst formation. Marginal osteophytes (unknown cause).

1315, 1316. Arthrosis of the ankle joint complicating rheumatoid arthritis. Similar to the above case, but the osteosclerosis is less marked.

1317, 1318. Arthrosis of the ankle joint after healing of a septic arthritis.

1319. Distal tibio-fibular synostosis.

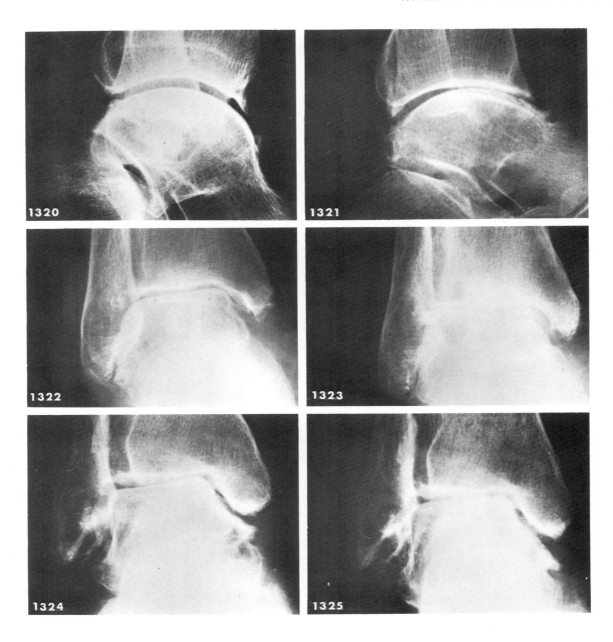

1320. Gout : sharp osteophytes.

1321 → 1323. Arthrosis complicating a chrondrocalcinosis. Same patient.

1321, 1322. Frontal and lateral views : anterior arthrosis.

1323. Frontal view, 3 years later : significant progression with large cyst-like bone lesions.

1324, 1325. Arthrosis complicating chondrocalcinosis : same patient, 3 years between the two radiographs : slight progression.

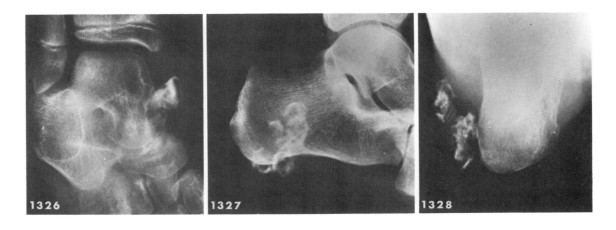

1326. Post-traumatic osteochondroma in a 10-year-old girl, under the medial malleolus.

1327, 1328. Ossification in the plantar soft tissues, probably of a hematoma.

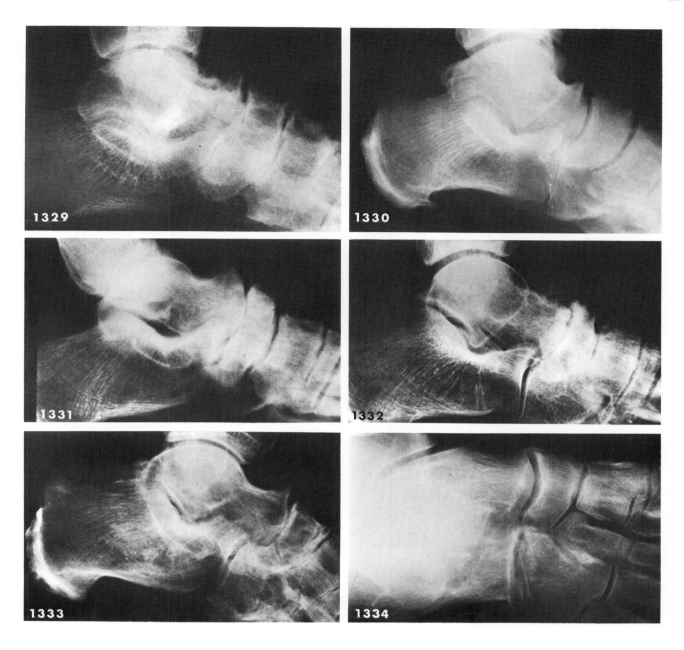

1329. Gout : narrowing of all the interarticular spaces of the foot ; spicular bone formation and osteophytes constituting the classical shape of the « spiked foot ».

1330. Gout : talonavicular sharp osteophytes, facing each other ; posterior and plantar calcaneal bony outgrowths ; subtalar arthrosis.

1331, 1332. Sequela of rheumatoid arthritis. Arthrosis of the talonavicular joint with marked dorsal osteophytosis.

1333. Arthrosis of the talonavicular, cuneonavicular and subtalar joints : narrowing of the posterior talocalcanean space.

1334. Arthrosis of the calcaneocuboid joint.

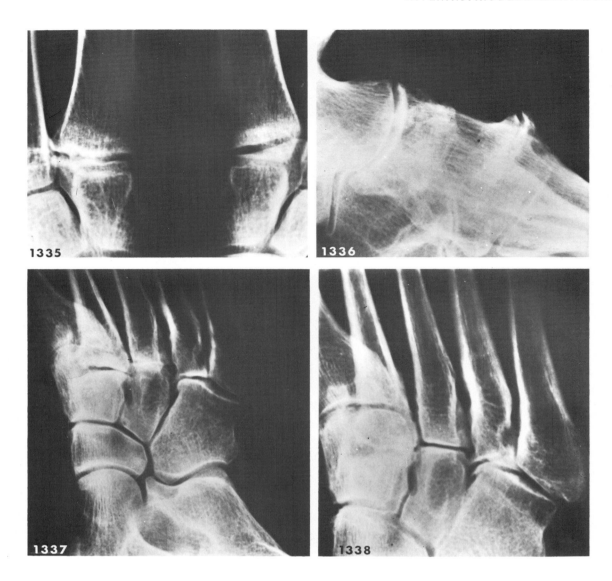

1335. Arthrosis of the left cuneo-first metatarsal joint with narrowing of the interarticular space.

1336. Arthrosis of the cuneo-first metatarsal joint. Osteophytes of the dorsum of the foot in a pes cavus varus.

1337, 1338. Arthrosis of the Lisfranc joint.

1337. Narrowing of the interarticular spaces.

1338. Magnified view : spur bone formation involving the fourth metatarsal.

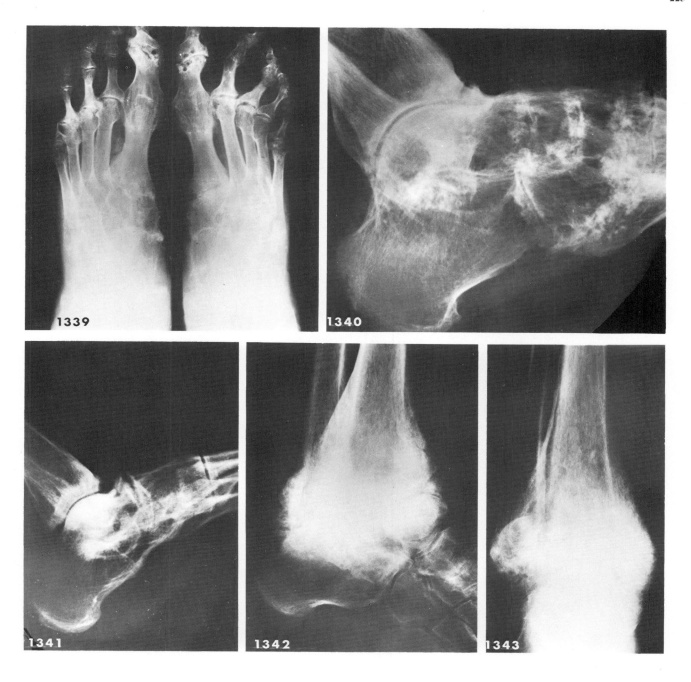

1339, 1340. Gout and diabetes. Complete or incomplete disappearance of numerous joint spaces. Osteolysis of left fifth toe, gouty lesions of the interphalangeal joints of both big toes. Articular and arterial calcifications.

1341. Arthrosis of the ankle and the talonavicular joints after healing of subtalar tuberculosis : disappearance of the subtalar, cuneonavicular and anterior tarsal joints.

1342, 1343. Tabes : dislocation of the ankle joint ; large tibial epiphysis with marked osteocondensation and periostosis : « arthrosis caricature ».

METATARSUS

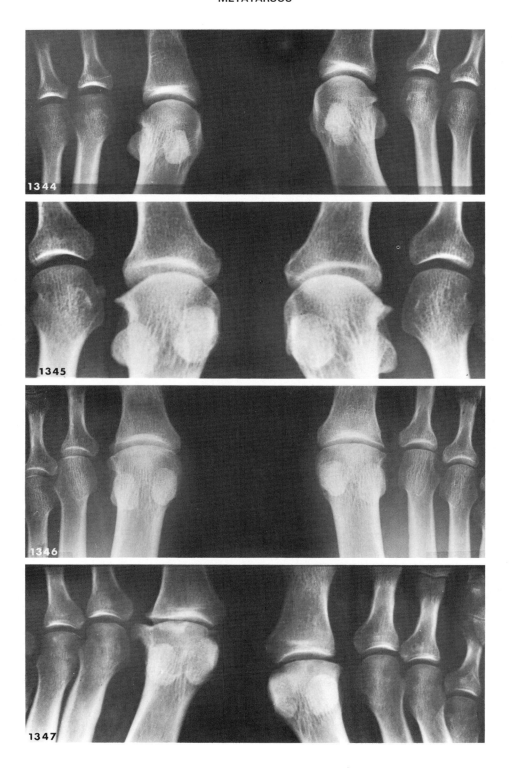

Hallux rigidus : this clinical definition applies to an arthrosis of the metatarsophalangeal and metatarsosesamoid joints of the great toe, without angulation, in contrast to the hallux valgus.

1344 → 1347. Hallux rigidus : early radiographic findings.

1344. Small spur bone formation on the lateral side of metatarsal condyle. No narrowing of the joint space.

1345. Same patient. Close-up view.

1346. Osteophytes, slight narrowing of the interarticular space.

1347. Right foot : subchondral cyst formation with fine osteosclerotic line of margination. Left foot : more advanced stage : large lateral osteophyte, narrowness of the joint space, erosion surrounded by an osteosclerotic area. Pagetoid appearance of the second and third metatarsals.

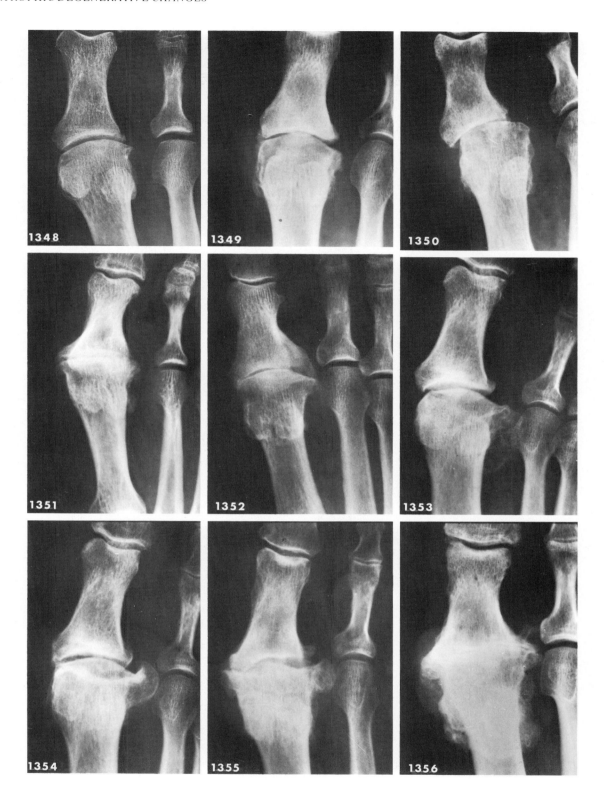

1348, 1349. Hallux rigidus : advanced stages.

1348. Narrowing of the joint space, lateral osteophytosis, cyst-like bone lesions.

1349. Marked narrowing of the joint space with osteosclerosis of both its margins and marginal osteophytes. Compare with next view.

1350. Chronic arthritis : erosions of the metatarsal head, narrowing of the joint space and dislocation, no osteophytes.

1351 → 1356. Hallux rigidus : advanced stages. **1351.** Marked narrowing of the joint space with destruction of the bone ends and osteophytes.

1352 → 1355. Various shapes of osteophytosis.

1356. Complete ankylosis : marked exostoses.

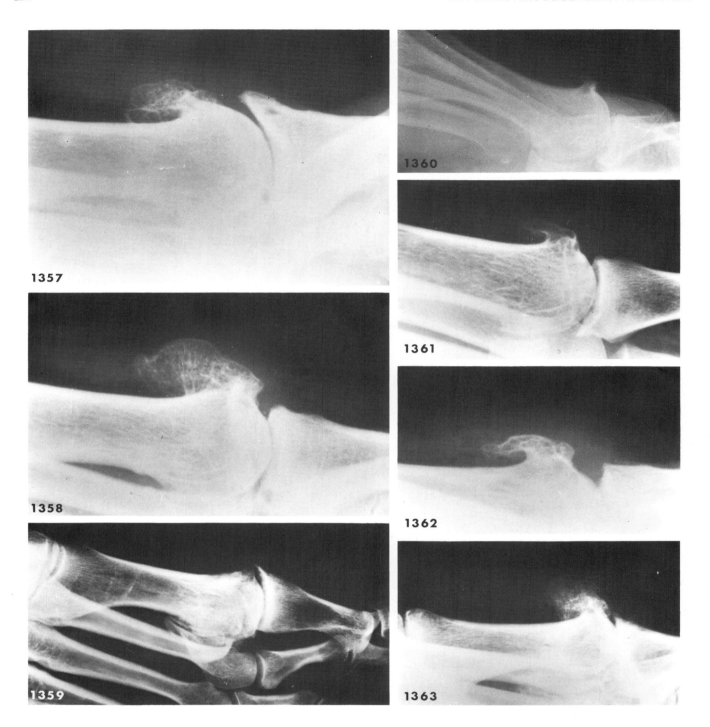

1357 → 1363. The exostosis associated with hallux rigidus is usually located on the dorso-lateral aspect of the first metatarsophalangeal joint. In contrast, hallux valgus is associated with an extosis growing externally on the side of the first metatarsal head (see **400**).

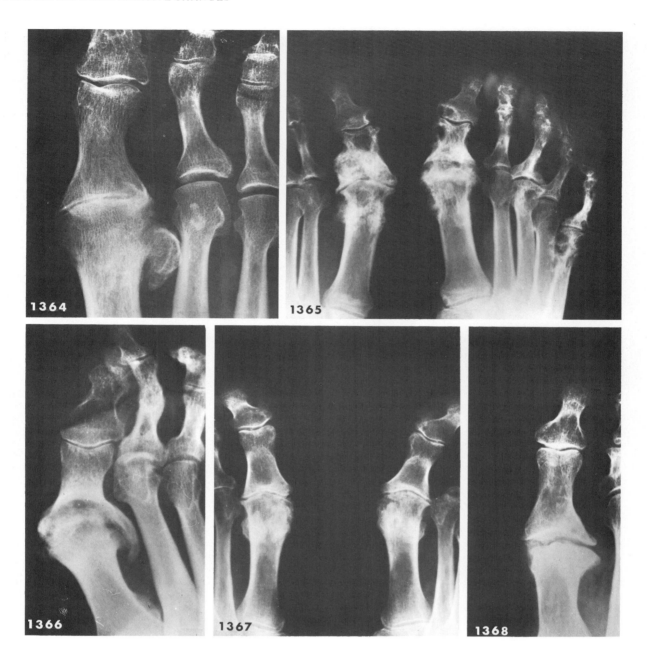

1364. Chondrocalcinosis : joint destruction, subluxation of the sesamoid bone, without metatarsophalangeal angulation.

1365. Gout : advanced stage of the metatarsophalangeal joint, lesions of both great toes. More characteristic gouty changes of the third and fifth digits are seen here.

1366. Diabetes : remodeling of the phalangeal base surrounding the lysis of the first metatarsal head. At the level of the second toe, dislocation of the metatarsophalangeal joint and ankylosis of the proximal interphalangeal joint.

1367. Rheumatoid arthritis : arthrosis complicating an arthritis of both first metatarsophalangeal joints without dislocation.

1368. Arthrosis after surgical resection of the first metatarsal head.

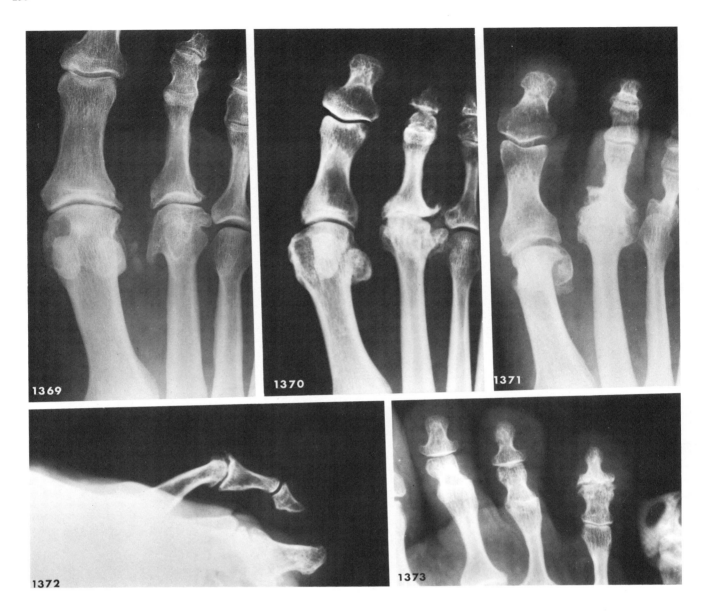

1369. Arthrosis of the second metatarsophalangeal joint associated with hallux rigidus.

1370. Arthrosis of the second metatarsophalangeal joint, sequela of a juvenile aseptic necrosis (Freiberg disease).

1371. Arthrosis of the second metatarsophalangeal joint, due to overloading, after surgical resection of the metatarsal head.

1372. Arthrosis of the proximal interphalangeal joint of the second toe, after septic arthritis.

1373. Arthrosis of the distal interphalangeal joint of the fourth toe after septic arthritis.

Note the bandage for digital corn of the fifth toe.

EXOSTOSES OR OSTEOCHONDROMAS

The solitary exostosis occurs in males as well as in females, appears during childhood, and constitutes cartilaginous tissue, springing from the epiphyseal cartilage. Radiologically the osteochondroma is well-defined with sharp borders and is formed by a compact bone and a spongy substance in continuity with the normal bone through its sessile or pediculate base of implantation.

Noticeable calcifications surrounding the exostosis, visible cyst-like areas of osteolysis at the level of its pedicle, or a restarting of growth in an adult are ominous findings of infrequent malignant degeneration (1 % of cases).

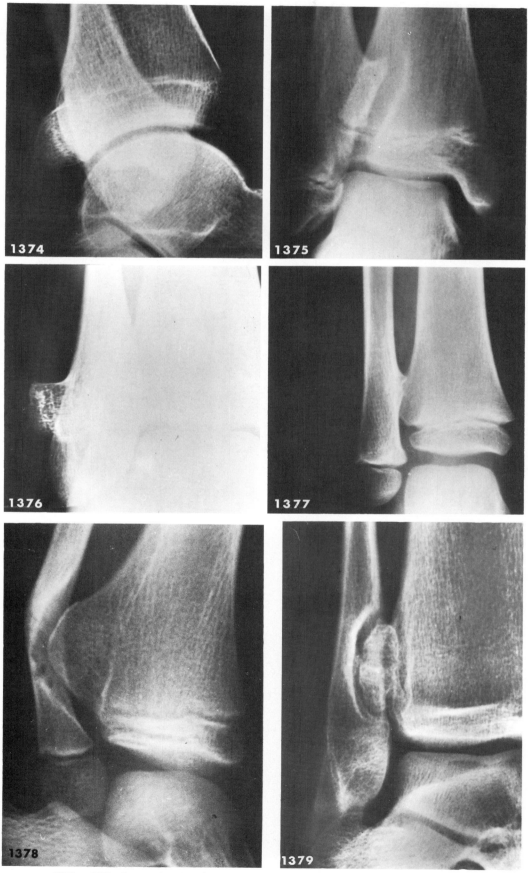

1374 → 1379. Peroneal and tibial exostoses. When the exostosis grows between tibia and fibula, it may dig a cavity or induce a diastasis.

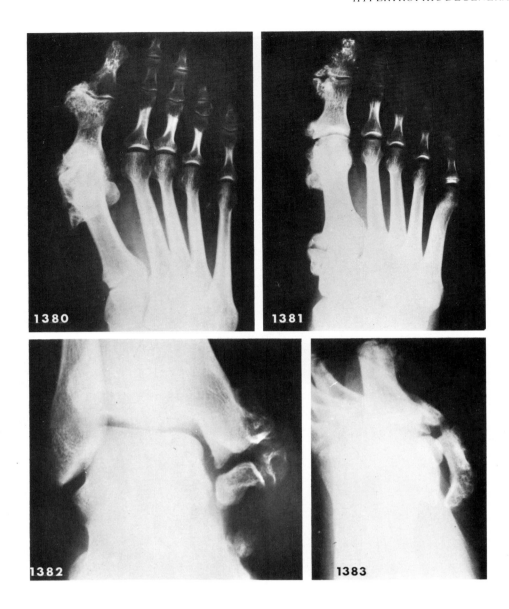

1380. Arthrosis of the interphalangeal and metatarsophalangeal joints of the great toe : osteophytosis, narrowed joint spaces.

1381 → 1383. Osteogenesis along the medial aspect of the foot from the tibial malleolus to the phalangeal tuft of the great toe, and occurring as exostoses and paraarticular bone formation (see **1383** the encircling of the sesamoid bone), without involvement of the joint spaces. Unknown cause (see the scintigram of this same case **247, 248**).

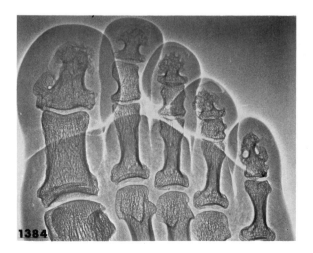

1384. Acromegaly.

Anchor-like hyperostosis of the tufts of the distal phalanges.

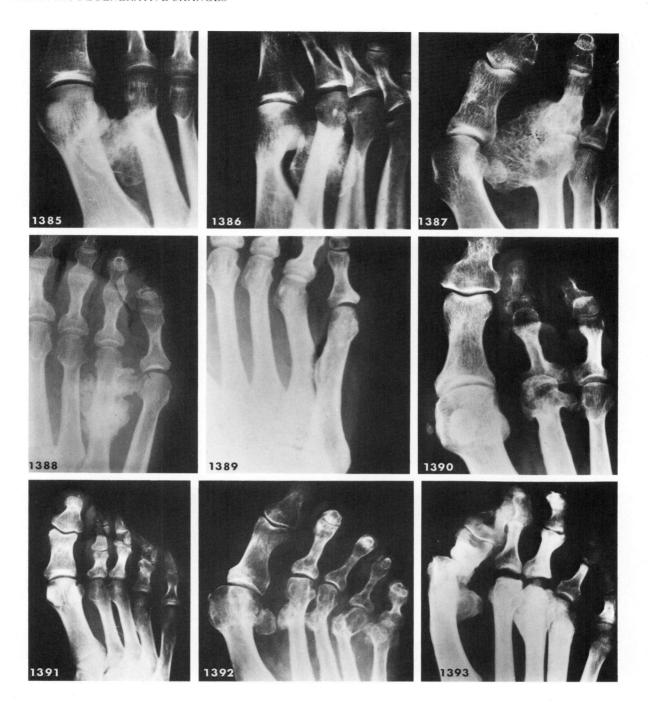

1385 → 1387. Solitary exostosis of the second metatarsal (various shapes).

1388. Exostosis of the shaft of the fourth metatarsal : exuberant callus-like appearance. Necessity of various radiographic projections to show the base of its implantation on the bone.

1389. Diaphyseal exostosis of the fifth metatarsal with air in the soft tissues (per-operative radiograph).

1390. Second metatarsophalangeal joint : osteophyte or osteochondroma. Note also the calcifying bursitis along the medial side of the first metatarsophalangeal joint.

1391. Hereditary multiple exostoses (diaphyseal aclasis) : autosomal dominant inherited chondrodysplasia, involving especially men, characterized by multiple osteochondromas and tending to malignancy in 20 % of the cases. Numerous small sessile exostoses. Brachyphalanges are frequently associated.

1392. Callus of fracture.

1393. Postoperative sequelae : osteophytosis, periostosis and osteosclerosis.

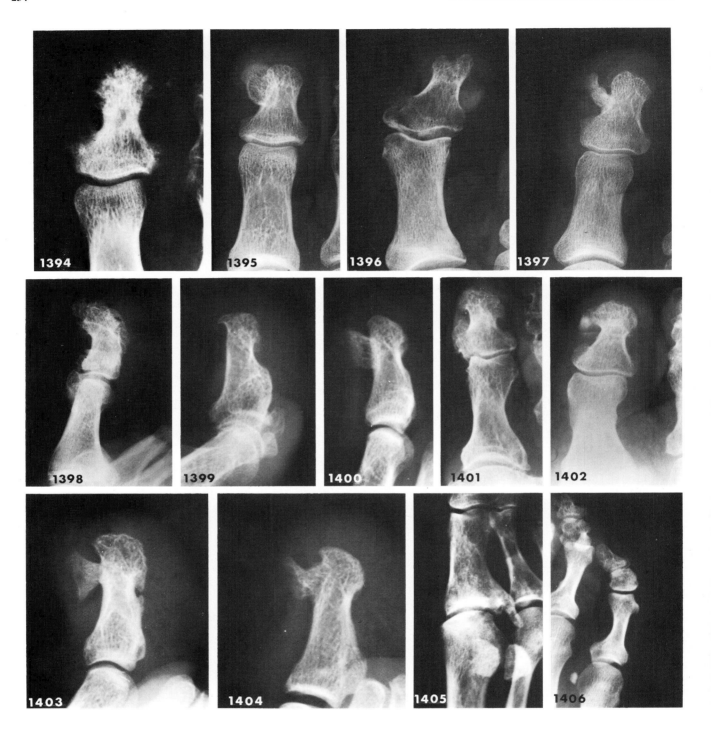

1394 → 1404. Exostosis of the distal phalanx of the great toe.

1394. Psoriasis : exhuberant osteophytosis of the distal phalanx of the great toe (pagoda-like).

1395. Subungual exostosis.

1396. Bifid end of the phalanx. Internal exostosis or normal variant.

1397. True exostosis.

1398. Periarticular and plantar new bone formation (same case as **1381**).

1399, 1400. Subungual exostosis.

1401. Exostosis of the phalangeal base.

1402. Opacity simulating an exostosis : therapeutic ointment for a mycosis, especially the nail fold.

1403, 1404. Subungual exostosis.

1405. Plantar exostosis of the base of the proximal phalanx.

1406. Lateral horn of the head of the proximal phalanx of the fifth toe.

15

SOFT TISSUES

TENDONS

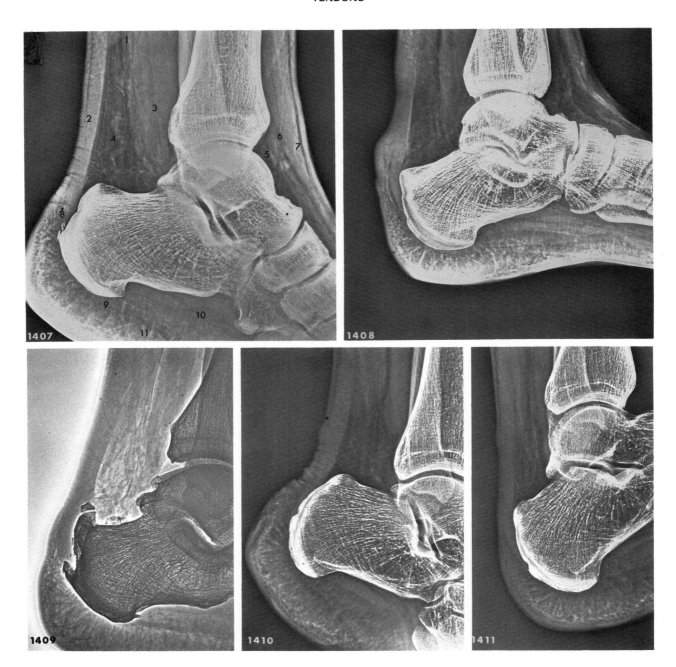

1407. Normal radiographic appearance of the soft tissues of the ankle on a lateral xeroradiograph. 1 : soleus muscle ; 2 : Achilles tendon ; 3 : flexor digitorum muscles ; 4 : pre-Achilles fat pad : a triangular radiolucent adipocellular tissue (Kager triangle) ; 5 : anterior bilocular adipocellular radiolucent space ; 6 : extensor tendons ; 7 : tendon of the tibialis anterior muscle ; 8 : site of the sub-Achilles bursa ; 9 : site of the plantar synovial bursa of Lenoir ; 10 : plantar muscles and aponeurosis ; 11 : rete plantaris of Lejars.

1408. Calcaneal posterior bursitis (Haglund disease).

1409. Bursitis opposite to the armoured posterior aspect of the calcaneus, with plantar and posterior calcaneal spurs.

1410. 1411. Normal radiographic appearance of the Kager triangle on a stress film with the foot in plantar and dorsi flexion. Note the small subcutaneous nodule.

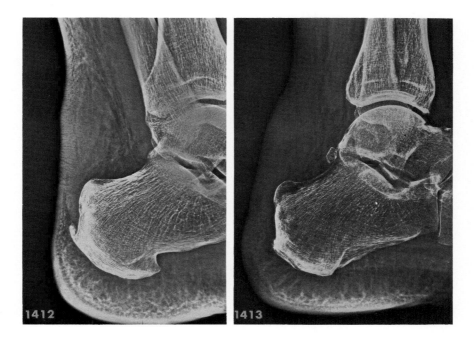

1412. Rupture of the Achilles tendon deforming its posterior margin and obscuring the Kager triangle.

1413. Old rupture of the Achilles tendon : disappearance of individual structures of the soft tissues.

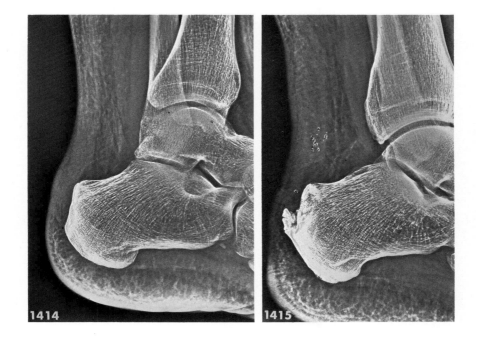

1414. Rupture of the Achilles tendon : ill-defined anterior side of the Achilles tendon. Kager triangle is obscured.

1415. Old rupture of the Achilles tendon : calcified scar.

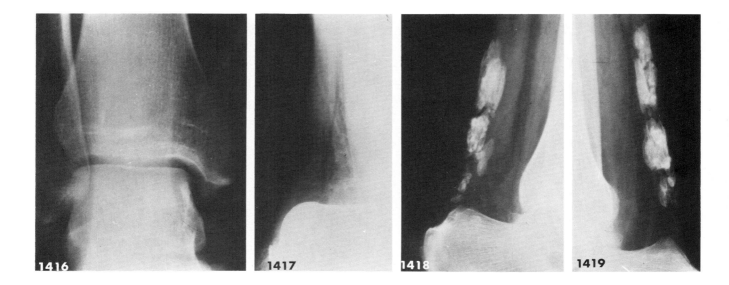

1416. Achilles tendon : one may see its borders on a frontal radiograph.

1417. Xanthomatous Achilles tendon : a xanthoma is a painless chronic tumor, varying in size, constituted by a tissue deposit of cholesterol, initially homogeneously radiolucent but which later may be calcified. It involves principally the Achilles tendon, bilaterally, and more or less symmetrically and it also affects the tendons of the extensor digitorum muscles. Similar deposits of cholesterol may be seen in the lungs and brain : cerebrotendinous xanthomatosis is an especially severe disease. Fusiform thickening of the tendon.

1418, 1419. Little disease (hypertonic congenital diplegia) : Achilles tenostosis.

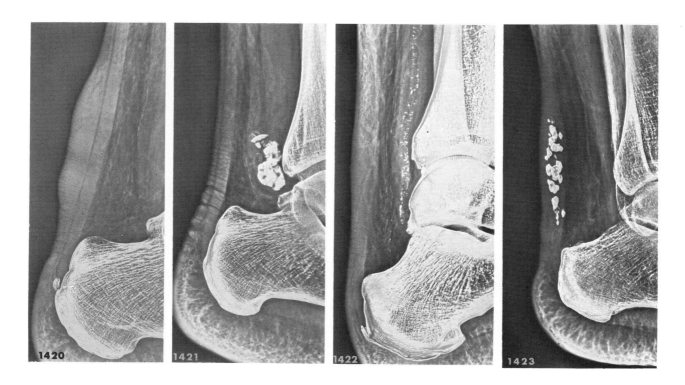

1420. Thickening of the skin simulating an Achilles tendinitis.

1421. Osteochondromatosis of the ankle joint.

1422. Achilles tendinitis. Calcified posterior tibial artery.

1423. Sequela of an Achilles tenonectomy for the purpose of lengthening it, 20 years previously.

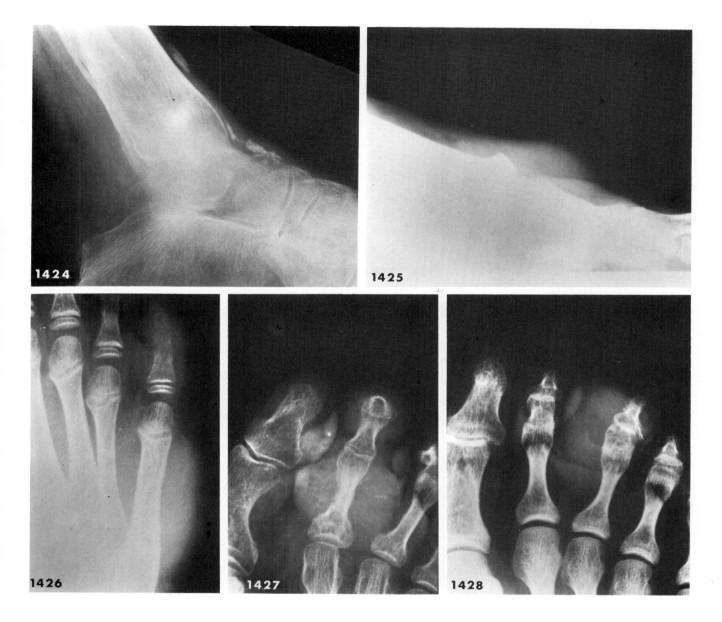

1424. Calcification in extensor tendons, unknown cause.

1425. Tendinous cyst : homogeneous increased density, without underlying bone lesions.

1426. Malignant synovioma : swelling of the soft tissues. Diaphyseal cyst-like lytic bone lesion of the fifth metatarsal (same cases as **961**).

1427. Giant cell tumor of Heurteau and Malherbe in the tendon sheath of the second toe : localized benign tenosynovitis expanding in the sole of the foot and deforming the phalangeal shaft without breaking the cortex.

1428. Benign nodular tenosynovitis : swelling of the soft tissues of the third toe and small cyst-like areas of osteolysis of the distal phalanges.

SYNOVIAL

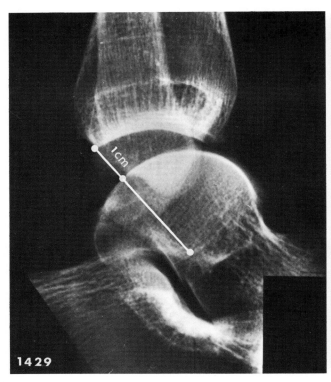

1429

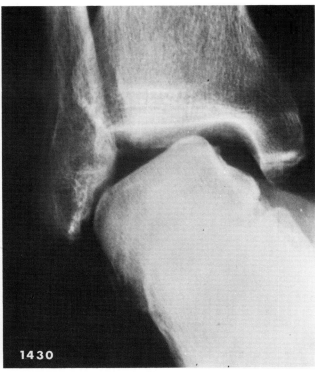

1430

1429, 1430. Ankle sprain : the ligamentous injuries can be brought out by stress radiography, mostly by anterior projection of the foot and stress varus of the ankle.

1429. Anterior projection : the distance between the third tibial malleolus and the talus on the line connecting this malleolus and the center of the talar head must be shorter than 1 cm (Castaing). A positive maneuver means that the anterior talofibular ligament, the strongest one, is injured. A posterior projection is useless, because of the third tibial malleolus protuberance.

1430. Stress varus : lateral gape of the joint, meaning an injury to the talofibular ligament. A stress valgus is useless because of the large size of the lateral malleolus.

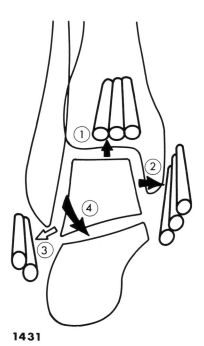

1431

1431. Diagram of the normal communications of the ankle joint cavity. 1 : synovial sheath of the tendons of the extensor muscles (6 %) ; 2 : synovial sheath of the tendons of the flexor muscles (15 %) ; 3 : synovial sheath of the tendons of peroneal and tibialis posterior muscle group (0 %, see **69**) ; 4 : subtalar joint cavity (12 %).

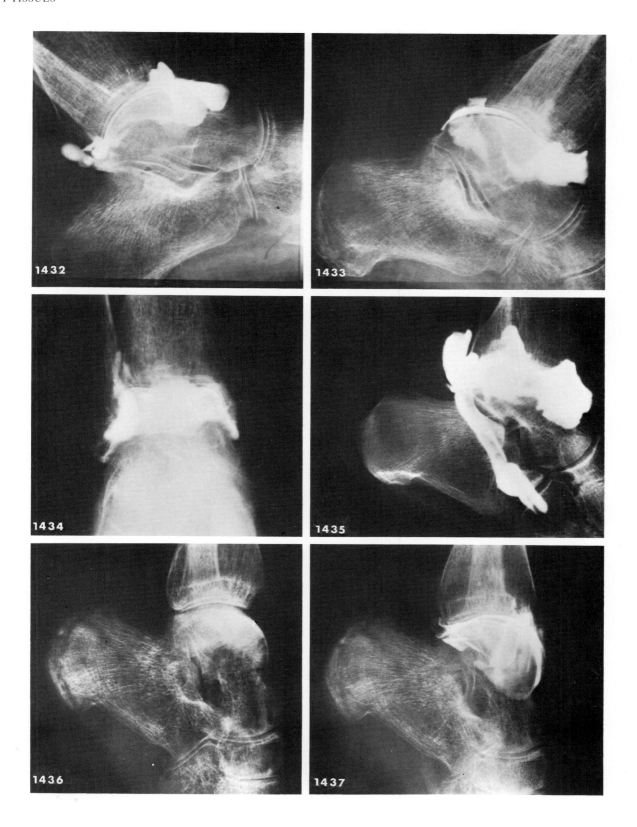

1432 → 1435. Normal arthrographic appearances of the ankle joint.

1432. Lateral radiograph with the foot in plantar flexion : distension of the posterior synovial cul-de-sac.

1433. Lateral radiograph with the foot in dorsal flexion : distension of the anterior synovial cul-de-sac.

1434. Frontal radiograph : the superior synovial cul-de-sac between the tibia and the fibula should not exceed 8 mm in height.

1435. Lateral radiograph : normal communication with the synovial sheath of the tendon of the tibialis posterior muscle.

1436, 1437. Retracted capsule : decreased volume without apparent anterior and posterior synovial recesses.

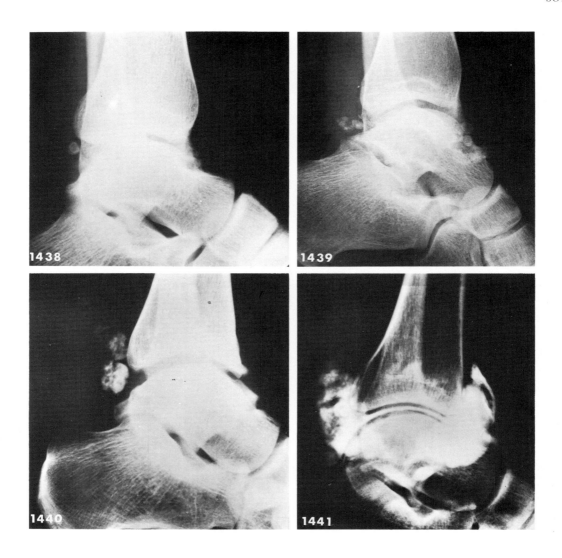

Synovial osteochondromatosis. Benign proliferative synovial metaplasia, usually monoarticular, affecting essentially men, with calcification of segments of synovial membrane. These synovial chondromas hang from the synovial membrane and occasionally may be completely separate, becoming free joint bodies and producing internal derangements.

1438 → 1443. Synovial osteochondromatosis of the ankle : the loose bodies lodge generally in the synovial cul-de-sac, forming ovoid more or less dense patchy opacities which may group into lobulated or granular mulberry-like calcified masses.

1438. Solitary osteochondroma in the posterior synovial recess.

1439. Multiple small osteochondromas. At the rear, they must be differentiated from an os trigonum (see **91**).

1440, 1441. Osteochondromatosis : arthrography proves the intraarticular site of the osteochondroma, but it is of most help when the joint mice are solely cartilaginous tissue and consequently radiolucent in the routine radiograph.

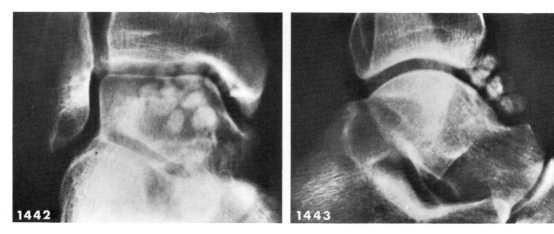

1442, 1443. Same patient. Multiple osteochondromas in the anterior synovial recess of the ankle.

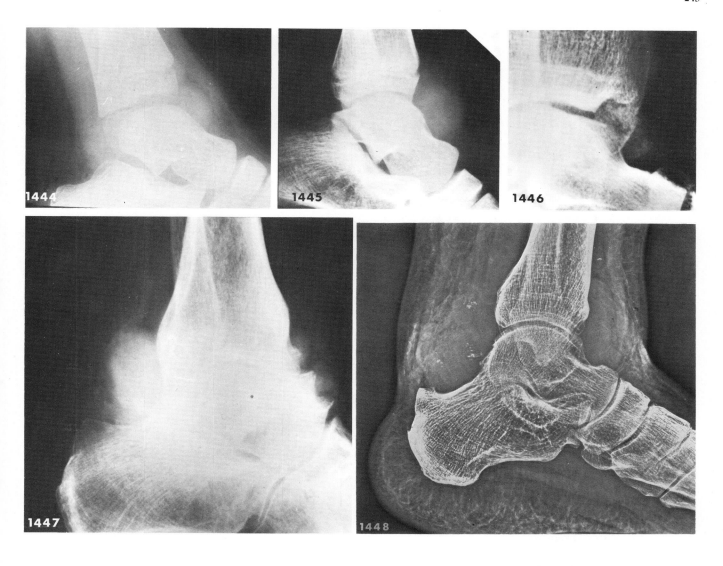

1444. Hemarthrosis due to a sprain of the ankle : the round supratalar opacity in the soft tissues is formed by the distended anterior synovial sac.

1445. Intraarticular effusion associated with villonodular synovitis of the ankle joint.

1446. Calcified gouty tophus.

1447. Two gouty tophi eroding the tibial and talar cortex. At the back, distended synovial sac or large tophus ?

1448. Likely synovioma of the ankle joint with calcifications inside.

SUBCUTANEOUS AND DEEP CONNECTIVE TISSUES

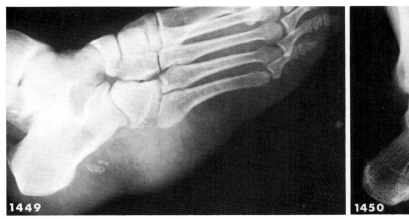 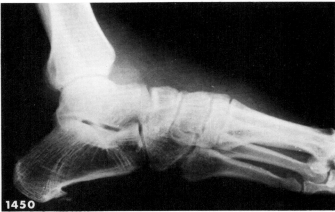

1449. Mycetoma : 2 years after the onset of the disease. Swelling and opacity of the soft tissues of the lateral aspect of the foot. Bones are spared *(Streptomyces somaliensis)*.

1450. Mycetoma : 4 years after the onset of the disease. Swelling of the soft tissues of the dorsum of the foot, fibrillar bone rarefaction of the whole tarsus. The bones are uninvolved *(Madurella mycetomi)*.

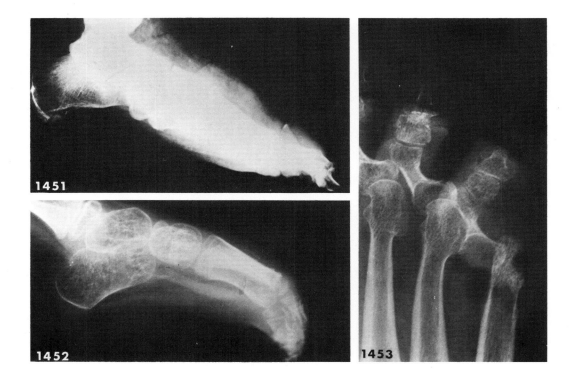

1451. Thyroid acropachy : edema and pachydermic swelling of the soft tissues with periosteal new bone formation.

1452. Arthrogryposis : plantar amyotrophy.

1453. Gas gangrene : radiolucent bubbles in the soft tissues and septic arthritis of the fifth metatarsal head.

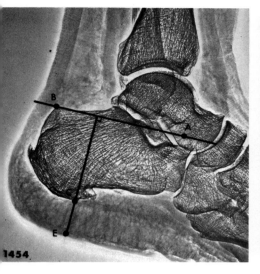
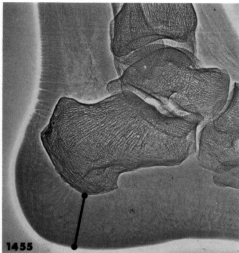
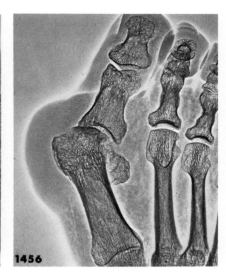

1454. Normal picture of a lateral xerograph of a calcaneus. Measurement of the thickness of the subcalcanean plantar pad by Kho's method. A : beak of the great apophysis of the calcaneus ; B : superior angle of the posterior tuber calcanei. The thickness CE of the soft tissues is measured on the perpendicular to the line AB passing through C, lowest point of the inferior aspect of the calcaneus. In a normal subject, CE may vary from 15 to 30 mm with an average of 21 mm.

1455. Acromegaly : CE = 30 mm by Kho's method. This measurement is helpful for the diagnosis. The thickness of the plantar pad enables one to monitor the treatment of the disease.

1456. Bursitis in a hallux valgus.

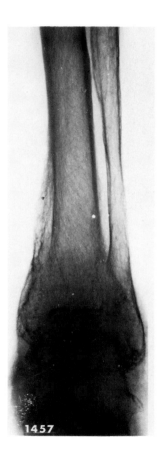
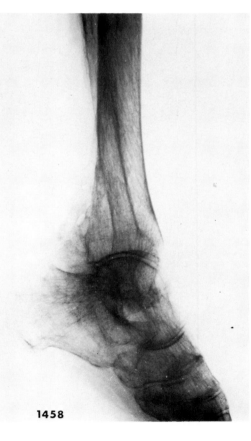
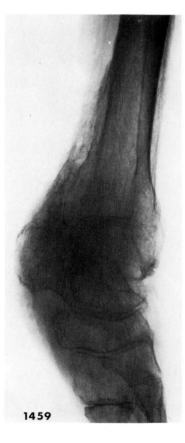

1457, 1458, 1459. Neurogenic para-osteoarthropathy : heterotopic ossification growing in the connective tissue, out of the muscles without involvement of the joints, and complicating a paralysis of intracranial origin or a long coma. This condition may be seen also in severe burns and tetanus.

Radiologically, the ossification is always situated outside of the articular capsule, drawing large irregular patches or tapes of calcification and often forming bridges across the joint, of which one sees the preserved intraarticular space. The ossification is exceptionally localized to the hands and the feet.

THICKENING OF HEEL PAD (greater than 22 mm)
Acromegaly
Dilantin therapy
Generalized edema
Infection of soft tissues (eg. mycetoma)
Myxedema, thyroid acropachy
Normal variant
Obesity
Trauma

SOFT TISSUE CALCIFICATIONS
Calcified bursitis

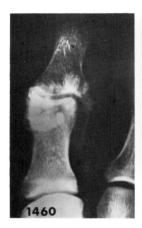 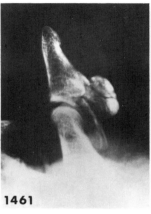 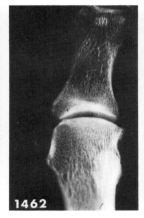 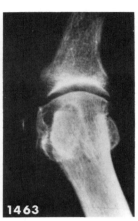

1460, 1461. Calcifying bursitis under the interphalangeal joint of the great toe.

1462, 1463. Calcifying bursitis opposite the first metatarsal head.

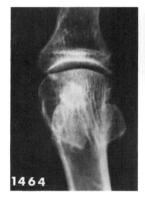 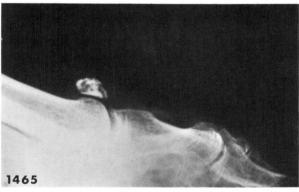

1464, 1465. Osteochondroma situated in the dorsal synovial recess of the first metatarsophalangeal joint.

CALCIFICATION OF ARTICULAR CARTILAGE

Acromegaly
Degenerative ; post-traumatic
Gout
Hemochromatosis
Hyperparathyroidism
Hypophosphatasia
Idiopathic
Ochronosis
Oxalosis
Pseudogout (calcium pyrophosphate arthropathy)
Wilson disease

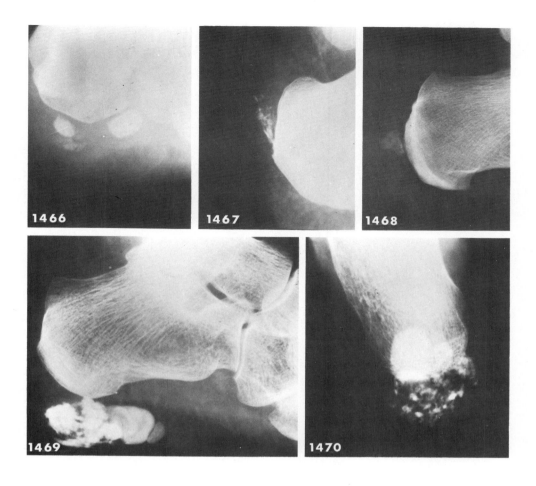

1466. Calcified bursitis at the level of the plantar aspect of the medial sesamoid.

1467. Calcified concretions of the Achilles tendon in a patient with chronic renal insufficiency.

1468. Calcified posterior calcaneal bursitis.

1469, 1470. Calcifying bursitis of Lenoir is synovial bursa (lateral and axial calcaneal views).

PERIARTICULAR OR INTRAARTICULAR CALCIFICATION

Charcot joint
Congenital stippled epiphyses (Conradi disease)
Degenerative arthritis, loose body, « joint mouse »
Dermatomyositis ; calcinosis universalis
Diabetes mellitus
Dysplasia epiphysealis hemimelica (Trevor disease)
Gout
Hematoma, traumatic or spontaneous
Hemochromatosis
Hyperparathyroidism, primary or secondary
Hypervitaminosis D
Hypoparathyroidism
Lupus erythematosus
Myositis ossificans
Ochronosis
Parosteal sarcoma
Pseudogout (calcium pyrophosphate arthropathy)
Rheumatoid arthritis
Scleroderma
Synovial osteochondromatosis
Synovioma
Synovitis, tendinitis (peritendinitis calcarea)
Tuberculosis
Tumoral calcinosis
Werner syndrome

Metabolic calcifications

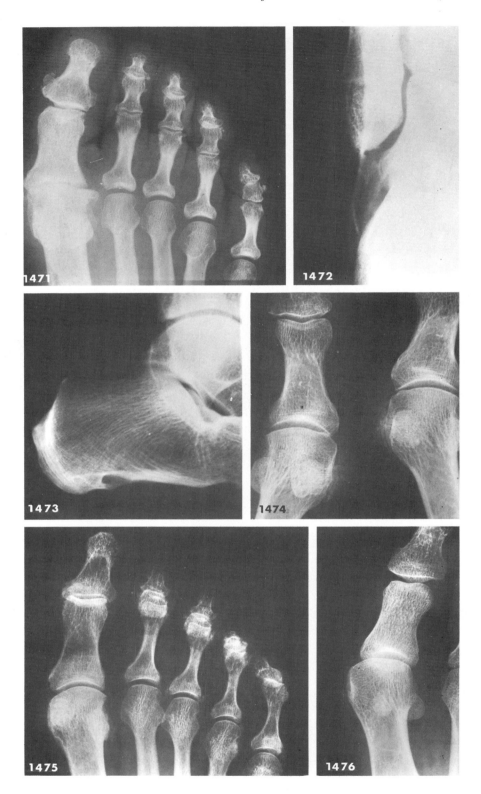

1471 → 1473. Calcifying polyperiarthritis.

1471. Tiny calcifications about the interphalangeal joints.

1472. Calcified calcaneofibular ligament.

1473. Posterior calcaneal calcification.

1474. Articular chondrocalcinosis : symmetrical periarticular calcifications at the first metatarsal head region.

1475, 1476. Articular chondrocalcinosis : periarticular calcifications about the metatarsophalangeal joints.

1475. In chronic renal insufficiency.

1476. In hyperparathyroidism.

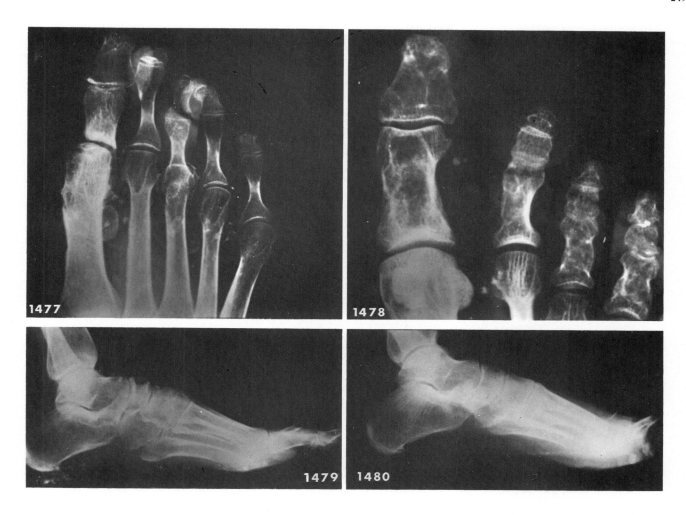

1477. Thibierge-Weissenbach syndrome. The progressive systemic sclerosis is a collagenosis characterized by the thickening of the dermic fibrous tissue with adhesion of the adjacent tissues, especially the skin, associated with various visceral disorders and involvement of the joints. The Thibierge-Weissenbach syndrome is a triad including scleroderma, Raynaud disease and calcinosis localized in the sclerogenic zones. Calcific opacities disseminated in the soft tissues of the forefoot.

1478. Maffucci-Kast syndrome : enchondromatosis and multiple cavernous hemangiomas with phleboliths.

1479. Thibierge-Weissenbach syndrome : calcium deposits in the sole of the foot.

1480. Calcinosis. A condition characterized by the deposition of calcium salts in nodular foci in subcutaneous and deep connective tissues without a disorder of calcium metabolism, but associated with collagen disease in 35 % of the cases.

CALCIFICATION IN THE MUSCLES AND SUBCUTANEOUS TISSUES

SYSTEMIC

Basal cell nevus S. (Gorlin)
Bone destruction with hypercalcemia
Congenital fibromatosis
Dermatomyositis ; calcinosis universalis
Ehlers-Danlos S.
Fat necrosis (pancreatitis ; Weber-Christian disease)
Fluorosis
Gout ; hyperuricemia
Homocystinuria
Hyperparathyroidism, primary and secondary
Hypervitaminosis D
Hypoparathyroidism, pseudohypoparathyroidism, pseudopseudohypoparathyroidism
Idiopathic hypercalcemia (eg, Wiliam S.)
Lupus erythematosus
Milk-alkali S.
Mucoviscidosis
Myositis ossificans progressiva
Osteoporosis (immobilization)
Paraplegia ; poliomyelitis
Parasites (eg. cysticercosis, guinea worms, loa-loa)
Post-carbon monoxide poisoning
Progeria ; Werner S.

Pseudoxanthoma elasticum
Scleroderma
Tumoral calcinosis
Vascular (see page 253)

NONSYSTEMIC

Avulsed fracture fragment
Burn, frostbite, electroshock
Epithelioma (pilo-matrixoma)
Foreign body granuloma
Healing infection or abscess (post-pyogenic myositis or fibrositis)
Idiopathic
Inoculation (eg, calcified sterile abscess ; antibiotic, bismuth, calcium gluconate, insulin, camphorated oil, or quinine injection ; BCG vaccination)
Leprosy (nerves)
Myositis ossificans, traumatic ; hematoma
Neoplasm, benign (eg, chondroma, fibromyxoma)
Neoplasm, malignant (eg, soft tissue osteosarcoma, chondrosarcoma, fibrosarcoma, liposarcoma, synovioma)
Scar
Volkman contracture

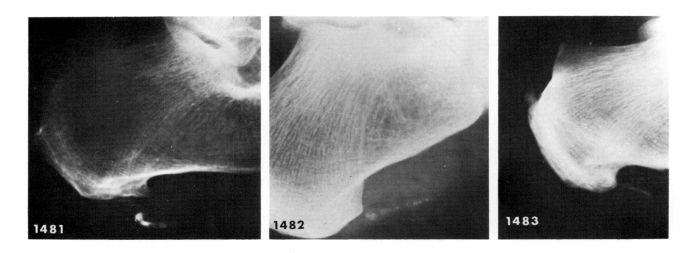

1481, 1482, 1483. Calcifications in the plantar aponeurosis :
various shapes.

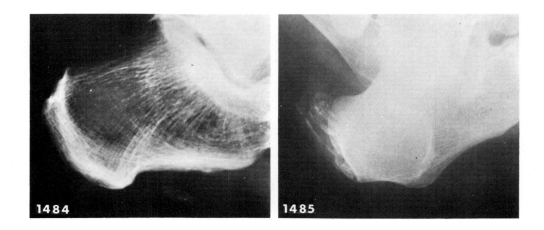

1484. Plantar aponeurotic ossification.

1485. Calcification of the Achilles tendon in a patient with chronic
renal insufficiency.

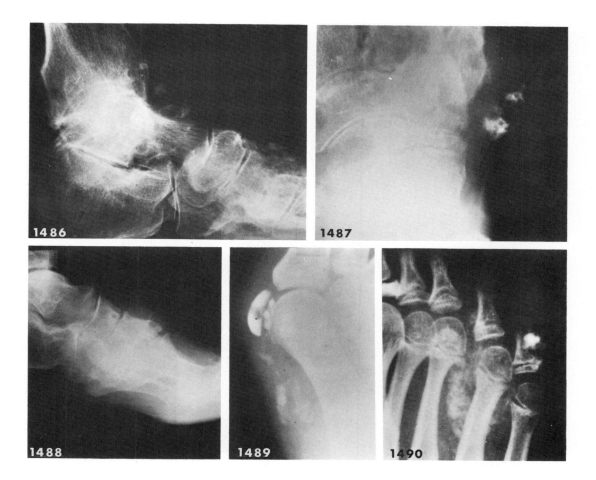

1486 → 1488. Gouty tophi : subcutaneous heterogeneous, more or less dense and circumscribed opacities, adjacent to cortical erosions of the adjoining bones, usually not calcified except in renal insufficiency associated with the gout.

1489. Calcific periarthritis of the metatarsophalangeal joint of the big toe, with a portion of the calcification located in the plantar soft tissues.

1490. Tumoral calcinosis (lipocalcinogranulomatosis) : a condition affecting most commonly Negroes, without reference to age, and characterized by large localized deposits of calcium salts. Radiologically, one sees irregular nodular dense masses. Tumoral calcinosis in the third intermetatarsal space in a 13-year-old child who was also affected by similar lesions at the level of both greater trochanters and of the posterior aspect of an elbow.

Note the conical epiphyses not necessarily associated with the disease.

Parasitic calcifications

1491, 1492. Dracunculosis : long interlaced calcified strands formed by the dead bodies of adult females of *Filaria medinensis*.

VESSELS

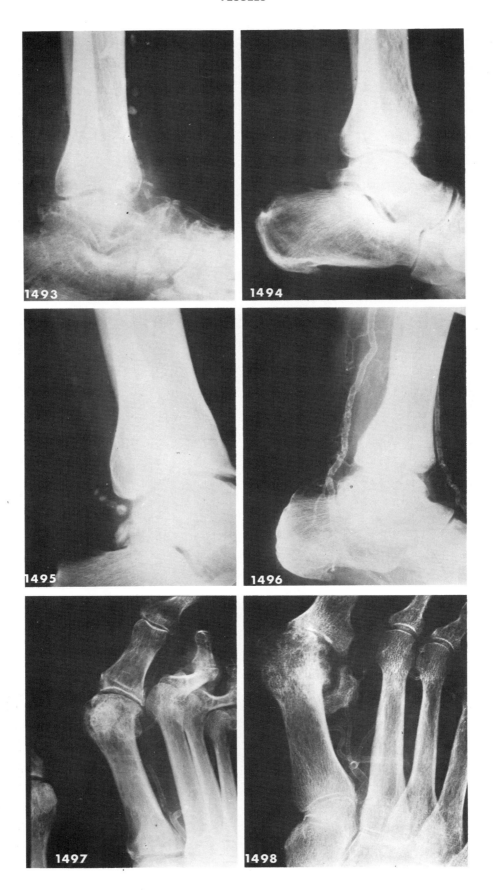

1493, 1494. Arterial calcifications. In the elderly, they may simply be a sign of atherosclerosis. In the young, they are often associated with diabetes.

1495. Pheboliths : small, round calcific concretions along the course of the veins.

1496 → 1498. Arterial calcification. Note the arthritis of the first metatarsophalangeal joint (**1497, 1498**).

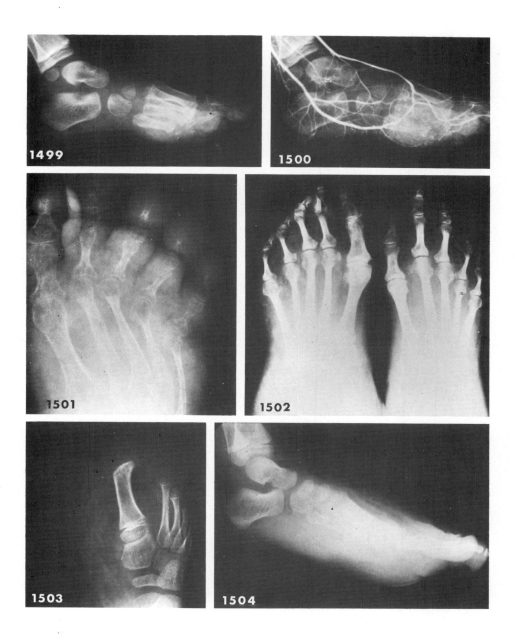

1499, 1500. Cavernous angioma in the sole of the foot of a 3-year-old child.

1499. Routine radiograph : swelling of the soft tissues of the fifth metatarsal.

1500. Angiogram, arteriolocapillary phase : slightly hypervascular tumor displacing the plantar metatarsal arteries.

1501. Venous angioma of the leg and the foot in a 22-year-old man. Swelling and increased opacity of the soft tissues. Diffuse osteoporosis, concentric osteolysis of the metatarsal shaft. No visible calcifications.

1502. Klippel-Trenaunay-Weber syndrome : a condition characterized by segmental aplasia of the deep venous network, angiomatous hypertrophy of the superficial veins with or without arteriovenous aneurysm, and hypertrophy of the skeleton and the soft tissues in the same zones.

1503. Macropodia and thoracic lymphangioma in a 6-year-old girl : marked swelling of the soft tissues and aphalangia.

1504. Klippel-Trenaunay-Weber syndrome.

VASCULAR CALCIFICATION

Aneurysm
Arteriosclerosis
Buerger disease
Burn, frostbite
Gout, hyperuricemia
Hemangioma ; arteriovenous malformation
Homocystinuria
Hyperparathyroidism, primary or secondary
Hypervitaminosis D
Hypoparathyroidism
Idiopathic hypercalcemia
Immobilization syndrome
Milk-alkali syndrome
Mucoviscidosis
Phleboliths (eg, normal, varicose veins, hemangioma, Maffucci syndrome, postradiation)
Premature atherosclerosis : familial hyperlipemia, generalized arterial calcification of infancy, progeria, secondary hyperlipemia (Cushing syndrome, diabetes mellitus, glycogen storage disease, hypothyroidism, lipodystrophy, nephrotic syndrome, renal homotransplantation), Werner syndrome.
Pseudoxanthoma elasticum
Raynaud disease
Sarcoidosis

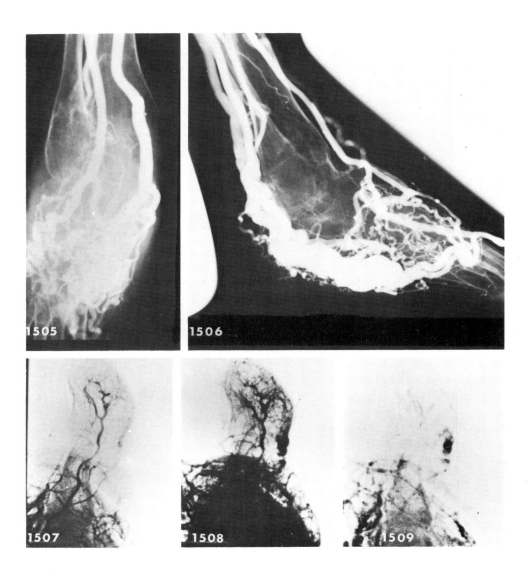

1505, 1506. Arteriovenous aneurysm of the foot following ankle arthrodesis : **1505.** Frontal arteriographic
projection ; **1506.** Lateral arteriographic projection.
Note the aneurysmal sac, the early and abundant venous
return (arteries and veins show simultaneously on the
same radiograph), the large diameter of arteries, the
distal vascular depletion due to the arteriovenous shunt,
explaining the trophic disorders of the toes which have
healed after the surgical treatment of the fistula.

1507 → 1509. Angioma in the plantar region of the great
toe. Angiography. Succession of filling phases : arterial
phase (**1507**) ; capillary phase (**1508**) ; venous phase with
persistent opacification of the angioma (**1509**).

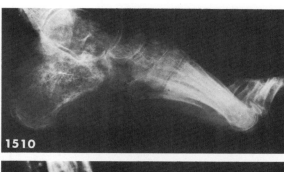

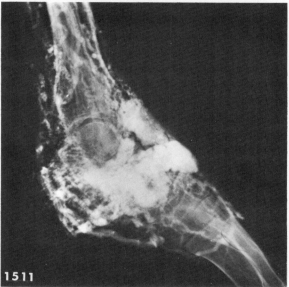

1510, 1511. Congenital arteriovenous fistula : diffuse bone rarefaction of the tarsus. The arteriogram shows a large aneurysmal sac in the dorsum of the foot.

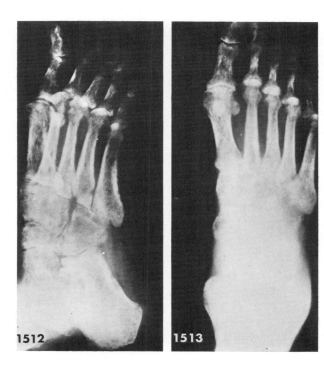

1512, 1513. Arteritis and algodystrophy. The isolated algodystrophy rarely complicates an arteritis.

LYMPHATIC VESSELS

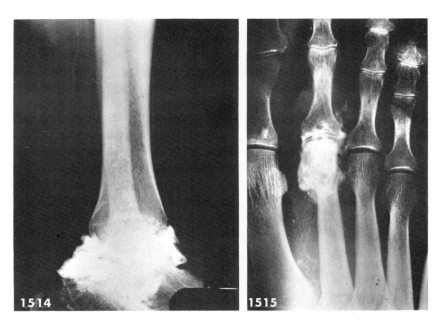

1514, 1515. The filling of the lymphatic vessels during arthrography is a sign of inflammatory arthritis.

1514. Arthrography of the ankle joint before synviorthesis in rheumatoid arthritis.

1515. Similar case at the level of the first metatarsophalangeal joint.

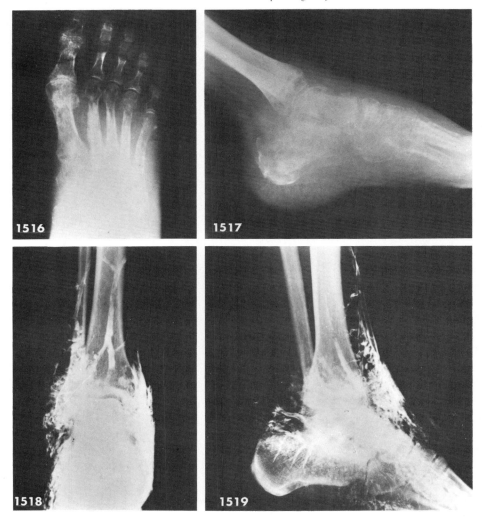

1516 → 1519. Elephantiasis : chronic lymphedema giving the involved limb an elephant-like leg shape, due to obstructed circulation in the lymphatic vessels by congenital abnormalities or various acquired diseases, eg cancer, fibrosis after radiotherapy, scars, thrombophlebitis, filariasis.

1516, 1517. The lymphatic stasis distends the intraosseous lymphatic vessels producing an osteoporosis of the whole foot with cystic bone rarefaction. **1518, 1519.** Reflux of the contrast medium during the lymphography.

NERVES

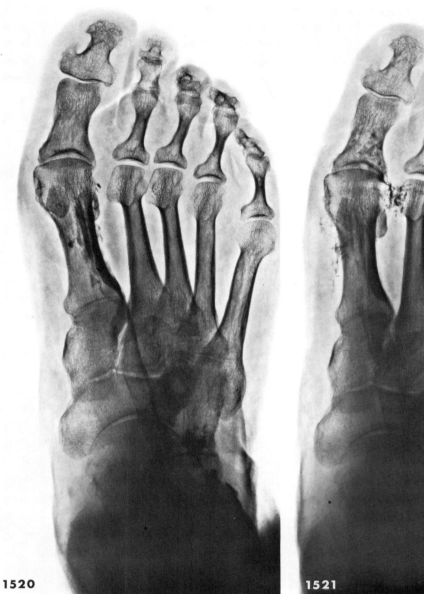

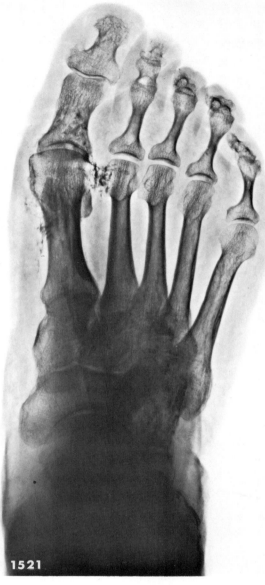

1520

1521

1520, 1521. Morton disease : neuroma of the digital nerve along its metatarsal course (generally in the third space), developing opposite the metatarsal head and bringing excruciating pain during motion or under pressure.

Neurography : a method proposed by G.Y. Gaizler and J. Komar, from Budapest, and showing the swelling of the nerve.

1520. Picture taken immediately after injection of the contrast agent at the level of the nerve.

1521. A neuroma of the first metatarsal space is still visible half an hour later.

STUDY OF THE PLANTAR WEIGHT-BEARING SURFACE

Numerous methods are proposed for the study of the plantar surface pressing on the ground, and its relation to the skeleton of the foot. Some use radiological techniques, others use only graphical or mechanical devices. Some interesting examples are cited.

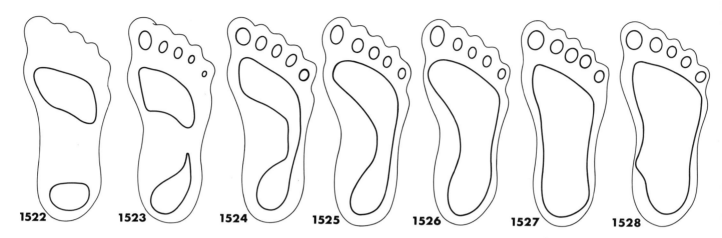

Reproduction of a footprint by the classical method : life-size footprints, identical to the picture given by the podoscope, may be printed on paper after an inking-roller has been pressed against the skin. One may also record the footprint on a photographic film after swabbing the skin with a developer and direct development with the fixer.

1522 → 1528. Patterns of footprints, normal and pathologic.

1522 → 1524. Pes cavus.

1525. Normal picture.

1526 → 1528. Flat foot.

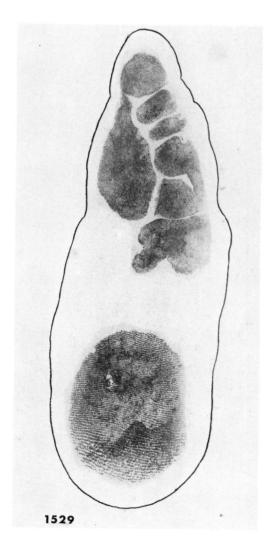

1529. Plantar print of the foot of a Chinese woman (**482**).

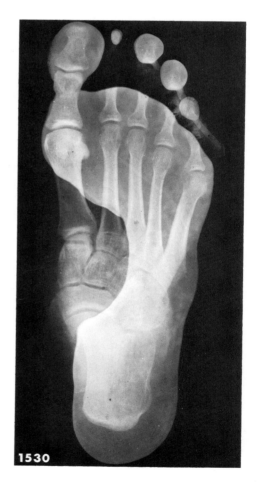

1530. Radiophotopodography (Roig-Puerta and A. Villadot). With the printing method on photographic film, exposure to X-rays superimposes the picture of the skeleton and the plantar print. The pressure zone is thus qualitatively, if not quantitatively, determined. Right foot, normal.

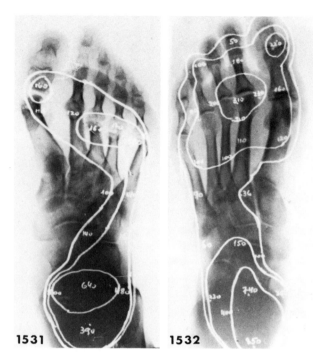

1531, 1532. Baroradiophotopodography (I. Stroescu) : superimposition on the radiophotopodograph of lines of equal plantar pressures, measured by electromechanical devices.

1531. Baroradiophotopodograph : right foot. Hyperpressure at the level of the second and third metatarsal heads.

1532. Baroradiophotopodograph : left foot. Hyperpressure at the level of the second and third metatarsal heads.

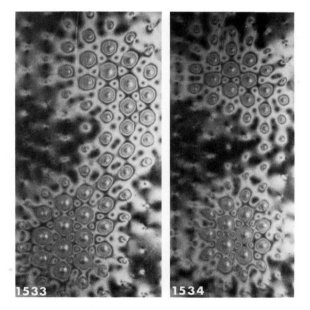

1533 → 1534. Photoelastopodometry (A. Leduc). The patient is standing on a plate of birefringent material put on a podoscope and lighted by polarized light. The zones of equal plantar pressure appear as isochromatic stripes. To obtain a quantitative evaluation of the pressures, a carpet containing small steel balls is laid between the patient's feet and the birefringent plate : the diameter and the color of each concentric circle are in proportion to the load exerted on each ball.

1533. Photoelastopodogram of a normal right foot.

1534. Photoelastopodogram of a right pes cavus.

1535 → 1542. Podostatigraphy (G. Pisani) : superimposition on the same film of the radiograph of the skeleton of the foot and the plantar print, the foot being placed on a bag filled with mercury, which delineates its outlines. Pressopodostatigraphy : by injecting an increasing volume of air, one may progressively balance the different plantar pressures, thus making the isobaric zones visible each time.

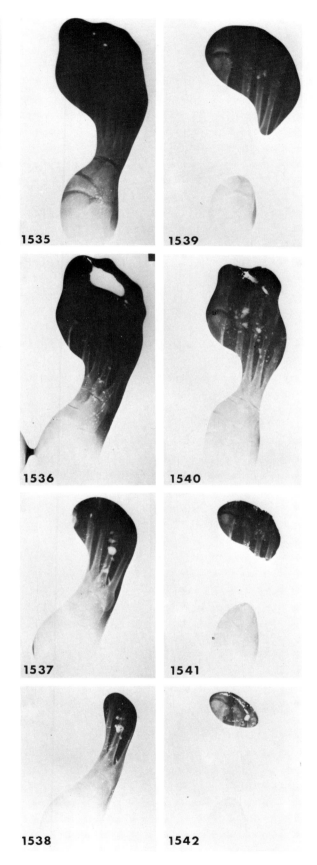

1535. Podostatigraph of a normal foot.

1536 → 1538. Pressopodostatigraphic seriography of a normal foot. The maximal pressure is exerted along the fourth ray : calcaneus, cuboid, fourth metatarsal.

1539. Podostatigraph of a pes cavus.

1540 → 1542. Pressopodostatigraphic seriograph of a pes cavus : maximal pressure is exerted at the metatarsal heads level.

BIBLIOGRAPHY

Anatomy - Evolution

ALBARET P., PILLET J., GUNTZ M. — Etude radio-anatomique des artères du pied. *Bull. Assos. Anat.*, 1975, *59*, 305-324.

ANTHONY J. — L'homme debout. Ses origines préhistoriques. *Ann. Podol.* 1973, 8 (2), 3-7.

CHANZY M., DUCLOS J.M., CHEVROT A., ALEXANDRE J.H. — Anatomie radiologique du calcaneum normal. *Sem. Hop. Arch. Anat. Pathol.*, 1972, 20 (4), 377- 384.

COBEY J.C. — Posterior roentgenogram of the foot. *Clin. Orthop.*, 1976, 118, 202-207.

EDWARDS E.A. — Anatomy of the small arteries of the foot and toes. *Acta Anat.*, 1960, *41*, 81-96.

GARNERI L. — Anatomia radiografica della sotto astragalica. *Minerva Ortop.*, 1977, *28*, 12, 731-732, 12 fig., (bibliogr.).

HAEGEL P. — Le pied humain. Anatomie comparée, embryologie, morphologie. *Ann. Podol.* 1973, 8 (1), 16-23.

HALL. M.C. — The trabecular patterns of the normal foot. *Clin. Orthop.*, 1960, 16, 15-25.

KEATS T. — *An atlas of normal developmental Roentgen anatomy.* Year Book Medical Publisher, 1977.

MESCHAN I. — Radiology of the normal foot. *Seminars in Roentgenol.*, 1970, 5 (4), 327-341.

PETERSON L., GOLDIE I.F. — The arterial supply of the talus. A study on the relationship to experimental talar fractures. *Acta. Orthop. Scand.*, 1975, *46* (6), 1026-1034.

RESNICK D. — Radiology of the talo-calcaneal articulations. Anatomic considerations and arthrography. *J. Am. Podiatry Assoc.*, 1964, 64 (6), 392-398.

VILADOT A. — L'évolution du pied. *Actualités de médecine et de chirurgie du pied - 9*, Toray-Masson, Barcelone, 1976, 37-53.

Bone growth
Epiphysoses Apophysoses

DENIS A. — A propos de la maladie de Freiberg ou deuxième maladie de Köhler (ostéonécrose primitive juvénile de la tête du deuxième métatarsien). 1965, *Rev. Rhum. 32*, 247.

KÖHLER A. — A typical disease of the second metatarso-phalangeal joint. *Am. J. Roentgenol.*, *1923, 10*, 705.

LAVAL-JEANTET M. — Appositions sous-périostées avec aspect de double contour radiographique des os longs du nourrisson. *Presse Méd.*, 1961, *68*, 2623-2626.

LEFEBVRE J., KOIFMAN A. — Etude de l'apparition des points osseux secondaires et détermination de l'âge osseux. *Arch. Fr. Pédiat.*, 1956, *13*, 1101-1105.

NAHUM H. SAUVEGRAIN J. — Croissance osseuse. *Encyclop. Méd.-Chir. (Paris)* 1965, 30900 A 10 - 30900 B 50.

WELLINGER CL. — Les ostéochondrites juvéniles de la cheville et du pied. *Rhumatologie* 1976, 279-288.

WHALEN J.P., WINCHESTER P., KROOK L., DISCHE R., NUNEZ E. — Mechanisms of bone resorption in human metaphyseal remodeling. A roentgenographic and histologic study. *Am. J. Roentgenol.*, 1971, *112*, 526-531.

X-Ray technics

BLONDIN-WALTER M. — Radiographie de la voute métatarsienne antérieure. *J. Radiol. Electrol.* 1949, *30*, 9-10, 543-544.

CALLAGHAN J.E., PERLY E. E., HILL R.0. — The ankle arthrogram. *J. Assoc. Canad. Radiol.*, 1970, *21*, 74-84.

CECILE J.P., CHERMET J. — Artériographie du pied. *Encycl. Med.-Chir.*, 1977, 5, 1-10.

DELAHAYE R.P., JOLLY R. — Pied. Technique radiologique et aspects normaux. *Encycl. Med.-Chir.*, Paris, Radiodiagnostic 30400 A 10 et 30400 A 20.

DJIAN A., ANNONIER Cl., DENIS A., BAUDOIN P. — Radiopodométrie. *J. Radiol. Electrol.*, 1968, *49*, 769-772.

DJIAN A., ANNONIER Cl. — Exploration radiologique du pied. *Journées de podologie, Paris.* Expansion Scientifique Française, Paris, 21-28.

DOSSA J. — Explorations arthrographiques du pied. *Rhumatologie*, 1976, *28*, 5, 165-169.

FREIBERGER R.H., HERSH A., HARRISON M.O. — Radiology of the normal foot. *Seminars in Roentgenol.*, *1970, 5*, 341-354.

GAUNEL C., LOUYOT P., TREHEUX A. — New radiological data on plantar statics. *J. Radiol. Electrol.*, 1971, *52*, 8, 528-529.

GOERGEN T.G., RESNICK D. — Peroneal tenography in previous calcaneal fractures. *Radiology*, 1975, 115, 211-213.

GORDON R.B. — Arthrography of the ankle joint. Experience in on hundred seven studies. *J. Bone and Joint Sarg.*, 1970, *52 A*, 16-23, 1631.

HJELMSTEDT A., SAHLSTEDT B. — Simultaneous arthrography of the talocrural and talonavicular joints to children. III. Measurements on normal feet. *Acta Radiol.*, 1977, *18*, 5, 513-522.

LEDUC A. — La fotoelastopodoscopia. *Chir. del Piede Ital.* 1977, *1*, 3-4, 417-422.

MAZAS L. — Techniques d'exploration radiologique standard de la statique du pied. *Rhumatologie*, 1976, *28*, 5, 146-149.

MAZZINARI S. — Podostatigrafia. *Ann. Podol.*, 1976, *9*, 245-248.

MEHREZ M. EL GENEIDY S. — Arthrographie de la cheville. *J. Bone Joint. Surg.*, 1970, 2, 308-312, 11 fig.

MEYER J.M., TAILLARD W. — L'arthrographie de l'articulation sous-astragalienne dans les syndromes douloureux post-traumatiques du tarse postérieur. *Rev. Chir. Orthop.*, 1974, *60*, 321-330.

ROIG-PUERTA. VILADOT A. — Exploration du pied creux par radiophotopodogramme. *Podologie*, 1962, 1, 36-44.

SIMON L., CLAUSTRE J. — Méthodes actuelles d'exploration radiographique du pied. *Colloque régional de pathologie locomotrice, Montpellier*, 3-4 octobre 1975. *Rhumatologie*, 1976, *28*, 5, 143.

STRŒSCU I. — La valeur de la baropodographie dans le diagnostic et dans la prévention des déformations du pied. *Ann. Podol.*, 1973, 8 2, 29-38.

VENNING P. — Sources of error in the production and measurement of standard radiographs of the foot. *Brit. J. Radiol.*, 1951, 24, 18-26.

Normal variants

BADGLEY C.E. — Coalition of the calcaneus and the navicular. *Arch. Surg.* 1927, 15, 75.

BECKLY D.E., ANDERSON P.W., PEDEGANA L.R. — The radiology of the subtalar joint with special reference to talo-calcaneal coalition. *Clin. Radiol.*, 1975, *26*, 3, 333-341.

BIGONGIARI L. — Pseudotibiotalar slant : A positioning artifact. *Radiology*, 1977, *122*, 699.

CONWAY J.J., COWELL H.R. — Tarsal coalition : Clinical significance and roentgenographic demonstration. *Radiology*, 1969, 92 : 799.

DEL SEL J.M., GRAND N.E. — Cubo-navicular synostosis. *Bone and Joint Surgery*, 1959, 41B, 149.

GREGERSEN H.N. — Naviculocuneiform coalition. *J. Bone and Joint Surg.*, 1977, *59*, 1, 128-130.

KAYE J.J., GHELMAN B., SCHNEIDER R. — Talocalcaneo navicular joint arthrography for sustentacular-talar tarsal coalition. *Radiology*, 1975, *115*, 3, 730-731.

KEATS T. — *An atlas of normal Roentgen variants, that may simulate disease.* Year Book Medical Publisher, 1974.

KOHLER A., ZIMMER E.A. — *Borderlands of the normal and early pathologic in skeletal roentgenology.* Grune and Stratton, New York and London, 1968.

MURAT J., DEVEZE F., GUILLET R. — Fausses fractures : le pied (limites du normal et du pathologique dans la radiographie osseuse). *Cah. Méd. Lyon.*, 14 mai 1971, *47*, 19, 2003-2014, 16 fig., bibliogr.

ROBINSON H.M. — Symetrical reversed plantal calcaneal spurs in children. A normal variant. *Radiology*, 1976, *119*, 1, 187-188.

WEINSTEIN S.L., BONFIGLIO M. — Unusual accessory (bipartite) talus simulating fracture. A case report. *J. Bone Joint Surg.*, 1975, 57, 8, 1161-1163.

YANKLOWITZ B.A., JAWOREK T.A. — The frequency of the interphalangeal sesamoïd of the hallux. A retrospective roentgenographic study. *J. Am. Podiatry Assoc.*, 1975, *65*, 11, 1058-1063.

Foot disorders : generalities

BONNET J., GARRETA L., DUCLOUX J.-M. — Les lacunes calca-
néennes. *Ann. Radiol.*, 1968, *11*, 3-4, 171-184, 21 fig., bibliogr.

BRAUN S., PANAHI F. — Le pied rhumatismal. *Gaz. Med. Fr.*, 1968,
75, 1, 77-94.

DE DONCKER E., KOWALSKI C. — Cinésiologie et rééducation du pied,
Masson,Paris, 1978.

ESTANOVE B. — Abord radiologique de la pathologie du pied. *Cah.
Méd. Lyon*, 20 avril 1973, *49*, 16, 1671-1680, 17 fig.

FORRESTER D.M., NESSON J.W. — *The radiology of joint disease.*
W.B. Saunders Company. Philadelphia, London, Toronto, 1973.

GIANNESTRAS N.J. — *Foot Disorders — Medical and Surgical
Management*, 2nd ed. Lea and Febiger, Philadelphia, 1973.

HOERR N.L., PYLE S.I. FRANCIS C.C. — Radiographic Atlas of
Skeletal Development of the Foot and Ankle. Charles C. Thomas.
Springfield, III., 1962.

KLERNERMAN L. OSMOND-CLARKE H. — *The foot and its disorders.*
Blackwell Scientific Publication, Oxford - London - Edinburgh,
Melbourne.

LELIEVRE J. — *Pathologie du pied.* Masson, Paris, 1971.

MAROTEAUX P. — Nomenclature internationale des maladies osseuses
constitutionnelles. *Ann. Génét.* (Paris), 1971, 14, 73.

MAROTEAUX P. — *Maladies osseuses de l'enfant.* Flammarion
Médecine-Sciences, Paris, 1974.

MURRAY O., JACOBSON G. — *The radiology of skeletal disorders.*
Churchill and Livingstone. Edinburgh, London, 1972.

REEDER M.M. — Tropical diseases of the foot. *Seminars in
Roentgenol.*, 1978, *5*, 4, 378-391.

RITCHIE G.W., KEIM H.A. — A radiographic analysis of major foot
deformities. *Canad. Med. Assos. J.*, 1964, *91*, 840. *Seminars in
Roentgenology. The Foot.* M70, *1*, 4. Henry M. Stratton.

SIMON L. et Coll. — Le pied inflammatoire. Maloine, Paris, 1977.

TEMPLETON A.W., McALISTER W.H., ZIM I.D. — Standardization of
terminology and evaluation of osseous relation-ships in congenital-
ly abnormal fect. *Am. J. Roentgenol.*, 1965, *93*, 374.

TRIAL R. — *Traité de radiodiagnostic. Os. Pathologie générale.*
Masson, Paris, 1969.

TRIAL R., LAVAL-JEANTET M., PLAINFOSSE M.C. — *Traité de
radiodiagnostic. Rhumatologie, articulations, parties molles.* Masson, Paris, 1976.

Arthritides

AVILA R., PUGH D.G., SLOCUMB C.H., WINKELMANN R.K. —
Psoriatic arthritis : A roentgenologic study. *Radiology*, 1960, *75*,
691.

BERENS D.L., LIN R.K. — *Roentgen diagnosis of rhumatoid arthritis.*
C.C. Thomas, Springfield, 1969.

BERENS D.L., LOCKIE L.M., LIN R., NORCROSS B.M. — Roentgen.
changes in early rheumatoid arthritis. *Radiology*, 1964, *82*, 645.

BRAUN S., CHATIGNOUX G., PANAHI F. — Pathologie rhumatismale du
calcaneum, *Concours Méd.,* 1970, *92*, 6, 1225.

BRAUN S. — Le pied dans les grands rhumatismes inflammatoires,
chroniques. *Rhumatologie*, 1975, *27*, 2, 47-56.

CAROIT M. — Les lésions ostéo-articulaires de la sarcoïdose. *Encycl.
Méd. Chir.*, Paris. App. locomoteur, 1972, 14027 C 10.

COSTE F., BRAUN S., MOUTOUNET J., PANAHI F. — Rheumatoid
forefoot, 1968, *Ann. Radiol.* (Paris), *11*, 1.

COSTE F., LAURENT F., BASSET F. — Polychondrite, polyarthrite et
syndrome de Gougerot Sjögren. *Rev. Rhum.*, 1961, *28*, 498-503.

DEBEYRE N., DENIS A. — Le pied douloureux inflammatoire
(polyarthrite rhumatoïde et pelvispondylite rhumatismale). *1re
Journée de podologie médico-chirurgicale du Centre Viggo Peter-
sen.* Expansion scientifique française, Paris, 1966, p. 32.

DOLAN D.L., LEMMON G.B., TEITELBAUM S.L. — Relapsing polychondritis. *Am. J. Med.*, 1966, 41, 285-299.

DRYLL A. — Psoriasis et rhumatismes inflammatoires du pied. *2e
Journée de podologie médico-chirurgicale du Centre Viggo Peter-
sen.* Expansion scientifique française, Paris, 1967, p. 36.

GREEN N., OSMER J.C. — Small bone changes secondary to systemic
lupus erythematosus. *Radiology*, 1968, *90*, 118-120.

LAAKSONEN A.L. — A prognostic study of juvenile rheumatoid
arthritis ; analysis of 554 cases. *Acta Paediatr. Scand.*, Suppl.,
1966, 166.

LAPLANE R., FONTAINE J.L., LAGARDÈRE S., PAQUELIN F., NAVARRO
J. — La polychondrite chronique atrophiante de l'enfant. *Nouv.
Presse Méd.*, 1973, *2*, 1045-1048.

MARTEL W. — Acute and chronic arthritis of the foot. *Seminars in
Roentgenol.*, 1970, 5, 4, 391-407.

MARTEL W. — Radiologic manifestations of rheumatoid arthritis with
particular reference to the hand, wrist and foot. *Med. Clin. N.
Am.*, 1968, *52*, 655.

MARTELL W., HOLT J.F., CASSIDY J.T. — Roentgenologic manifestations of juvenile rheumatoid arthritis. *Am. J. Roentgenol. Radium
Ther. Nucl. Med.*, 1962, *88*, 400.

NORGAARD F. — Earliest roentgen changes in polyarthritis of the
rheumatoid type. *Radiology*, 1969, *92*, 299.

RAPPOPORT A.S., SOSMAN J.L., WEISSMAN B.N. — Lesions resembling gout in patients with rheumatoid arthritis. *Am. J. Roentgenol.*, 1976, *126*, 1, 41-45.

RESNICK D. — Roentgen features of the rheumatoid mid- and
hindfoot. *J. Can. Assoc. Radiol.*, 1976, *27*, 99-107.

RESNICK D. — The interphalangeal joint of the great toe in
rheumatoid arthritis. *J. Can. Assoc. Radiol.*, 1975, *26*, 255-262.

RESNICK D. — Bony proliferation of terminal toe phalanges in
psoriasis « the ivory » phalanx. *J. Can. Assoc. Radiol.*, 1977, *28*, 3,
187-189.

RESNICK M.D., MITCHELL L., FEINGOLD D.P.M., JOHN-CURD M.D.,
GEN-NIWAYAMA M.D., THOMAS G., GOERGEN M.D. — Calcaneal
abnormalities in articular disorders : rheumatoid arthritis, ankylosing spondylitis, psoriatic arthritis and Reiter syndrome. *Radiology*, 1977, *125*, 2, 335-367.

ROTES-QUEROL J., ROIG ESCOFFET D. — Début de l'arthrite rhumatoïde. *Rev. Rhum.*, 1968, *35*, 21-30.

RUBENS-DUVAL A., VILLIAUMEY J., KAPLAN G., BISSON M., RONDIER
J. — Arthropathies de l'avant-pied à forme destructive au cours de
la spondylarthrite ankylosante. *Rev. Rhum.*, 1966, *33*, 562.

SERRE H., SIMON L., CLAUSTRE J. — L'atteinte du pied dans la
spondylarthrite ankylosante. *Ann. Podol.*, 1973, *8*, 1, 125-139.

SCHWEIZER A. Th., KANAAR P. — Sarcoidosis with polyarthritis in a
child. *Arch. Dis. Child.*, 1967, *42*, 671-674.

SIEGELMAN S.S., JACOBSON H.G. — The foot in acquired systemic
diseases. *Seminars in Roentgenol.*, 1970, *5*, 4, 436-450.

SILVER T.M., FARBER S.J., BOLE G.G., MARTEL W. — Radiological
features of mixed connective tissue disease and scleroderma-
systemic lupus erythematosus overlap. *Radiology*, 1976, *120*, 2,
269-275.

TUFFANELLI D.L., WINKELMANN R.K. — Systemic scleroderma :
Clinical study of 727 cases. *Arch. Dermatol.*, 84, 359-371.

VERHAEGHE A., LEMAITRE G., LEBEURRE R., — Les calcanéites de la
spondylarthrite ankylosante. *Rev. Rhum., Mal. Ostéoaortic.*, 1961,
28, 504-507.

VIDIGAL E., JACOBY R.K., DIXON A.S.J., RARLIFF A.H., KIRKUP J. —
The foot in chronic rheumatoid arthritis. *Ann. Rheumat. Dis.*,
1975, *34*, 4, 292-297.

WESTON W.J. — Positive contrast arthrography in rheumatoid arthritis.
Austral. Radiol., 1968, *12*, 141-147.

WRIGHT V. — Psoriasic arthritis (a comparative study of rheumatoid
arthritis and arthritis associated with psoriasis). *Ann. Rheum. Dis.*,
1961, *20*, 123-132.

Degenerative joint disease

ARLET J., RUFFIÉ R. — Etude sur les arthroses tibio-tarsiennes et sur
les arthroses astragalo-calcanéennes et astragalo-scaphoïdiennes.
Etiologie. Signes cliniques et radiologiques. *Rev. Rhum.*, 1961, *28*,
368.

BINGOLD E.C., COLLINS D.H., — Hallux rigidus. *J. Bone and Joint
Surg.*, 1950, *32B*, 214-222.

ESSEL L., BONNEY G. — Hallux rigidus in the adolescent. *J. Bone and
Joint. Surg.*, 1958, 40B, 3, 668-673.

KESSEL L., BONNEY G. — Hallux rigidus in the adolescent. *J. Bone
and Joint Surg.*, 1958, 40B, 668.

MEARY R., FICAT C. — L'arthrose de la première métatarso-
phalangienne. Traitement chirurgical. Etude de 92 cas. *Rev. Chir.
Orthop.*, 1975, 61, 507-515.

REGNAUD B., LEROUX M.J. — L'hallux rigidus. *Ann. Podol.*, 1965, 4,
45-60.

SABATIER J., BERTRAND P. — Les arthroses du pied (Hallux valgus
excepté). *Rhumatologie*, 1975, *27*, 2, 57-60.

Infective osteo-arthritides

BEZÈS H. — Mycoses osseuses. *Encyclop. Méd.-Chir.* Paris, Os,
articulations, 14.020 A 10.

BEZÈS H. — Lésions osseuses du pian. *Encyclop. Méd.-Chir.*, Paris,
14, 021 A 10, p. 3-4.

BOULET P., SERRE H., MIROUZE J., OLIVIER J. — Ostéopériostite tibio-péronière au cours d'une brucellose chronique. *Rev. Rhum.*, 1955, *22*, 344-346.

CHARTRES J.C., COCKSHOTT P. — Radiological aspects of some parasitic diseases. *In* Middlemiss M. (Ed.), *Tropical Radiology.* Intercontinental Médical Bool Corp., New York, 1961, 115-127.

COCKSHOTT P. — Mycetoma. *In :* Middlemiss H. (Ed.), *Tropical Radiology.* Intercontinental Medical Book Corp., New York, 1961, 38-51.

COLWILL M. — Osteomyelitis of the metatarsal sesamoids. *J. Bone and Joint Surg.*, 1962, 51B, 464-468.

CREMIN B.J., FISHER R.M. — The lesions of congenital syphilis. Part. I. The early or perinatal lesions. *Br. J. Radiol.*, 1970, *43*, 333-341.

CREMIN B.J., FISHER R.M., LEVINSOHN M.W. — Multiple bone tuberculosis in the young. *Br. J. Radiol.*, 1970, *43*, 638-645.

DAVIS J.A., BLUESTONE R. — Tuberculous arthritis of first toe skeletal radiology, 1979, 4, 1, 37-39.

DELAHAYE R.P., ALLAIN Y.M., MAJER L., PLAINFOSSE M.C. — Arthrites infectieuses. In : *R. Trial. Traité de radiodiagnostic.* Masson, Paris, 1976.

DELAHAYE R.P., BOURSIQUOT P., CREN M. — Les aspects radiologiques des lésions osseuses du plan. *J. Radiol. Electrol.*, 1968, *49*, 1-2, 41-48.

DELAHAYE R.P., DESTOMBES P., MOUTOUNET J. — Les aspects radiologiques des mycétomes. *Ann. Radiol.*, 1962, *5*, 11-12, 817-838, bibliogr.

DELAHAYE R.P., LAURENT H., MASSOUBRE A. — Les aspects radiologiques de l'hydatidose osseuse (à propos de 4 observations). *J. Radiol. Electrol.*, 1967, *48*, 5, 269-276.

EDEIKEN J., DE PALMA A.F., MOSKOWITZ H., SMYTHE V. — « Cystic » tuberculosis of bone. *Clin. Orthop.*, 1963, *28*, 163.

FEIGIN R.D., MCALISTER W.H., VENUSTO H.S.J., MIDDELKAMP J.N. — Osteomyelitis of the calcaneus. *Am. J. Dis. Child.*, 1970, *119*, 61.

GAENSLEN F.J. — Split-heel approach in osteomyelitis of os calcis. *J. Bone and Joint Surg.*, 1931, *13*, 759-772.

GHARBI H.A. et Coll. — Les localisations rares de l'hydatidose chez l'enfant. *Ann. Radiol.*, 1977, *20*, 1, 151-157.

HOUKOM S.S. — Tuberculosis of the ankle joint ; an end-result study of 25 cases. *Surg. Gynecol. Obstet.*, 1943, *76*, 438.

LEVIN E.J. — Healing in congenital osseous syphilis. *Am. J. Roentgenol.*, 1970, *110*, 591-597.

MARTINI M. — Tuberculose osseuse et ostéo-articulaire du membre supérieur, du cou de pied et du pied. *Encycl. Méd. Chir.*, Paris, App. locomoteur, 1977, 14185 E 10.

MARTINI M., BOUDJEMAA A., BOULAHBAL F. — Les ostéites tuberculeuses. *Rev. Chir. orthop.*, 1972, *58*, 595-608.

RYCKEWAERT A., LEMAIRE V., AMBROSINI C., SÈZE S. DE. — Arthrites bactériennes aiguës suppurées après injections intra-articulaires de dérivés cortisoniques. *Rev. Rhum.*, 1973, *40*, 189-193.

TARDOS R., TOMARI V.A. — Aspect actuel de la syphilis osseuse en Algérie. *J. Radiol. Electrol.*, mai 1962, *43*, 5, 288-298, 12 fig.

WHITEHOUSE W.M., SMITH W.S. — Osteomyelitis of the feet. *Seminars in Roentgenol.*, 1970, 5, 4, 367-378.

Virus arthritides

AMOR B. — Le pied dans le syndrome de Fiessinger-Leroy-Reiter. *In :* *Le pied inflammatoire*, sous la direction de L. SIMON. Maloine, Paris, 1977, 1 vol. p. 63-72.

BRAUN S. — Le pied dans les grands rhumatismes inflammatoires chroniques. *Rhumatologie*, 27, 21-56, 1975.

DOURY P., PATIN S. — Le pied dans le syndrome de Fiessinger-Leroy-Reiter. *Rhumatologie*, 1978, *30*, 7, 233-237.

PETERSON C.C.Jr., SILBIGER M.L. — Reiter's syndrome and psoriatic arthritis : This roentgen spectra and some interesting similarities. *Am. J. Roentgenol.*, 1967, 101, 860.

RUDOLPH A.J., SINGLETON E.B., ROSENBERG H.S., SINGER D.B., PHILLIPS C.A. — Osseous manifestations of the congenital rubella syndrome. *Am. J. Dis. Child.*, 1965, *110*, 428-433.

Metabolic, endocrine and toxic osteo-arthropathies

BOHRER S.P., UDE A.C. — Hell pad thickness. *Skeletal Radiol.*, 1978, *3*, 2, 108-112.

BRAILSFORD J.F. — The radiology of gout. *Br. J. Radiol.*, 1959, *32*, 472.

CHEVROT A., PALLARDY G., LEDOUX-LEBARD G. — Lésions osseuses de l'hyperthyroïdie. *J. Radiol. Electrol.*, 1978.

DODDS W.J., STEINBACH H.L. — Primary hyperparathyroidism and articular cartilage calcification. *Am. J. Roentgenol.*, 1968, *104*, 884-891.

DORFMANN H., SOLNICA J., DI MENZA C. et SÉZE S. DE. — Les arthropathies des hémochromatoses. *Sem. Hôp. Paris*, 1969, *45*, 517-523.

DOYLE F.H. — Some quantitative radiological observations in primary and secondary hyperparathyroidism. *Br. J. Radiol.*, 1966. 39, 161.

GONTICAS S.K., IKKOS D.G., STERGIOU L.H. — Evaluation of the diagnostic value of heelpad thickness in acromegaly. *Radiology*, 1969, *92*, 304-307.

GOODING C.A., BALL J.A. — Idiopathic juvenile osteoporosis. *Radiology*, 1969, *93*, 1349.

HIOCO D. — L'ostéomalacie. *Symposium du centre du métabolisme phospho-calcique, Paris, 1967*, Masson, Paris, 1967, 1 vol.

HIOCO D. — L'ostéoporose. *Symposium du centre du métabolisme phospho-calcique, Paris, 1963*, Masson, Paris, 1963, 1 vol.

HOUANG M.T.W., BRENTON D.P., RENTON P., SHAW D.G. — Idiopatic juvenile osteoporosis. *Skeletal Radiol.*, 1978, 3, 1, 17-23.

JOHNSON C., GRAHAM B.C., KINGSBURY-CURTIS F. — Roentgenographic manifestations of chronic renal disease treated by periodic hemodialysis. *Am. J. Roentgenol.*, 1967, *101*, 915-926.

LAVAL-JEANTET M., SCALA H. — Chondrocalcinose articulaire diffuse. *J. Radiol. Electrol.*, 1963, *44*, 793-796.

LEFEBVRE J., GUY E. — Rachitisme. *Encyclop. Méd.-Chir., Paris*, Radiodiagnostic, t. II, 31, 135 A 10.

LEFEBVRE J., GUY E. — Scorbut infantile. Maladie de Barlow. Avitaminose C. *Encyclop. Méd.-Chir., Paris*, Radiodiagnostic, t. II, 31, 134 C 10.

LOOSER E. — Uber pathologische Formen von Infraktionen und Callusbildungen bei Rachitis und Osteomalakie und anderen Knockenerkrankungen. *Zentralbl. Chir.*, 1920, *47*, 1470.

LOTE J.T., GOUGEON J. — Ostéopathies endocriniennes de l'adulte. *Encyclop. Méd.-Chir.*, Radiodiagnostic, t. II, 31, 175 A 20.

LOUYOT P., MATHIEU J., GAUCHER A., MATHIEU-GILLE T. — Signes radiologiques de l'ochronose alcaptonurique. *J. Radiol. Electrol.*, 1962, *43*, 892-894.

MCCARTY D.J. — Crystal deposition disease. *J. Am. Med. Ass.*, 1965, *193*, 129-132.

MCCARTY D.J., HASKIN M.E. — The roentgenographic aspects of pseudogout (articular chondrocalcinosis). An analysis of 20 cases. *Am. J. Roentgenol.*, 1963, *90*, 1248.

MARTEL W. — The overhanging margin of bone : A roentgenologic manifestation of gout. *Radiology*, 1968, *91*, 755.

MARTEL W., CHAMPION C.K., THOMPSON G., CARTER T. — A radiologically distinctive arthropathy in some patients with the pseudogout syndrome. *Am. J. Roentgenol.*, 1970.

MILKMAN L.A. — Multiple spontaneous idiopathic symmetrical fractures. *Am. J. Roentgenol.*, 1934, *32*, 622.

MINDELZUN R., ELKIN M., SCHEINBERG I.H., STERNLIEB I. — Skeletal changes in Wilson's disease. A radiological study. *Radiology*, 1970, *94*, 127-132.

PARLEE D.E., FREUNDLICH I.M., MCCARTY D.J. — Comparative study of roentgenographic techniques for detection of calcium pyrophosphate dihydrate deposits (pseudogout) in human cartilage. *Am. J. Roentgenol. Radium Ther. Nucl. Med.*, 1967, *99*, 688.

PINET E., PINET A., BARRIÈRE J., BOUCHE B., BOUCHE M.M. — Les ostéopathies fluorées endémiques condensantes du Souf (Sud-Algérien). *Ann. Radiol.*, 1961, *4*, 7, 589-612.

POPPEL M.H., ZEITEL B.E. — Roentgen manifestations of milk drinker's syndrome. *Radiology*, 1956, *67*, 195.

POUREL J., LOUYOT P., DIEBOLD P., BAUMGARTNER J. — Stéatonécrose disséminée à déterminations articulaires, osseuses et mésentériques. *J. Radiol. Electrol.*, 1970, *51*, 423-426.

SCANLON G.T., CLEMETT A.R. — Thyroid acropachy. *Radiology*, 1964, *83*, 1039-1042.

SCHABEL S.I., KORN J.H., RITTENBERG G.M., LEMAN R.B. — Bone infarction in gout. *Skeletal Radiol.*, 1978, *3*, 1, 36-47.

SERRE H., SIMON L., GIVAUDAND A., BENAMARA M. — La radiographie du pied dans le diagnostic de la goutte. *Ann. Radiol.*, 1962, 5, 649-655.

SORIANO M., MANCHON F. — The radiological aspects of a new type of bone fluorosis, periostitis deformans. *Radiology*, 1966, 87, 1089-1094.

STEINBACH H.L., RUSSELL W. — Measurement of the Heel-Pad as an Aid to Diagnosis of Acromegaly. *Radiology*, 1964. 82, 418-422.

TAYBI H., KEELE D. — Hypoparathyroidism ; review of the literature and report of 2 cases in sisters, one with steatorrhea and intestinal pseudo-obstruction. *Am. J. Roentgenol. Radium Ther. Nucl. Med.*, 1962, *88*, 432.

TEMPLETON A.W., JACONETTE J.R., ORMOND R.S. — Localized osteosclerosis in hyperparathyroidism. *Radiology*, 1962, *78*, 955-958.

VANDENDORP F., DU BOIS R., LOCQUET G. — Squelette et myxœdème congénital. *J. Radiol. Electrol.*, 1959, *40*, 787-791.

WEISSENBACH R.J., FRANÇON F. — Un aspect radiographique du pied goutteux : le « pied hérissé ». *Rev. Rhum.*, 1938, *5*, 870.

WELLER M.P., EDEIKEN J., HODES P.J. — Renal osteodystrophy. *Am. J. Roentgenol. Radium. Ther. Nucl. Med.*, 1968, *104*.

ZIMMERMAN H.B. — Osteosclerosis in chronic renal disease ; report of 4 cases associated with secondary hyperparathyroidism. *Am. J. Roentgenol. Radium. Ther. Nucl. Med.*, 1962, *88*, 1152.

Neurogenic osteo-arthropathies

ARNOTT G., PETIT H., MERLEN J.F., BENOIT M., FOURLINNIE J.C. — Syndrome of the tarsal scaphoid reveling latent diabetes. *Rev. Neurol.* (Paris), 1971, *124*, 3, 233-243.

AZERAD E., LUBETZKI J., STUHL L., SLOTINE M. — Etude radiologique des ostéopathies du diabète sucré. Le pied diabétique. *Ann. Radiol.*, 1963, *6*, 421-436.

BANSON B.B., LACY P.E. — Diabetic microangiopathy in human toes ; with emphasis on the ultrastructural change in dermal capillaries. *Am. J. Pathol.*, 1964, *45*, 41.

BÉNASSY J. — L'ostéogénèse neurogène. *Rev. Rhum.*, 1961, *28*, 234-239.

BIDART Y. — Immobilité et ostéomes. *Ann. Méd. Phys.*, 1970, *13*, 341-348.

BLOCH-MICHEL M., CAUCHOIX J., BOURDON R. — Les arthropathies du tabès et de la syringomyélie. *Rev. Prat.*, 1960, *10*, 2015-2040.

BOULET P., MIROUZE J., PÉLISSIER M. — Le squelette du pied dans le diabète sucré. *Rev. Rhum.*, 1955, *22*, 115-127.

BUREAU Y., BARRIÈRE H., LITOUX P., BUREAU B. — Les ostéoarthropathies neurotrophiques. *Presse Méd.*, 1967, *73*, 547-549.

BUREAU Y., BARRIÈRE H., KERNÉIS J.P., FERRON A. DE. — Acropathies ulcéro-mutilantes pseudo-syringomyéliques non familiales des membres inférieurs (à propos de 2 à 3 observations). *Presse Méd.*, 1957, *65*, 2127-2132.

CÉCILE J.P., DESCAMPS C., REGNIER G. et coll. — L'arthrographie du pied diabétique. *J. Radiol. Electrol.*, 1973, *54*, 4, 313-318.

CHARCOT J.M. — Sur quelques arthropathies qui paraissent dépendre d'une lésion du cerveau ou de la moelle épinière. *Arch. Physiol. Normale et Pathol.*, 1868, *1*, 161-178.

DEROT M., RATHERY M. — Syndrome du scaphoïde tarsien. *Le Diabète*, 1967, *15*, 131-138.

FAGET G.H., MAYORAL A. — Bone changes in leprosy, A clinical and roentgenological study of 505 cases. *Radiology*, 1944, *42*, 1.

GEOFFROY J., HOEFFEL J.C., POINTEL J.P., BROUIN P., DEBRY G., MARTIN J. — Les lésions ostéo-articulaires chez le diabétique. Etude systématique de 1501, dossiers radiologiques. *J. Radiol. Electrol.*, 1978, *59*, 10, 557-562.

GOUGEON J., SEIGNON B. — Ostéoarthropathies nerveuses. *Encycl. Méd.-Chir.*, Paris, 1978, App. Locomoteur, 14285 A 10.

JOHNSON A.C., JAMES A.E., REDDY E.R., JOHNSON S. — Relation of vascular and osseous changes in leprosy. *Skeletal Radiol.*, 1978, *3*, 1, 36-41.

KRAFT E., SPYROPOULOS E., FINBY N. — Neurogenic disorders of the foot in diabetes mellitus. *Am. J. Roentgenol.*, 1975, *124*, 1, 17-24.

LINQUETTE M., FOSSATI P., FOURLINNIE J.C. — Le pied et l'angiopathie diabétique. Intérêt de la radiographie osseuse. *Rev. Fr. Endocrinol. Clin.*, 1974, *15*, 4, 321-329.

MENANTEAU B., ÉTIENNE J.C., DEFAUT P., SÉGAL M. — Acropathies ulcéro-mutilantes. Intérêt de l'étude angiographique. *Ann. Radiol.*, 1973, *16*, 9-10, 649-653 (bibl.).

NEWMAN H., CASEY B., DU BOIS J.J., GALLACHER T. — Roentgen features of leprosy in children. *Am. J. Roentgenol.*, 1972, *114*, 2, 402-410.

RAVAULT P.-P., MAITREPIERRE J., RIFFAT G. — Le pied décalcifié douloureux idiopathique. *Rev. Rhum.*, août 1959, *26*, 8, 393-407, 7 fig., bibliogr.

RÉNIER J.-C. — Algodystrophies du membre inférieur et leur traitement. *Rev. Prat.*, 21 déc. 1958, *8*, 33, 3835-3843, 2 fig., bibliogr.

RUFFIE R., FOURNIER A., MANSAT CH. — Le pied douloureux œdémateux décalcifié. *Ann. Podol.*, 1964, *3*, 177-187.

SEIGNON B., HIBON J., GOUGEON J. — Acropathie ulcéro-mutilante et arthropathie du diabète sucré. Etude radio-clinique comparée de deux séries de 10 cas. *Rev. Rhum. Mal. Ostéo-artic.*, 1974, *41*, 333-339.

SEIGNON B., MENANTEAU B., HIBON J., GOUGEON J. — Acropathie ulcéro-mutilante et arthropathie du diabète sucré. Etude artériographique. *Rev. Rhum. Mal. Ostéo-artic.*, 1974, *41*, 341-347.

SERRE H., SIMON L., CLAUSTRE J. — Les algodystrophies réflexes du pied. *Ann. Podol.*, 1966, *6*, 265-283.

SIEGELMAN S.S., HEIMANN W.G., MANIN M.C. — Congenital indifference to pain. *Am. J. Roentgenol.*, 1966, *97*, 242-247.

SILVERMAN F., GILDEN G. — Congenital insensitivity to pain. A neurologic syndrom with bizarre skeletal lesions. *Radiology*, 1959, *72*, 176-190.

THÉVENARD A. — L'acropathie ulcéro-mutilante familiale. *Rev. Neurol.*, 1972, *74*, 193-212.

WARTER J.P., KEMPF F., MANTZ J.M., TEMPE J.D. — Aspects radiologiques de l'ossification para-ostéoarticulaire, complication fréquente du tétanos (13 observations personnelles). *J. Radiol. Electrol.*, 1968, *49*, 227-230.

WASTIE M.L. — Radiological changes in serial X-rays of the foot and tarsus in leprosy. *Clin. Radiol.*, 1975, *26*, 2, 285-292.

Osteo-arthropathies occuring in blood diseases

BEACHLEY M.C., PECK LAU B., RICHARD KING E. — Bone involvement in Hodgkin's disease. *Am. J. Roentgenol.*, 1972, *114*, 559-563.

BISMUTH V., BÉNACERRAF R. — Etude radiologique des manifestations osseuses des anémies hémolytiques héréditaires. *Ann. Radiol.*, 1967, *10*, 559-574 et 723-736.

BOHRER S.P. — Acute long bone diaphyseal infarcts in sickle cell disease. *Br. J. Radiol.*, 1970, *43*, 685.

BOUVET J.P. — Sclérose tubéreuse de Bourneville. *Encyclop. Méd.-Chir.*, Paris, 1978, App. locomoteur, 14023 T 20.

BUSY J., LOTE J., PALLARDY G. — Etude radiologique des localisations osseuses de la maladie de Hodgkin. *J. Radiol. Electrol.*, 1958, *39*, 4, 239-247, 32 fig.

CAFFEY J. — Colley's anemia ; a review of the roentgenographic findings in the skeleton. *Am. J. Roentgenol. Radium Ther. Nucl. Med.*, 1957, *78*, 381.

CLARISSE P.T., STAPLE T.W. — Diffuse bone sclerosis in multiple myeloma. *Radiology*, 1971, *99*, 327.

ENGELS E.P., SMITH R.C., KRANTZ S. — Bone sclerosis in multiple myeloma. *Radiology*, 1960, *75*, 242-247.

FAURÉ CL. — Manifestations ostéo-articulaires et musculaires de l'hémophilie. *Encycl. Méd.-Chir.*, Paris, Radiol., 1968, 31375 A 10.

FOURNIER A.M., PADOVANI J., DENIZET D. — La neuro-fibromatose de Recklinghausen, son polymorphisme radio-clinique. *J. Radiol. Electrol.*, 1963, *44*, 513-522.

FUCILLA I.S., HAMANN A. — Hodgkin's disease in bone. *Radiology*, 1961, *77*, 53-60.

GODEFROY D., GALMICHE J.M., CHEVROT A., PALLARDY G. — Sarcoïdose osseuse et pulmonaire chez une fillette de 12 ans. Etude radiologique. *J. Radiol. Electrol.*, 1976, *57*, 1, 97-102.

GODIN E., CAPESIUS P., KEMPF F. — Acro-ostéosclérose au cours de la maladie de Besnier-Boeck-Schaumann. *J. Radiol. Electrol.*, 1977, *58*, 2, 115-118.

JUHL J.H., WESENBERG R.L., GWIN J.L. — Roentgenographic findings in Fanconi's anemia. *Radiology*, 1967, *89*, 646-653.

LEIGHTMAN D.A., BIGONGIARI L.R., WICKS J.D. — Tibiotalar slant in sickle cell anemia. *Skeletal radiology*, 1978, *3*, 2, 99-101.

MC BRINE C.S., FISCHER M.S. — Acrosclerosis in sarcoidosis. *Radiology*, 1975, *2*, 279-281.

MESZAROS W.T., GUZZO F., SCHORSCH H. — Neurofibromatosis. *Am. J. Roentgenol.*, 1966, *98*, 557-569.

O'HARA A.E. — Roentgenographic osseous manifestations of the anemias and the leukemias. *Clin. Orthop.*, 1967, *52*, 63-83.

PAPILLON J., CROIZAT P., CHASSARD J.L., REVOL L., BOTHIER F., COSTE — Les localisations osseuses de la maladie de Hodgkin. *J. Radiol. Electrol.*, 1964, *45*, 3-4, 109-116, 13 fig.

PAVLICA P., STASI G., TONTI R., VENEZIANO S., VIGLIETTE G. — L'ostéo-sclérose phalangienne dans la sarcoïdose. *J. Radiol. Electrol.*, 1977, *58*, 10, 603-604.

PITT M.J., MOSHER J.F., EDEIKEN J. — Abnormal periosteum and bone in neurofibromatosis. *Radiology*, 1972, *103*, 143-146.

POUYANNE L., REBOUL J., GENESTE R., DELORME G., BOUYSSOU P. — Radiodiagnostic du granulome éosinophile des os. *J. Radiol. Electrol.*, *1957*, 38, 3-4, 230-235, 13 fig.

PROUX CH.. MABILLE J.P. — Une localisation de la maladie de Hodgkin au niveau des os longs des membres inférieurs. *J. Radiol. Electrol.*, 1961, 42, 6-7, 400-401, 2 fig.

SHAUB M., ROSEN. R., BOSWELL W., GORDONSON J. — Tibiotalar slant : A new observation in sickle cell anemia. *Radiology*, 1975, 117, 551.

SIMMONS C.R., HARLE T.S., SINGLETON E.B. — The osseous manifestations of leukemia in children. *Radiol. Clin. North Am.* 1968, 6, 115.

SVOBODA M., MALY VL. — Les altérations articulaires dans l'hémophilie. Images radiologiques, tomographiques et agrandies directement. *J. Radiol. Electrol*, 1958, 39, 610-616.

THOMAS L.B., FORKNER C.E., FREI E., BESSE B.E., STABENAU J.R. — The skeletal lesions of acute leukemia. *Cancer*, 1961, 14, 608-621.

VANDENDORP P., DUBOIS R., MARGERIN M. — Aspects radiologiques des arthrites hémophiliques. *J. Radiol. Electrol.*, 1962, 43, 422-426.

WEISSENBACH R.J., LIÈVRE J.A. — Sur la myélomatose décalcifiante diffuse. *Rev. Rhum.*, 1948, 15, 221-224.

WILLSON J.K.V. — The bone lesions of childhood leukemia. A survey of 140 cases. *Radiology*, 1959, 72, 672-681.

Post-traumatic osteo-arthropathies

CAYLA J., RONDIER J. — Algodystropies réflexes des membres inférieursd'origine vertébro-pelvienne. *Rhumatologie*, 1973-25, 2.

DELAHAYE R.P., DOURY P., PATTIN S., METGES P.J., MINE J. — Les fractures de fatigue des métatarsiens. *Rev. Rhum.* Mal. Ostéoartic., 1976, 43, 12, 707-713.

DELAHAYE R.P., JOUFFROY J., LAURENT H., LOZE P.C. — Les fractures de fatigue. *J. Radiol. Electrol.*, 1966, 47, 525-534.

DENIS A. — Fracture de fatigue du métatarse. Encycl. Med. Chir. Paris 1971, App. locomoteur, 15740 E 10.

DEVAN W.T., CARLTON D.C. — The march fracture persists. A report of 145 cases during 15 month period at an infantry Basic Training Center. *Am. J. Surg.*, 1954, 87, 227-231.

DEVAS M.B., SWEETNAM D.R. — Stress fractures of the fibula. A review of fifty cases in athletes. *J. Bone and Joint Surg.*, 1956, 38 B, 818-829.

FESSARD C., MAROTEAUX P., LAMY M. — Le syndrome de Silverman. « Fractures multiples du nourrisson » (étude de seize observations). *Arch. Fr. Pédiat.*, 1967, 24, 651-665.

GOLDMANN A.B., KATZ M.C., FREIBERGER R.H. — Capsulite adhésive post-traumatique de la cheville. Diagnostic arthrographique. *Am. J. Roentgenol.*, 1976, 127, 585-588.

LEABHART J.W. — Stress fracture of the calcaneus. *J. Bone and Joint Surg.*, 1959, 41 A, 1285-1290.

PIETRON K., KOSLOWSKI K., BOROCH Z. — Fractures de contrainte des métatarsiens chez l'enfant. *Ann. Radiol.*, 1972, 15, 149-152.

RIFFAT G., BÉRARD E., JACQUOT F. — Algodystrophie réflexe du pied. *Rhumatologie*. 1973, 25, 2.

SCHNEIDER H.J., KING A.Y., BRONSON J.L., MILLER E.H. — Stress injuries and developmental change of lower extremities in Ballet Dancers. *Radiology*, 1974, 113, 627-632.

SERRE H., SIMON L., CLAUSTRE J. — La réadaptation du pied algodystrophique. *Rhumatologie*, 1973, 23, 2.

SILVERMAN F.N. — Unrecognized trauma in infants, the battered child syndrome, and the syndrome of Ambroise Tardieu. Rigler lecture. *Radiology*, 1972, 104, 337-353.

STEIN R.E., STELLING F.H. — Stress fracture of the calcaneus in a child with cerebral palsy. *J. Bone and Joint Surg.*, 1977, 59, 1, 131.

SUDECK P. — Uber die akute entzundliche Knochen atrophie. *Arch. F. Klin. Chir.*, 1900, 62, 147.

WILSON E.S., KATZ F.N. — Stress fractures : an analysis of 250 consecutive cases. *Radiology*, 1969, 92, 481-486.

Foot in standing

BEDOUELLE J. — Malformations congénitales du pied. *Encycl. Méd. Chir. Paris.* Radiodiagnostic. 15255 B 10.

BREWERTON D.A., SANDIFER P.H., SWEETNAM D.R. — The aetiology of pes cavus. *Br. Med. J.*, 1963, 2, 659-661.

CARLIOZ H., POUS J.G. — Le *pied bot varus équin. Cahiers d'enseignement de la SOFCOT.* Expansion Scientifique Française, Paris, 1976.

CHIGOT P.L., GUIBAL A.M. — Maladie amniotique. *Encycl. Méd. Chir.*, Paris, 1974, App. locomoteur, 15200 B 10.

CHOLMELEY J.A. — Hallux valgus in adolescents. *Proc. Royal Soc. Med.*, 1958, 51, 903-906.

DAVIS L.A., HATT W.S. — Congenital abnormalities of the foot. *Radiology*, 1955, 64, 818-825.

DENIS A. — Pied plat valgus statique. *Encycl. Méd. Chir.*, Paris, 1974, App. locomoteur, 15730 F 10.

DUCROQUET R., DUCROQUET J., DUCROQUET P. — *La marche et les boiteries. Etudes des marches normales et pathologiques.* Masson, Paris, 1965.

EYRE-BROOK A.L. — Congenital vertical talus. 1967, *J. Bone and Joint Surg.*, 1967, 49 B, 618.

FREIBERGER R.H., HERSH A., HARRISON M.O. — Roentgen examination of the deformed foot. *Seminars Roentgenol.*, 1970, 5, 4, 341-353.

GAUNEL CH.. LOUYOT P., TREHEUX A. — Etude radiologique des désaxations en pronation ou supination du pied. *Rev. Rhum. Mal. Ostéo-artic.* 1971, 38, 10, 591-598.

GAUNEL C., LOUYOT P., TREHEUX A. — Etude radiologique du pied creux. *Rev. Rhum. Mal. Ostéo-artic.* 1971, 28, 10, 581-589.

GIANNESTRAS N.J. — Foot Disorders. Medical and Surgical Management. London, 1967. Henry Kimpton.

HAINES R.W., McDOUGALL A. — The anatomy of hallux valgus. *Bone and Joint Surg.*, 1954, 36B, 272.

HOLLINGSWORTH R.P. — An X-ray study of valgus ankles in spina bifida children with valgus flat foot deformity. *Proc. Royal Soc. Med.*, 1975, 66, 8, 481-484.

JACKSON B.T., KINMONTH J.B. — Pes cavus and lymphoedema. An unusual familial syndrome. *J. Bone Joint Surg.*, 1970, 52, 3, 518-520.

JOHNSON J.C. — Peroneal spastic flatfoot syndrome. *South Med. J.*, 1976, 69, 6, 807-809.

JUDET J., LAUGIER A., POULIQUEN J.Cl. — Les pieds congénitaux. *Actual. Chir. Orthop.* F2, 1976, 13, 106-139.

KITE J.H. — Congenital metatarsus varus. *J. Bone and Joint Surg.* 1965, 49A, 388-397.

LAMY L., WEISSMAN L. — Congenital convex pes valgus. *J. Bone and Joint Surg.*, 1939, 21, 79.

LLOYD-ROBERTS G.C., SPENCE A.J. — Congenital vertical talus. *J. Bone and Joint Surg.*, 1958, 40B, 33-41.

LUNDBERG B.J., SULJA T. — Skeletal parameters in the hallux valgus foot. *Acta Orthop. Scand.*, 1972, 43, 6, 576-582.

McCORMICK D.W., BLOUNT W.P. — Metatarsus adductovarus. 'Skewfoot'. *J. Am. Med. Ass.*, 1949, 141, 449.

MARTORELL-MARTORELL J. — Concept et études de la métatarsalgie et son traitement. *Ann. Podol.*, 1973, 8, 2, 237-270.

MEARY R. — Symposium sur le pied creux essentiel. *Rev. Chir. Orthop.*, 1967, 53, 389-467.

MEARY R. — Symposium sur le pied plat. *Ann. Orthop. de l'Ouest*, 1969, 1, 57-71.

MOTTRAM M.E., PYLE I.R. — Mandarin feet. *Am. J. Roentgenol.*, 1973, 118, 2, 318-319.

ONO K., HAYASHI H. — Residual deformity of treated congenital club foot. A clinical study employing trontal tomography of the hind part of the foot. *J. Bone Joint Surg.*, 1974, 56, 8, 1577-1585.

POZNANSKI A.K. — Foot manifestations of the congenital malformations syndromes. *Seminars Roentgenol.*, 1970, 5, 4, 354-367.

REGNAULD B. — Déformations majeures de l'avant pied. *Chir. Del Piede Ital.*, 1978, 2, 3, 121-136.

SIMON L., CLAUSTRE J. — Les métatarsalgies (Hallux valgus excepté). *Rhumatologie*, 1975, 27, 2, 61-73.

VOUTEY H. — Pieds contracturés et pieds péroniers spastiques. *Ann. Podol.*, 1971, 7, 74-80.

YALE I. — Practical considerations on bone pathology at the first metatarsophalangeal joint. *J. Am. Podiatry Assoc.*, 1974, 64, 10, 821-825.

YORAM BEN-MENACHEM BUTLER J.E. — Arteriography of the foot in congenital deformities. *J. Bone Joint Surg.*, 1974, 56, 8, 1625-1630.

Soft tissues

AUQUIER L., SIAUD J.R. — Tendinites nodulaires du tendon d'Achille. *Rev. Rhum.* 1971, 38, 373.

BENASSY J. — Talalgies et forage du calcaneum. *Rhumatologie*, 1975. 27, 3, 127-129.

BLERY M., PAMIER S., BARRE J.L. — Etude radiologique de l'arthrogrypose. *J. Radiol. Electrol.*, 1977, 58, 10, 597-602.

BLOMQVIST G. — Xanthoma of the Achilles tendon. *Acta Radiol.*, 1962, 57, 45-48.

BOURREL P., REY A., BLANC J.F., PALINACCI J.C., BOURGES M., GIRAUDEAU P. — Syndrome du canal tarsien. A propos de 15 cas purs et de 100 cas associés à la lèpre ou au diabète. *Rev. Rhum. Mal. Ostéo-artic.*, 1976, *43*, 12, 723-728.

BROWNE S.G. — Ainhum : a clinical and etiological study of 83 cases. *Ann. Trop. Med.*, 1961, 55, 314.

CASTAING J., DELPLACE J. — A propos de 62 cas de rupture du tendon d'Achille. *Ann. Orthop. Ouest*, 1972, 4, 25.

COLE G.J. — Ainhum. An account of fifty four patients with special reference to aetiology and treatment. *J. Bone and Joint Surg.*, 1965, *47B*, 43-51.

DENIS A. — Tendinites nodulaires du tendon d'Achille. *Rev. Rhum. Mal. Ostéoartic.* 1971, *38*, 470.

FETTERMAN L.E., HARDY R., LEHRER H. — The clinico-roentgenologic features of ainhum. *Am. J. Roentgen.*, 1967, *100*, 512.

FICAT P. — Le syndrome du tunnel tarsien. *Podologie*, 1966/67, *5*, 22.

FIELDS M.L., GREENBERG G.H., BURKETT L.L. — Roentgenographic measurement of skin and heel pad thickness in the diagnosis of acromegaly. *Am. J. Med. Sci.*, 1967, *254*, 162.

FOURNIE A., PUTOIS J. — Tumeurs des gaines et des tendons. *Ann. Podol.*, 1966-67, *5*, 177-184.

GAUTHIER G., DUTERTRE P. — La maladie de Morton : syndrome canalaire : 74 cas opérés sans résection du névrome. *Lyon Méd.*, 1975, *223*, 917-921.

GAYLER B.W., BROGDON B.G. — Soft tissue calcification in the extremities in systemic disease. *Am. J. Med. Sci.* 1965, *249*, 590.

GERSTER J.C., HAUSER H., FALLET G.H. — Xeroradiographic technics applied to assessment of Achilles tendon in inflammatory or metabolic diseases. *Ann. Rheum. Dis.*, 1975, *34*, 6, 479-488.

GONTICAS S.K., IKKOS D.G., STERGIOU L.H. — Evaluation of the diagnostic value of heel pad thickness in acromegaly. *Radiology*, 1969, *92*, 304.

GOODMAN L.R., SHANSER J.D. — The pre-Achilles fat pad : An aid to early diagnosis of local or systemic disease. *Skeletal Radiol.*, 1977, *2*, 81-85.

HILBISH T.F., BARTTER F.C. — Roentgen findings in abnormal deposition of calcium in tissues. *Am. J. Roentgen.* 1963, *87*, 1128.

KECK C. — The tarsal-tunnel syndrome. *J. Bone Joint Surg.*, 1962, *44A*, 180.

LABROUSSE C., LATHELIZE H., ANDRIEU J., DESPROGES-GOTTERON R. — Les talalgies. *Rhumatologie*, 1975, *27*, 2, 75-78

LOTKE P.A. — Ossification of Achilles tendon. *J. Bone and Joint Surg.*, 1970, *52 A*, 157-160.

MAROTEAUX P. — La myosite ossifiante. *Rev. Rhum.*, 1965, *32*, 512-513.

MELMED E.P. — Spontaneous bilateral rupture of the calcaneal tendon during steroid therapy. *J. Bone and Joint Surg.*, 1965, *47 B*, 104-105.

MORNET J., DOLIVEUX P. — La maladie des tendons d'Achille et sa complication : la rupture (maladie de Jacques Delarue). *Rev. Rhum. Mal. Ostéo-artic.*, 1973, *40*, 10, 607-611.

MORRIS M.-A. — Morton's Metatarsalgia. Clinical orthopoedics and related. *Research*, 1977, *127*, 203-207.

MORTON T. — A peculiar and painful affection of the fourth metatarso-phalangeal articulations. *Am. J. Med. Sciences*, 1876, 71, 37-45.

POZNANSKI A.K., LA ROWE P.C. — Radiographic manifestations of the arthrogrypsosis syndrome. *Radiology*, 1970, *95*, 353.

PRICE E.W. — Studies on plantar ulcers of leprosy. *Lepr. Rev.*, 1959, *30*, 98, 180.

PUCKETTE Jr. S.E., SEYMOUR E.O. — Fallibility of the heel pad thickness in the diagnosis of acromegaly. *Radiology*, 1967, *88*, 982.

RESNICK D. — Calcaneal abnormalitis in articular disorders : rheumatoïd arthritis, ankylosing spondylitis. Reiter's syndrome. *Radiology*, 1977, *125*, 355-366.

ROBINSON H.M. — Symmetrical reversed plantar calcaneal spurs in children. *Radiology*, 1976, *119*, 187-188.

SEMAT P., CHAPIRO E. — Le syndrome de Thibierge-Weissenbach. *J. Radiol. Electrol.*, 1971, *52*, 27-30.

SERRE H., SIMON L., CLAUSTRE J. — Le syndrome douloureux aigu du 2ᵉ espace inter-métatarsien. *Rev. Rhum.*, 1972, *39*, 495-503.

SEWELL J.R., LIYANAGE B., ANSELL B.M. — Calcinosis in juvenile dermatomyositis. *Skeletal Radiol.*, 1978, *3*, 3, 137-143.

SINGLETON E.B., HOLT J.F. — Myositis ossificans progressiva. *Radiology*, 1954, *62*, 47.

SNEIDER P. — Xanthoma of the calcaneus. *Br. J. Radiol.*, 1963, *36*, 222-223.

STEINBACH H.L., RUSSELL W. — Measurement of the heel pad as an aid to diagnosis of acromegaly. *Radiology*, 1964, *82*, 418.

STRAUSS J., VOUTEY H., PERRIN M. — Les ténosynovites au niveau du pied. *Rhumatologie*, 1975, *27*, 2, 79-86.

TROISIER O. — Tendinites et ténosynovites du pied. *Ann. Podol.*, 1966-1967, *5*, 149-153.

VOUTEY H., STRAUSS J. — Synovites subaiguës des articulations métatarso-phalangiennes. *Ann. Podol.*, 1973, *8*, 1, 157-162.

Vascular bone lesions

ASKAR O., KASSEM K.A. — A clinicoradiological study of the varicose foot. *J. Cardio-vascul. Surg. Ital.*, 1975, *16*, 1, 71-78.

AUQUIER L., PAOLAGGI J.B. — Deux observations d'ostéonécrose non traumatique de l'astragale. *Rev. Rhum.*, 1967, *34*, 43.

BESSON J., WELLINGEN C. — L'ostéochondrite disséquante de l'astragale. *Rev. Rhum.*, 1967, *34*, 552.

BLOM J.M.H., STRIJK S.P. — Lesions of the trochlea tali (fractures ostéochondrales et ostéochondrite dissécante de la trochlée de l'astragale). *Radiol. Clin.* (Suisse), 1975, *44*, 5, 387-396.

BRISMAR J., GOETHLIN J. — Phlebography and thrombosis of the deep veins of the foot. *J. Radiol. Electrol.*, 1972, *45*, 531, 199-202.

CAYLA G. — L'ostéonécrose de l'astragale. *Actual. Rhum.*, 1972, *9*, 229.

CHENEY W.D. — Acro-osteolysis. *Am. J. Roentgenol. Radium Ther. Nucl. Med.*, 1965, *94*, 595.

CAYLA G., DENIS A. — Nécrose de l'astragale. *Encycl. Med. Chir.*, Paris, 1973, App. locomoteur, 15741 D 10.

DENIS A. — Les ostéonécroses aseptiques du pied chez l'adulte. *Actual. Rhum.*, 1968, *5*, 47.

DENIS A. — L'ostéo-nécrose aseptique des sésamoïdes du 1ᵉʳ orteil (Maladie de Renander). *Rhumatologie*, 1975, *27* 2, 113-117.

FONTAINE R., BOLLACK C., CHADDAD F. — Les lésions des artérioles et métartérioles étudiées au niveau des orteils dans les artérites des membres inférieurs de nature artérioscléreuse. *Presse Méd.*, 1967, 75.

FONTAINE R., WARTER P., WEIL F., TUCHMANN L., SUHLER A. — Les altérations des os de la jambe déclenchées par les troubles circulatoires veineux des membres inférieurs. *Journ. Radiol. Electrol.*, 1964, *5*, 219-225, 11 radios, 5 tabl., 15 réf.

GALLY L., ARVAY N. — Les lésions osseuses dans les troubles circulatoires et trophiques des membres. *Journ. Radiol. Electrol.*, 1950, *31*, 11-12, 690-694, 6 fig.

GERLER R.D., WALKER L.A., MACHARD J.L., WEENS H.S. — Osseous changes in chronic pancreatitis. *Radiology*, 1965, *85*, 494-500.

GOTHLIN J., ZURBRINGEN S. — Frequency of thrombosis and post-thrombotic conditions of the foot at phlebography. *Acta Radiol. Diagnosis*, 1975, *16*, 1, 107-112.

MALAN E. et Coll. — Les courts-circuits artério-veineux en pathologie vasculaire du pied. *Ann. Podol.*, 1965, *4*, 109-127.

ROSENFELD M. — A propos de l'ostéochondrite de l'astragale. *Rev. Rhum. Mal. Ostéo-artic.*, 1972, *39*, 2, 123-127.

SERVELLE M. — Pathologie vasculaire. Les affections artérielles. T. 1 et 2. Masson, Paris, 1973.

WELLINGER C., BESSON J. — L'ostéochondrite dissécante de l'astragale. *Ann. Podol.*, 1973, *8*, 1, 163-173.

Bone lesions caused by physical agents

GRALINO B.J., PORTER J.M., ROSCH J. — Angiography in the diagnosis and therapy of frostbite. *Radiology*, 1976, *119*, 2, 301-305.

MOULY R. — Les radiodermites du pied. *Ann. Podol.*, 1973, *8*, 2, 110-121.

PAILHERET J.-P. — Brûlures et gelures du pied. *Ann. Podol.*, 1973, *8*, 2, 88-92.

SAPIN-JALOUSTRE J. — Les pieds gelés. *Ann. Podol.*, 1964, *3*, 117-152.

TISCHLER J.M. — The soft-tissue and bone changes in frosbite injuries. *Radiology*, 1972, *102*, 3, 511-513.

Bone and joint diseases of unknown origin

BEALS R.K., BIRD C.B. — Carpal and tarsal osteolysis. A case report and review of the literature. *J. Bone Joint Surg.*, 1975, *57 A*, 5, 681-686.

CAFFEY J., SILVERMAN W.A. — Infantile cortical hyperostoses ; preliminary report on new syndrome. *Am. J. Roentgenol.*, 1945, *54*, 1-16.

CLAUSTRE J., BLOTMAN F., SIMON L. — Les atteintes du pied au cours de la maladie osseuse de Paget. *Rev. Rhum. Mal. Ostéo-artic.*, 1976, *43*, 1, 45-49.

COURY CH. — *L'hippocratisme digital, l'ostéopathie hypertrophiante pneumique .et les autres dysacromélies apparentées.* Baillières, Paris, 1960, 1 vol., 230 p.

FAURE CL. — Diagnostic radiologique des hyperostoses cortico-périostées du tout jeune nourrisson. *Concours Méd.*, 1969, *91*, 3799-3810.

FIRAT D., STUTZMAN L. — Fibrous dysplasia of the bone. Review of 24 cases. *Am. J. Med.*, 1968, *44*, 421-429.

FOURNIER A.M. — Pachydermopériostose. *J. Radiol. Electrol.*, 1973, *54*, 5, 417-423.

GILLET J., IMANI F., BENZAKOUR M., CUIGNARD J. — L'hyperostose corticale infantile (Maladie de Caffey) à propos de 2 observations. *Ann. Radiol.*, 1974, *17*, 7, 707-711.

GIRARD J., MAZABRAUD A. — Un cas particulier de dysplasie fibreuse à localisations osseuses et tendineuses. *Journ. Radiol. Electrol.*, 1957, *38*, 11-12, 1143-1146, 4 fig., bibliogr.

GORHAM L.W., STOUT A.P. — Massive osteolysis (acute spontaneous absorption of bone, phantom bone, disappearing bone). *J. Bone and Joint Surg.*, 1955, *37 A*, 985.

KOHLER E., BARBITT D., HUIZENGA B., GOOD T.A. — Hereditary osteolysis. A clinical, radiological and chemical study. *Radiology*, 1973, *108*, 1, 99-105.

LAINE R., LEGRAND J. — Ostéopathie hypertrophiante pneumique de Pierre Marie. *Journ. Radiol. Electrol.*, 1965, *46*, 3-4, 147-152, 5 fig.

LICHTENSTEIN L. — Polyostotic fibrous dysplasia. *Arch. Surg.*, 1938, 36, 874.

LICHTENSTEIN L., JAFFE H.L. — Fibrous dysplasia of bone. *Arch. Pathol.*, 1942, *33*, 777.

LION G. — Ostéo-arthropathie hypertrophiante pneumique. *J. Belge Radiol.*, 1960, *43*, 5, 417-444.

PAJEWSKI M., VURE E. — Late manifestation of infantile cortical hyperostosis (Caffey's disease). *Br. J. Radiol.*, 1967, *40*, 90-95.

RESNICK D., SHAUL S.R., ROBINS J.M. — Diffuse idiopathic skeletal hyperostosis (Dish) : fore Stier's disease with extraspinal manifestations. *Radiology*, 1975, *115*, 3, 513-524.

ROSENBAUM H.D. — Geographic variation in the prevalence of Paget's disease of bone. *Radiology*, 1969, *959*.

SCHWARTZ D.T., ALPERT M. — The malignant transformation of fibrous dysplasia. *Am. J. Med. Sci.*, 1964, *247*, 1-19.

URSING B. — Pachydermoperiostosis. *Acta Med. Scand.*, 1970, *188*, 157-160.

Malignant bone tumors

CHAVANNE G., CALLE R., GRICOUROFF G. — A propos de quelques observations de cancers osseux induits par radiothérapie externe. *Symposium ossium.* Londres, 1968.

CHAVANNE G., CALLE R., SCHLIENGER P. — A propos des chondro-sarcomes osseux (étude radioclinique de 44 observations). *J. Radiol. Electrol.* (Paris), 1971, *52*, 425-438.

COMITE NEERLANDAIS DES TUMEURS OSSEUSES. — *Tumeurs osseuses bénignes et malignes.* 2 tomes. Mouton et Maloine, Paris, 1978.

CUNNINGHAM M.P., ARLEN M. — Fibrosarcome médullaire de l'os. *Cancer*, 1968, *21*, 31-37.

DAHLIN D.C. — *Bone tumors, General aspects and analysis of 2 276 cases.* Thomas C.C., Springfield, 1957.

DAHLIN D.C., COVENTRY M.B., SCANLON P.W. — Ewing's sarcoma. A critical analysis of 165 cases. *J. Bone Joint Surg.*, 1961, *43 A*, 185-192.

DAHLIN D.C., SALVADOR A.H. — Chondrosarcomas of bones of the hands and feet. A study of 30 cases. *Cancer* (U.S.A.), 1974, *34*, 3, 755-760.

EDEIKEN J., FARRELL C., ACKERMAN L.V., SPJUT H.J. — Parosteal sarcoma. *Am. J. Roentgenol. Radium Ther. Nucl. Med.*, 1971, *111*, 579.

KITTREDGE H.D. — Arteriography in Ewing's tumor. *Radiology*, 1970, *97*, 609-610.

MASSELOT J., BERGIBON C., TCHERNIA G., TOURNADE M.F., MARKO-VITS P. — Etude radioclinique des métastases du néphroblastome. *Ann. Radiol.*, 1972, *15*, 1-12.

MULVEY R.B. — Peripheral bone metastases. *Am. J. Roentgenol.*, 1964, *91*, 155.

NORMAN A. — Tumor and tumor-like lesions of the bones of the foot. *Seminars Roentgenol.*, 1970, *5*, 4, 407-419.

RIDINGS G.R. — Ewing's tumor. *Radiol. Clin. N. Amer.*, 1964, *2*, 315-325.

VAN RONNEN J.R. — Diagnostic radiologique de l'ostéosarcome. Classification des types radiologiques. Fidélité du diagnostic radiologique. L'examen radiologique peut-il remplacer la biopsie ? *Ann. Radiol.*, 1970, *13*, 465-482.

VOHRA V.G. — Roentgen manifestation in Ewing's sarcoma ; a study of 156 cases. *Cancer*, 1967, 20, 727-733.

Benign bone tumors

APPENZELLER J., WEITZNER S. — Intraosseous lipoma of os calcis. Case report and review of literature of intraosseous lipoma of extremities. *Clin. Orthop. Relat. Res.*, 1974, *101*, 171-175.

BOURREL P., PALINACCI J.C., FERRO R., DELATTE P., VEILLARD J.M. — Les exostoses chez les jeunes militaires (à propos de 72 cas). *Méd. et armées*, 1976, *4*, 7, 651-656.

BUSSIERE J.L., LOPITAUX R., LEROY V. — Kystes synoviaux intra-osseux. *Rhumatologie*, nov. 1977, 331-336.

CHANG C.H., PIATT E.D., THOMAS K.E., WATNE A.L. — Bone abnormalities in Gardner's syndrome. *Amer. J. Roentgenol.*, 1968, *103*, 645-652.

CHEVROT A., d'IZARN J.J., PALLARDY G., FOREST M. — Tumeurs glomiques et kystes épidermoïdes des phalanges. *J. Radiol. Electrol.*, 1976, *57*, 8-9, 645-647.

DELRIEU F., AMOR B., OBADIA J.P., LEVY P. — Ostéome ostéoïde de l'astragale. A propos de deux cas. *J. Radiol. Electrol.*, 1972, *53*, 5, 437-439.

DENIS A. — Deux observations d'ostéome ostéoïde du tarse. *Rev. Rhum.*, 1976, *43*, 305-306.

FELDMAN F., HECHT H.L., JOHNSTON A.D. — Chondromyxoid fibroma of bone. *Radiology*, 1970, 94, 249-260.

FOREST M., VINH T.S. — Tumeurs glomiques. Kystes épidermoïdes. Chirurgie orthopédique. Tumeurs bénignes osseuses. Dystrophie pseudo-tumorale. *Monogr. Ann. Chir.*, 1974, 98-99, 100-101.

FOWLES S.J. — Osteoid osteoma. *Br. J. Radiol.*, 1964, *37*, 245-252.

FREIBERGER R.H., LORTMAN B.S., HELPERN M., THOMPSON T.C. — Osteoid osteoma : a report on 80 cases. *Am. J. Roentgenol.*, 1959, *82*, 194-205.

GROUPE ROBERT MEARY. — Tumeurs bénignes osseuses et dystrophies pseudo-tumorales. *Monogr. Ann. Chir.*, 1974.

HALLIDAY D.R., DAHLIN D.C., PUGH D.G., YOUNG H.H. — Massive osteolysis and angiomatosis. *Radiology*, 1964, *82*, 637.

HOLM CL. — Primary synovial chondromatosis of the ankle. *J. Bone Joint Surg.*, 1976, *58*, 6, 878-880.

JAFFE H.L. — Benign osteoblastoma. *Bull. Hosp. Joint Dis.*, 1956, *17*, 141.

JAFFE H.L., LICHTENSTEIN L. — Benign chondroblastoma of bone : a reinterpretation of the so-called calcifying or chondromatous giant-cell tumor. *Am. J. Pathol.*, 1942, *18*, 969-983.

KUBICZ S. — Aspect radiologique du kyste osseux anévrysmal chez l'enfant. *Ann. Radiol.*, 1970, *13*, 211-218.

LEFEBVRE J., NEZELOF C., FAURE C., HUC M., ERRERA A. — Les lacunes corticales métaphysaires des os longs chez l'enfant et l'adolescent. Rapports avec le fibrome non ostéogénique. A propos de 32 observations. *J. Radiol. Electrol.*, (Paris), 1956, *37*, 300-307.

MARTINI M. et Coll. — Un cas de synovite villo-nodulaire pigmentaire de l'articulation tibio-tarsienne. *Rev. Chir. Orthop.*, 1970, *56*, 6, 571-575. .

MARTINI M., GOT G., CHLAP Z. — Quatre nouveaux cas d'ostéome ostéoïde du col de l'astragale. *Rev. Chir. Orthop.*, 1976, *61*, 651-657.

MEARY R., ABELANET R., FOREST M., LE CHARPENTIER Y., TOMENO B., LANGUEPIN A., NEZELOF CH., LESEC G. — Les chondroblastomes bénins des os. Etude anatomo-clinique et ultra-structurale à propos de 11 observations. *Rev. Chir. Orthop.*, 1975, *61*, 717-734.

MERCIER R., BRESSON P., VIALLET J.F., VANNEUVILLE G. — Intérêt de l'artériographie dans les tumeurs glomiques sous-unguéales. *J. Radiol. Electrol. Méd. Nucl.*, mai 1970, *51*, 5, 303-304.

MERLE D'AUBIGNE R., THOMINE J.M. — Les tumeurs osseuses à cellules géantes. *Rev. Prat.*, (Paris), 1969, *19*, 2163-2174.

MURPHY F.P., DAHLIN·D.C., SULLIVAN R.C. — Articular synovial chondromatosis. *J. Bone Joint Surg.*, 1962, *44*, 8.

PALLARDY G., GALMICHE J.M., CHEVROT A., CORREAS G., BIDON J., FOREST M. — Tumeurs à cellules géantes. Etude radiologique à propos de 89 observations. *J. Radiol. Electrol.*, 1976, *57*, 8-9, 637-640.

PIATKOWSKI S., WARDA E. — L'ostéome ostéoïde au niveau du calcaneum. *Rev. Chir. Orthop.*, 1973, *59*, 609-613.

POUSSA M., HOLMSTROM T. — Intraosseous lipoma of the calcaneus. Report of a case. *Acta Orthop. Scand.*, 1976, *47*, 5, 570-574.

QUENEAU P., DOLOMIER F., BOUSQUET G., PICAULT C. — La maladie exostosante. A propos de 16 observations. Revue de la littérature. *Rhumatologie*, 1978, *30*, 6, 183-191.

REILLY B.J., DAVIDSON J.W., BAIN H. — Lymphangiectasis of the skeleton. A case report. *Radiology*, 1972, *103*, 385-386.

RIGAULT P., KLISOWSKI H. — Les fibromes non ossifiants de l'extrémité inférieure du tibia chez l'enfant et l'adolescent. Rapport de 5 cas et revue de la littérature. *Rev. Chir. Orthop.*, 1969, *55*, 533-541.

SMITH J.H., PUGH D.G. — Roentgenographic aspects of articular pigmented villonodular synovitis. *Am. J. Roentgenol.*, 1962, *87*, 1145-1156.

SMITH R.W., SMITH C.F. — Solitary unicameral bone cyst of the calcaneus. A review of twenty cases. *J. Bone Joint Surg.*, 1974, *56*, 1, 49-56.

SOREFF J. — Aneurysmal bone cyst of the talus. *Acta Orthop. Scand.*, 1976, *47*, 3, 356-360.

TRIFAUD A., BUREAU H., PAYAN H. — *Tumeurs bénignes des os.* Masson, Paris, 1959.

TRIFAUD A., FAYSSE R., PAPILLON J. — Les tumeurs à myéloplaxes des os ou tumeurs osseuses à cellules géantes. *Rev. Chir. Orthop.*, 1956, *42*, 413-513.

TRISTANT H., TOURAINE R., FUNES P. DE, NICK J., MIGNOT B., LAVAL-JEANTET M. — Syndrome de Mafucci et angiomes des membres. *J. Radiol. Electrol.*, 1971, *52*, 413-416.

TURCOTTE B., PUGH D.G., DAHLIN D.C. — The roentgenologic aspects of chondromyxoid fibroma of bone. *Am. J. Roentgenol.*, 1962, *87*, 1085-1095.

Constitutional bone diseases
1) Osteochondrodysplasia

ALBERS-SCHÖNBERG H. — Röntgenbilder einer seltenen Knochenerkrankung. *Münch. Med. Wschr.*, 1904, *51*, 365-368.

BUCHIGNANI J.S., COOK A.J., ANDERSON L.G. — Roentgenographic findings in familial osteodysplasia. *Am. J. Roentgenol.*, 1972, *116*, 3, 602-608.

CAFFEY J. — Chondroectodermal dysplasia (Ellis-Van Creveld disease). Report of three cases. *Am. J. Roentgenol.*, 1952, *68*, 875-886.

CAMURATI M. — Di un raro caso di osteite simmetrica ereditaria degli arti inferiori. *Chir. Organi Mov.*, 1922, *6*, 622-665.

ENGELMANN G. — Ein Fall von Osteopathia hyperostotica (Sclerosis) multiplex infantilis. *Fortschr. Röntgenstr.*, 1929, *39*, 1101-1106.

ENGFELDT B., FAJERS C.M., LODIN H., PEHRSON M. — Studies on osteopetrosis. III. Roentgenological and pathologic-anatomical investigations on some of the bone changes. *Acta paediatr.* (Upsala), 1960, *49*, 391-408.

GREEN A.E., Jr., ELLSWOOD W.H., COLLINS J.R. — Melorheostosis and osteopoikilosis, with a review of the literature. *Am. J. Roentgenol.*, 1962, *87*, 1096-1111.

HAINES J.O., ROGERS S.C. — Oculo-dento-digital dysplasia. A rare syndrome. *Br. J. Radiol.*, 1975, *48*, 575, 932-936.

LAMY M., MAROTEAUX P. — Le nanisme diastrophique. *Presse méd.*, 1960, *68*, 1977-1980, 18 fig.

LEDOUX-LEBARD R., CHABANEIX, DESSANE — L'ostéopœcilie, forme nouvelle d'ostéite généralisée. *J. Radiol. Electrol.*, 1916, *2*, 133-134.

LE MAREC B., SENEGAL J. et coll. — Epiphyses ponctuées et aberrations chromosomiques. *Ann. Radiol.*, 1976, *19*, 6, 599-607.

LERI A., LIEVRE J.A. — La mélorhéostose, l'hyperostose d'un membre « en coulée ». *Presse Méd.*, 1928, *36*, 801-805.

LIEVRE J.A. — La fragilité osseuse constitutionnelle (étude de 25 familles comportant 53 malades). *Rev. Rhum.*, 1959, *8*, 420-432.

MAROTEAUX P., GILLES M. — Etude radiologique de l'osteogenesis imperfecta. *Ann. Radiol.*, 1965, *8*, 571-583.

MAROTEAUX P., LAMY M. — The malady of Toulouse-Lautrec. *J. Am. Med. Ass.*, 1965, *191*, 715-717.

MAROTEAUX P., LAMY M. — La pycnodysostose. *Presse Méd.*, 1962, *70*, 999-1002.

MURRAY R.O., CREDIE J.M.C. — Melorheostosis and the sclerotomes : a radiological correlation. *Skeletal Radiology.* 1979, *4*, 2, 57-71.

PORAK C., DURANTE G. — Les micromélies congénitales : achondroplasie vraie et dystrophie périostale. *Nouv. Iconogr. Salpêt.*, 1905, *18*, 481-538.

RUELLE M., DUBOIS J.L. — A propos de deux cas familiaux de sclérose diaphysaire multiple (syndrome de Camurati-Engelmann). *Rev. Rhum.*, 1964, *7*, 345-348.

STOVER C.N., HAYES J.T., HOLT J.F. — Diastrophic dwarfism. *Am. J. Roentgenol*, 1963, *89*, 914-922, 13 fig.

VOORHOEVE N. — L'image radiologique non encore décrite d'une anomalie du squelette. *Acta Radiol.*, 1924, *3*, 407-427.

WALKER N. — Pyle's disease or cranio-metaphyseal dysplasia. *Ann. Radiol.*, 1966, *9*, 197-207.

WORTH H.M., WOLLIN D.G. — Hyperostosis corticalis generalisata congenita. *J. Canad. Ass. Radiol.*, 1966, *17*, 67-74.

2) Dysostoses

APERT E. — De l'acrocéphalosyndactylie. *Bull. Soc. Méd. Hôp. Paris*, 1906, *23*, 1310-1330.

BEDOUELLE J. — Aplasies congénitales du péroné. *Encycl. Méd. Chir.*, Paris, 1955. Radiodiagnostic, 15206 B 10.

BEDOUELLE J. — Aplasies congénitales du tibia. *Encycl. Méd. Chir.*, Paris, 1955. Radiodiagnostic, 15207 B 10.

CHENEY W.D. — Acro-osteolysis. *Am. J. Roentgenol.*, 1965, *94*, 595-607.

HARLE T.S., STEVENSON J.R. — Hereditary symphalangism associated with carpal and tarsal fusions. *Radiology*, 1967, *89*, 91-94.

KARCHINOW K. — Congenital diplopodia with hypoplasia or aplasia of the tibia. A report of 6 cases. *J. Bone Joint Surg.*, 1973, *55*, 3, 604-611.

MAROTEAUX P., BOUVET J.P., BRIARD M.L. — La maladie des synostoses multiples. *Nouv. Presse Méd.*, 1972, *1*, 45, 3041-3047.

MURRAY I.P.C. — Bone scanning in occupational acro-osteolysis. *Skeletal Radiol.*, 1978, *3*, 3, 149-154.

MUSALLAM S.S., POLEY J.R., RILEY H.D., Jr. — Apert's syndrome (Acrocephalosyndactyly). A description and a report of 7 cases. *Clin. Pediatr.*, 1975, *14*, 11, 1054-1062.

PETIT P., BEDOUELLE J. — Anomalies de volume des membres. *Encycl. Méd. Chir.*, Paris, 1955. Radiodiagnostic, 15200 D 10.

POZNANSKI A.K. — Foot manifestations of the congenital malformation syndromes. *Seminars Roentgenol.*, 1970, *5*, 354-366.

POZNANSKI A.K., GALL J.C., Jr., STERN A.M. — Skeletal manifestations of the Holt-Oram syndrome. *Radiology*, 1970, *94*, 45-53.

POZNANSKI A.K., STERN A.M., GALL J.C. Jr. — Radiographic findings in the hand-foot-uterus syndrome (HFUS). *Radiology*, 1970, *95*, 129.

WILDERVANCK L.S., GOEDHARD G., MEIJER S. — Proximal symphalangism of fingers associated with fusion of os naviculare and talus and occurrence of two accessory bones in the feet (os paranaviculare and os tibiale externum) in an European-Indonesian-Chinese family. *Acta Genet.* (Basel), 1967, *17*, 166-177.

3) Metabolic abnormalities

ABLOW R.C., HSIA Y.E., BRANDT I.K. — Acrodysostosis coinciding with pseudohypoparathyroïdism and pseudo-speudo-hypoparathyroïdism. *Am. J. Roentgenol.*, 1977, *128*, 1, 95-99.

AGUS S., GOLDBERG M. — Pathogenesis of uremic osteodystrophy. *Radiol. Clin. N. Amer.*, 1972, *10*, 545-556.

ALAVI S.M., KEATS T.E. — Toxopachyostéose diaphysaire tibiopéronière, syndrome de Weismann-Netter. *Am. J. Roentgenol.*, 1973, *118*, 314-317.

CAFFEY J. — Chronic poisoning due to excess of vitamin A; description of clinical and roentgen manifestations in 7 infants and young children. *Pediatrics*, 1950, *5*, 672-687 ; *Am. J. Roentgenol.*, 1951, *65*, 12-26.

GREENFIELD G.B. — Roentgen appearance of bone and soft tissue changes in chronic renal disease. *Am. J. Roentgenol.*, 1972, *116*, 749-757.

HUNTER C. — A rare disease in two brothers. *Proc. Royal Soc. Med.*, 1917, *10*, 104-116.

HURLER G. — Ueber einen Typ multipler Abartungen, vorwiegend am Skelettsystem. *Z. Kinderheilk.*, 1919, *24*, 220-234.

LACHMAN R., CROCKER A., SCHULMAN J., STRAND R. — Radiological findings in Niemann-Pick disease. *Radiology*, 1973, *108*, 659-664.

LANGER L.O., Jr., CAREY L.S. — The roentgenographic features of the KS mucopolysaccharidosis of Morquio (Morquio-Brailsford's disease). *Am. J. Roentgenol.*, 1966, *97*, 1-20.

LEFEBVRE J., GUY E. — Scorbut infantile. Maladie de Barlow. Avitaminose C. *Encycl. Méd.-Chir.*, Paris, 1956, 31134 C 10.

LEFEBVRE J., GUY E. — Rachitisme. *Encycl. Méd.-Chir.*, Paris, 1959, 31135 A 10.

LEFEBVRE J., MICHEL J.R., ROYER P. — Les aspects radiologiques des altérations métaphysaires au cours de troubles métaboliques phosphocalciques. *Ann. Radiol.*, 1960, *3*, 213-240.

MCPHERSON R.I., KROEKER M., HOUSTON C.S. — Hypophosphatasia. *J. Can. Ass. Radiol.*, 1972, *23*, 16-26.

MAROTEAUX P., HORS-CAYLA M.C., PONT J. — La mucolipidose de type II. *Presse Méd.*, 1970, *78*, 179-181.

MAROTEAUX P., LAMY M., FOUCHER M. — La maladie de Morquio. Etude clinique, radiologique et biologique. *Presse Méd.*, 1963, *71*, 2091-2094.

MORQUIO L. — Sur une forme de dystrophie osseuse familiale. *Arch. Méd. Enf.*, 1935, *38*, 5-24.

NOLTE K., SPRANGER J. — Early skeletal changes in mucolipidosis III. *Ann. Radiol.*, 1976, *19*, 1, 151-159.

STEINBACH H.L., RUDHE U., JONSSON M., YOUNG D.A. — Evolution of skeletal lesions in pseudo-hypoparathyroïdism. *Radiology*, 1965, *85*, 670-676.

STEINBACH H.L., YOUNG D.A. — The roentgen appearance of pseudo-hypoparathyroïdism (PH) and pseudo-pseudohypoparathyroïdism (PPH). Differentiation from other syndromes associated with short metacarpals, metatarsals, and phalanges. *Am. J. Roentgenol.*, 1966, *97*, 49-66.

VOUTEY H. — Maladie de Refsum-Thiebaut. *Ann. Podol.*, 1971, *7*, 310-314.

4) *Primary disturbances of growth*

BOURGEOIS S., ROBERT P. — Deux cas de syndrome de Klippel-Trenaunay. *J. Radiol. Electrol.*, 1956, *37*, 915-918, 8 fig.

FAURE C., LASCAUX J.P., MONTAGNE J.Ph. — Le syndrome de Larsen. *Ann. Radiol.*, 1976, *19*, 6, 629-636.

FREEMAN E.A., SHELDON J.H. — Cranio-carpo-tarsal dystrophy. An undescribed congenital malformation. *Arch. Dis. Childh.*, 1938, *13*, 277-283.

KLIPPEL M., TRENAUNAY P. — Du nævus variqueux ostéo-hypertrophique. *Arch. Gén. Méd.*, 1900, *77*, 641-672.

LANGE C. DE — Sur un type nouveau de dégénération (Typus amstelodamensis). *Arch. Méd. Enf.*, 1933, *36*, 713-719.

MACLEOD P.M., FRASER C. — Congenital contractural arachnodactyly. *Am. J. Dis. Child.*, 1973, *126*, 810-813.

MARFAN A.B. — Un cas de déformation congénitale des quatre membres, plus prononcée aux extrémités, caractérisée par l'allongement des os avec un certain degré d'amincissement. *Bull. Soc. Méd. Hôp.*, Paris, 1896, *13*, 220-226.

RIGGS W., Jr., SEIBERT J. — Cockayne's syndrome. Roentgen findings. *Am. J. Roentgenol.*, 1972, *116*, 623-633.

ROSEN R.S., CIMINI R., COBLENTZ D. — Werner's syndrome. *Br. J. Radiol.*, 1970, *43*, 193-198.

SMITH D.W., LEMLI L., OPITZ J.M. — A newly recognized syndrome of multiple congenital anomalies. *J. Pediat.*, 1964, *64*, 210-217.

TAYBI H., RUBINSTEIN J.H. — Broad thumbs and toes and unusual facial features. A probable mental retardation syndrome. *Am. J. Roentgenol.*, 1965, *93*, 362-366.

5) *Chromosomal aberrations*

JAMES A.E., Jr., ATKINS L., FEINGOLD M., JANOWER M.L. — The « cri du chat » syndrome. *Radiology*, 1969, *92*, 50-52.

JAMES A.E., Jr., BELCOURT C.L., ATKINS L., JANOWER M.L. — Trisomy 13-15. *Radiology*, 1969, *92*, 44-49.

JAMES A.E., Jr., BELCOURT C.L., ATKINS L., JANOWER M.L. — Trisomy 18. *Radiology*, 1969, *92*, 37-43.

INDEX*

---

* Roman characters refer to figure numbers and italics refers to page numbers.

Imprimé par l'Imp. de Compiègne - rue N. Niepce - ZAC de Mercières - 60205 Compiègne - France
Dépôt légal : 2e Trim. 1981 - No d'impression : 42843